CLINICAL WONDERS OF ACUPUNCTURE-MOXIBUSTION

Compiled by: Zheng Qiwei and Qian Chunyi

Translated by: Du Wei, Hong Tao, Hu Ronghui, Huang Hui, Lu Xiaozhen, Wang Fang, Wang Yue and Zhang Yongmei

FOREIGN LANGUAGES PRESS   BEIJING

First Edition   2002

Home Page:
http://www.flp.com.cn
E-mail Addresses:
info@flp.com.cn
sales@flp.com.cn

ISBN 7-119-02982-7

Published by Foreign Languages Press
24 Baiwanzhuang Road, Beijing 100037, China

Distributed by China International Book Trading Corporation
35 Chegongzhuang Xilu, Beijing 100044, China
P.O. Box 399, Beijing, China

Printed in the People's Republic of China

CONTENTS

CONTENTS

PREFACE

Clinical Wonders of Acupuncture-Moxibustion is a monograph introducing the clinical experiences of acupuncture practitioners. The compilers have tapped the wisdom of acupuncture physicians from various generations, gathered the experience of other acupuncture professionals, and consulted hundreds of volumes of relevant Chinese and foreign documents. The writing of this book has also benefitted from many years' clinical and teaching experience gained by the compilers.

A total of 130 common and intractable diseases of internal medicine, surgery, gynecology, pediatrics, ENT and dermatology are included in the book. The names of the diseases are mainly those used in traditional Chinese medicine, while those of modern medicine are added only when necessary. Each section consists of three parts, i.e., "Introduction," "Clinical Experience," and "Remarks." The emphasis of the book is on "Clinical Experience," and nearly 2,000 instances of simple but applicable and markedly effective clinical experience are collected.

In writing the book, the compilers had the privilege of the instruction of Prof. Cheng Xingnong, a world-renowned acupuncture specialist and vice-president of the China Association of Acupuncture-Moxibustion. Prof. Cheng was our postgraduate studies tutor.

The book's Chinese edition, which came out in 1995, was an instant success. Before the publication of the English edition, the compilers revised it, but no doubt there will be some shortcomings, nevertheless. It is our sincere hope that acupuncture professionals engaged in clinical practice and education all over the world will not hesitate to offer their valuable comments and opinions.

CHAPTER ONE
INTERNAL MEDICINE

COMMON COLD

[INTRODUCTION]

The common cold is manifested by heightened sensitivity to cold, fever, headache, nasal obstruction with running nose and cough. It occurs in all seasons, but is especially prevalent in autumn. The etiology involves an invasion of pathogenic factors. Since the climates in the four seasons are so different, the normal clinical diagnostic division is into wind-cold and wind-heat categories. The treatment principle is to benefit the lung *qi*, eliminate the exterior syndrome and dispel the external wind. The points are selected from the Hand-Taiyin, Yangming and Foot-Taiyang meridians, i.e., Fengchi (GB20), Hegu (LI4), Quchi (LI 1) and Feishu (BL13). For the wind-cold type, moxibustion is applied, and for the wind-heat type, Yuji (LU10), Dazhui (GV14) and Waiguan (TE5) are added, and the bleeding technique using the three-edged needle is also applicable. In modern medicine, upper respiratory inflammation falls in this disease category.

[CLINICAL EXPERIENCE]

1. CONVENTIONAL ACUPUNCTURE

(1) Selecting Hegu (LI 4)

Technique: A one-*cun* filiform needle is inserted on the bilateral Hegu (LI 4) with the fever reducing technique, inducing the needling sensations to be distributed to the upper arm, and even to the neck and head, and sweating.

(2) Selecting Dazhui (GV14)

Technique: The patient is in a sitting position with the head slightly lowered. A 1.5-*cun* filiform needle is inserted with penetrating "heaven coolness" manipulation for 5 to 10 minutes. In 188 cases that were studied, the fever began to recede one hour after needling and in a period of six to 15 hours, the temperature became normal.

(3) Selecting Zusanli (ST36)

Technique: To needle Zusanli (ST36) laterally with the reinforcing method and remove the needle after the sensation of soreness, numbness will be distributed to the foot dorsum. One treatment is given only for preventing a common cold with a certain effect.

2. MOXIBUSTION

Points: Dazhui (GV14), Fengmen (BL12) and Feishu (BL13)

Technique: The patient is in a sitting position with arms crossed over the chest to completely expose the upper back, and the head slightly bowed. Each point is stimulated with a moxa stick for 5 to 10 minutes until the skin turns red. The treatment is given daily. The patient feels slight sweating, but the symptoms are relaxed and the nasal obstruction relieved after treatment. Most cases are cured after two to three treatments.

3. CUPPING

Points: Dazhui (GV14), Shanzhu (GV12), Dazhu (BL11), Fengmen (BL10) and Feishu (BL13)

Technique: The prone position is selected and the cups in moderate or big size are applied on the points for 20 minutes and no blisters happen. Such a method is for treating the common cold due to wind and cold, and the moving cupping method on the Governor Vessel and Bladder meridian is applicable. The cup is sucked on Dazhui (GV14) and moved down slowly along the Governor Vessel to Zhiyang (GV9) and back up to Dazhui (GV14), and this movement is repeated six to eight times until the skin is red or congested.

Finally, the cup is retained on Dazhui (GV14). The same method is also applied on Fengmen (BL10) along the Bladder meridian, between Fengmen (BL10) and Geshu (BL17) and finally the cup is retained on Fengmen (BL10) for 10 minutes. Before the moving cupping technique is applied, some cream should be applied on the skin to prevent skin injury.

4. BLEEDING METHOD

(1) Bleeding on Three Shang Points

Points: Shaoshang (LU11), Zhongshang (about 0.1 *cun* to the center of the nail root of the thumb dorsum) and Laoshang (about 0.1 *cun* lateral to the ulnar side of the thumbnail).

Technique: A three-edged needle is applied on the points bilaterally to achieve slight bleeding. The treatment is given once a day for epidemic common cold.

(2) Bleeding on Jinjin (Ex-HE12) and Yuye (Ex-HE13)

Points: Jinjin (Ex-HE12), Yuye (Ex-HE13), Quze (PC3) and Weizhong (BL40)

Technique: Bleeding method is applied on the points to achieve slight bleeding, once daily. The method is suitable for treating epidemic gastrointestinal common colds.

5. LASER THERAPY

Points: Fengchi (GB20), Dazhui (GV14), Feishu (BL13), Quchi (LI11), Hegu (LI4) and Yingxiang (LI20)

Technique: He-Ne laser, 1 to 30 mA is given, 20 to 30 mm away from the point once daily. The therapy is applied twice a day for severe cases. Each point is radiated for 2 to 5 minutes.

[REMARKS]

1. Acupuncture can receive a certain clinical effect.

2. The severely ill patient should rest in bed and the air in the room should be fresh and be capable of being changed regularly. The room should be sterilized with ultra-violet ray or boiled vinegar evaporation.

COUGH

[INTRODUCTION]

Coughs are divided into two categories: invasion of the external factor and internal injury. A cough due to invasion of external factors is related to wind cold or wind heat attacking the lung, resulting in the lung *qi* failing to disperse and dysfunction of the clearing and descending, and is manifested by a short duration of illness, severe coughing, associated with heightened sensitivity to cold, fever, nasal obstruction and superficial pulse. The treating principle is to disperse the wind and benefit the lung *qi* to stop the coughing. The points are selected from Hand-Taiyin and Yangming meridians, i.e., Feishu (BL13), Chize (LU5), Quchi (LI11), Lieque (LU7) and Hegu (LI4). A cough due to internal injury is related to a *yin* deficiency of the lung and kidney, and manifested as a dry cough with little sputum or bloodstained sputum, associated with tidal fever, along with night sweating. The treatment principle is to benefit the *yin* and clear away any heat. The points are Feishu (BL13), Gaohuangshu (BL43), Chize (LU5) and Zhaohai (KI6). For spleen deficiency involving the failure to transport and transform, and retention of phlegm in the lung, the symptoms are a cough with profuse thin and white sputum, chest tightness, epigastria and a poor appetite. The treatment for these symptoms is to strengthen the spleen to resolve the phlegm and regulate and tonify the lung *qi* with Feishu (BL13), Pishu (BL20), Taiyuan (LU9), Taibai (SP1), Fenglong (ST40) and Hegu (LI4). For liver fire burning the lung, the symptoms are paroxysmal cough leading to pain in the chest and the hypochondriac region, associated with a bitter taste in the mouth and a dry throat. The treatment is to clear away the liver fire and reduce the lung heat with Feishu (BL13), Yuji (LU10), Ganshu (BL18), Xingjian (LR2) and Yanglingquan (GB34). Coughing is commonly seen in respiratory inflection, bronchitis, bronchiectasis and TB.

[CLINICAL EXPERIENCE]

1. CONVENTIONAL ACUPUNCTURE

(1) Penetrating Puncture

Points: Shanzhong (CV17) and Hegu (LI4)

Technique: The patient is in a supine position. A No.30 2-*cun* long filiform needle is inserted from Shanzhong (CV17) downward along the presternum and penetrating to Jiewei (CV14), after which a lifting, thrusting and rotating technique is applied. Then Hegu (LI4) is stimulated. The needles are retained for 30 minutes. Such a method can treat all types of cough.

(2) Gentle Puncture

Points: Jinjin (Ex-HE12), Yuye (Ex-HE13), Yuji (LU10), Tiantu (CV22), Feishu (BL13) and Zhongwan (CV12).

Technique: Gentle puncture is applied on all the points. Except Jinjin (Ex-HE12) and Yuye (Ex-HE13), the needles are retained on the rest points for 20 minutes. Coughing due to lung *yin* deficiency is indicated.

2. MOXIBUSTION

(1) Sparrow-Pecking Moxibustion

Point: Feishu (BL13)

Technique: The patient is in a sitting position with both arms crossed over the chest. Sparrow-pecking moxibustion with moxa stick is applied on bilateral Feishu (BL13) simultaneously for 30 to 60 minutes each time until the skin turns purplish red. Moxibustion is given once daily. Chronic bronchitis is indicated.

(2) Moxibustion with Moxa Cone

Point: Taodao (GV8)

Technique: The patient is in a prone position. Taodao (GV8) is stimulated with moxa cone, 3 to 7 cones each time. The treatment is given once daily and 10 days in succession. Cough of a deficiency type is indicated.

(3) Moxibustion with Incense Thread

Points: Feishu (BL13), Fengmen (BL12) and Tiantu (CV22)

Technique: To burn the acupoint swiftly with incense thread, one burning on each point. Swift, correct and gentle pressing is required. Acute bronchitis and cough with itching throat are indicated. After the treatment is given once or twice, the therapeutic effects will be apparent.

3. ELECTRIC THERAPY

Points: Zhikexue, located 0.5 *cun* above Yuji (LU10), Feirexue, located 0.5 *cun* lateral to T3 and T4, Huxidian, located 1/3 inferior to the posterior border of sternocleidomastoid muscle, Kongzui (LU6).

Technique: Puncture the acupoints in the routine method, and then select the points for electric stimulation for chronic bronchitis based on clinical symptoms and constitution. For a simple cough, the positive electrode is on Zhikexue and the negative on Feirexue, for profuse sputum and a good constitution, the positive is on Kongzui (LU6) and the negative on Huxidian. The frequency is based on dense-sparse wave and the electric intensity is increased from weak to moderate. The treatment is given once daily and lasts 10 to 20 minutes each time. Six days make up one course. The second course is given if the case is not cured. The effective rate of treating chronic bronchitis is relatively high. Generally, with electric stimulation, the patient feels relief from chest tightness and breathes smoothly.

4. CATGUT-EMBEDDING METHOD

Points: Dingchuan (Ex-B1), Feishu (BL13), Shangzhong (CV17) and tender points on the back.

Technique: The patient is in a sitting position. No.0 surgical catgut, 1.5 to 2 cm long is embedded on a pair of points bilaterally in each treatment. Ten days later, the other points are replaced. Two to three treatments make one course. In the first treatment, Shanzhong (CV17) is embedded as the extra for chronic bronchitis, with the therapeutic effect recorded at 97%.

5. CUPPING

Points: Dazhui (GV14), Dazhu (BL11), Shenzhu (GV12), Feishu (BL13) and Shangzhong (CV17)

Technique: Four to six cups are applied in each treatment, and retained for 15 to 20 minutes. The treatment is given once daily and is good for stopping cough and resolving phlegm.

6. FINGER ACU-PRESSURE IN THE CHEST POINTS

Point: The lower borders of the first and fifth sternocostal joints

Technique: One to two pairs of points are selected in each treatment, pressed with the index or middle fingers for 10 to 15 minutes on each point. The treatment is given twice a day and 10 days make up one course.

7. HYDRO-ACUPUNCTURE

Points: Jiaji (Ex-B2) from C7 to T6

Technique: The placenta tissue liquid, 1 ml, is prepared. In each treatment, a pair of points is injected, 0.5 ml for each. The points are changed daily from up to down. The treatment is given once every two days and 10 treatments make up one course.

8. CONVENTIONAL ACUPUNCTURE

Point: Tinggong (SI19) penetrating to Internal Nose

Technique: A one-*cun* filiform needle is inserted from Tinggong (SI19), 0.2 to 0.3 *cun* deep and penetrated obliquely to the Internal Nose (auricular point) with the ear tragus left by the thumb and index finger. A constant pricking sensation is produced and the needle is retained for 10 to 15 minutes. The treatment is given daily and on one ear each time. The ears are punctured alternately. Ten days make up one course.

9. MEDICINAL APPLICATION ON ACU-POINT

Point: Shenque (CV8)

Technique: Gongdingxiang (Flos Caryophylli) 0.5 g, Rougui (Cortex Cinnamomi) 5 g, Mahuang (Herba Ephedrae) 5 g, Cangerzi (Frutus Xanthii) 3 g, Baijiezi (Semen Sinapis Albae) 4 g, and Banxia (Rhizoma Pinelliae) 3 g. All the herbs are ground into powder and stored. The umbilicus is sterilized with 75% alcohol, filled with herbal powder and covered to prevent leakage. The medicine is changed once every 48 hours. Ten compresses make up one course and five to seven days should elapse between two courses. A study of 200 cases of chronic bronchitis treated by this method revealed a total effective rate of 94.5%.

[REMARKS]

1. Certain short-term and long-term effects have been achieved for chronic bronchitis with moxibustion and medicinal application on acu-points.

2. Physical exercise or continuous moxibustion on Dazhui (GV14), Feishu (BL13) and Zusanli (ST36) may build up the constitution to prevent a recurrence of the cough.

ASTHMA

[INTRODUCTION]

The pathological location of asthma is in the lung, and related to the liver, spleen and kidney. In clinical work, asthma is divided into the categories of deficiency and excess. The excess is due to an invasion of wind and cold, improper diet, overeating greasy, sweet and fishy food, which results in a dysfunction of the spleen in terms of transportation and transformation, the production of phlegm that affects the lung; or is due to the liver *qi* attacking the lung. The excess type is manifested by harsh breathing with the mouth open and the shoulder raised, and is treated by the points in Hand-Taiyin and Yangming meridians, i.e., Dingchuang (Ex-B1), Lieque (LU7), Chize (LU5), Hegu (LI4) and Shanzhong (CV17) with reducing needling technique. Moxibustion is added for wind and cold type. The deficiency is due to insufficiency of lung *qi*, weakness of the spleen, stomach and kidney, and is manifested as asthmatic weak breathing, speaking in a low voice, lassitude, or more exhalation than inhalation. The treatment principle is to strengthen the anti-pathogenic *qi*, reducing the phlegm to relieve the asthma. The points include Feishu (BL13), Shenshu (BL23), Pishu (BL20), Dingchuan (Ex-B1), Gaohuangshu (BL43), Taiyuan (LU9), Zusanli (ST36) and Qihai (CV6), stimulated with reinforcing technique. Acupuncture and moxibustion are applied together. Bronchial asthma, chronic asthmatic bronchitis and allergic asthma fall in this disease category.

[CLINICAL EXPERIENCE]

1. CONVENTIONAL ACUPUNCTURE

(1) Puncturing Shuliao (GV25)

Technique: Shuliao (GV25) is punctured 0.2 to 0.3 *cun* deep, with swift rotation. The patient feels soreness and distension in the nose. The method is for acute attack of asthma manifested as a shortage of breath and being unable to lie down.

(2) Puncturing Yuji (LU10)

Technique: A one-*cun* filiform needle is inserted obliquely towards the palm center, about 0.5 *cun* deep, and retained for 20 to 30 minutes after the arrival of the needling sensation. The needle is rotated once every five minutes. The treatment is given once daily. In case of an attack, the treatment is given at any time and Yuji (LU10) of one side is punctured each time, the two sides being punctured alternately. Ten treatments make one course.

(3) Puncturing Tiantu (CV22)

Technique: The patient is in a sitting or lying position with the head slightly raised. A 1.5-*cun* filiform needle is inserted perpendicularly 0.2 *cun* deep, then the needle tip goes to the posterior of the sternum downward, 0.5 to 1.2 *cun* deep. The needle is retained for 20 minutes when a tense feeling appears under the needle. The needle is rotated several times during retention.

(4) Puncturing the Sensitive **Points** *on the Back*

Technique: The patient is in a sitting position, with the back exposed. Pain, soreness, distension, numbness sensitive points are detected with the thumb pressing on the first and second lines of the bladder meridian. In each treatment, four to six sensitive points are selected and given strong stimulation. The needles are retained for 20 minutes. The treatment is given once a day, or twice a day in times of attack. Ten treatments make one course.

2. MOXIBUSTION

(1) Indirect Moxibustion with Ginger

Points: ① Feishu (BL13) and Lingtai (GV10). ② Shenshu (BL23). ③ Tiantu (CV22) and Shanzhong (CV17)

Technique: The three group points are applied alternately daily. The ignited moxa cone (in the size of half of a date-stone) is placed on the acu-point isolated with a slice of fresh ginger, about 0.1 *cun* thick. Five to seven cones are required for each treatment on each point. A seven-day treatment makes up one course. The method is good for bronchial asthma.

(2) Scaring Moxibustion

Points: ① Tiantu (CV22), Lingtai (GV10) and Feishu (BL13). ② Fengmen (BL12) and Dazhui (GV14). ③ Dazhu (BL11) and Shanzhong (CV17). Supplementary points according to the differentiation of syndromes: for cold type, adding Zhongwan (CV12), Lieque (LU7) and Zusanli (ST36); for phlegm heat type, adding Lieque (LU7) and Fenglong (ST40); for the deficiency type, adding Shenshu (BL23) and Guanyuan (CV4); for facial edema, adding Shuifen (CV9) and Pishu (BL20).

Technique: The moxa cone, 0.6 to 0.8 cm in diameter and 1 to 1.2 cm high, is prepared. The point is sterilized and given a local anesthesia with procarine 0.5 to 1 ml. Then the garlic juice is applied on the point. Five to nine cones are required on each point in each treatment. Generally, moxibustion is given three times for an adult once a year. The best treatment duration is from Lesser Heat to White Dew by the lunar calendar. (The treatment can also be given in other times of year.) The three prescriptions are applied alternately in each treatment and modified based on the differentiation.

3. HYDRO-CUPPING

Point: Feishu (BL13)

Technique: The patient is in a sitting position with the back exposed. The big No.1 cup is applied containing half a cup of warm water. The cup is placed on the bilateral Feishu (BL13) swiftly after the ignited paper is thrown into the cup. After the cup is retained for about 15 minutes it will be removed slowly and carefully to prevent leakage. Generally, four to five administrations of cupping are required for asthma, five to six times for a severe case. For a case that proves difficult to treat, Wuyi (ST15) is also cupped bilaterally on the chest.

4. ELECTRIC ACUPUNCTURE

Points: Kongzui (LU6) and Chize (LU5)

Technique: The patient is in a supine position. Kongzui (LU6) and Chize (LU5) are punctured bilaterally. The up-down conductive sensation is required on Kongzui (LU6). The negative electrode is put on Kongzui (LU6) and the positive one on Chize (LU5). Two group wires are put on the bilateral points respectively. The electric stimulation lasts for 30 to 60 minutes. The treatment is given once daily. The method is good for relieving asthma and suitable for acute attacks.

5. AURICULAR THERAPY

Points: Main points: Lung, Trochia, Adrenal, Asthma Relieving and Ear-Shenmen. Supplementary points: Spleen, Kidney, Triple Energizer, Large Intestine, Asthma Point and Vagus Root.

Technique: Four to 5 points are selected and punctured on two ears alternately for each treatment. The needles are retained for one hour at least and the treatment is given once daily. Electric stimulation is applicable. The treatment is given once every two days until the symptoms are relieved. The seed-pressing therapy is applied to strengthen the effect in the recovery stage.

6. CUTANEAUS PUNCTURE

Points: The running course of the lung meridian of Hand-Taiyin, and the bilateral sternocleidomastoid muscles.

Technique: The patient is in a sitting position. The plum-blossom needle is used to tap the bilateral lung meridian and sternocleidomastoid muscles. Thirty minutes of tapping is required in each treatment until the skin turns slightly red. The method is applied during an asthma attack to bring relief.

7. NEEDLE-EMBEDDING METHOD

Point: Shanzhong (CV17)

Technique: A No.29 filiform needle, 1.5 *cun* long, is inserted from Shanzhong (CV17), subcutaneously straight down to Zhongting (CV16) and rotated for several seconds. The reducing technique is applied to produce a dispersed needling sensation. The needle is retained for 15 minutes. When asthma is relieved, the needle will be fixed with a plaster and embedded for two to five days. Generally, the needle-embedding method is applied once every seven days, and three treatments make up one course. The treatment is good for chronic asthma and effective for persistent non-curing cases.

8. CATGUT-EMBEDDING METHOD

Points: Feishu (BL13) and Dingchuan (Ex-B1)

Technique: The patient is in a sitting position. After routine sterilization, the catgut thread is embedded beneath the skin, 2 to 4 cm long, and fixed with a piece of gauze. The points on the bilateral sides are selected alternately. The method is applied once every two weeks, and three to four treatments make up a course.

9. HYDRO-ACUPUNCTURE

Point: Jiaji (Ex-B2) from C7 to T6

Technique: A pair of points are selected and injected with placenta tissue liquid 0.5-1 ml each time. The points change from up to down everyday. The treatment is given once a day or once every two days. Twenty treatments make up one course. The method is for the recovery stage.

10. LASER THERAPY

Points: Tiantu (CV22), Shanzhong (CV17), Feishu (BL13), Dingchuan (Ex-B1) and Chize (LU5)

Technique: Two to three points are selected and radiated with He-Ne laser, eight minutes on each point each time. The treatment is given once a day and 10 treatments make up one course. One week later, another course begins. The method is effective during asthma attacks.

11. MEDICINAL APPLICATION ON ACU-POINTS

(1) Application with Asthma Relieving Plaster

Points: Feishu (BL13), Xinshu (BL15) and Geshu (BL17)

Technique: Baijiezi (Semen Sinapis Albae) 21 g, Yuanhu (Rhizoma Corydalis) 21 g, Gansui (Radix Euphorbiae Kansui) 12 g and Xixin (Herba Asari) 12 g are prepared. All herbs are ground into powder, which is enough for a person for one year. The method is applied in the three 10-day periods of the hot season. Each time, the paste is mixed by 1/3 herbal powder and fresh ginger juice (each time, the juice is squeezed from 100 g fresh ginger) and separated into six pieces of paper or plastic cloth, 5 cm in diameter. The points bilaterally are compressed for four to six hours generally. The compress is removed earlier if burning or pain appears in the locality. The application is given once every 10 days, a total of three times successively in the first, second and third 10-day hottest periods in summer. The treatment is applied continuously for three years for acute attacks or in the recovery stage. The effect is especially good for cases due to cold of *yang* deficiency, manifested as white clean and thin sputum. It is reported that the effect is better if the application is given around noontime on a sunny day and worse on a cloudy or rainy day.

(2) Application with Fresh Maogen (Rhizoma Imperatae Cylindricae)

Point: Dazhui (GV14)

Technique: Three to five leaves of fresh Maogen (Rhizoma Imperatae Cylindricae) are ground into powder and mixed with ginger juice. The herbal paste is put on Dazhui (GV14) until blisters appear. The treatment is given once every 10 days, and three treatments make one course. Chinese herb therapy is applied in combination.

[REMARKS]

1. If the therapeutic effect is not satisfactory by acupuncture for acute attack of asthma for longer duration, comprehensive therapy with Chinese and Western medicine should be applied to control the attack rapidly.

2. All causes and allergies related to the onset of an asthma attack should be avoided to reduce the frequency of the attacks.

3. "To treat in summer for the attack in winter" is the principle of curing asthma. The patient should be told that the symptoms are treated for the attack and the root cause treated for the recovery. Good cooperation may maintain solid and long-lasting therapeutic effect.

APHONIA

[INTRODUCTION]

Aphonia is caused by invasion of pathogenic wind and heat leading to the lung *qi* failing to disperse; or mental depression, the liver *qi* stagnation being transformed into fire that affects the throat along the liver meridian; or *yin* deficiency of the lung and kidney resulting in lack of nourishment of the throat. The treatment principle is to benefit the lung *qi* to dispel the pathogenic factors and nourish *yin* to clear away the heat. The points are mainly selected from the Hand-Taiyin meridian, i.e., Futu (LI18), Tianding (LI17), Yuji (LU10) and Tongli (HT5). For wind cold involved, Hegu (LI4), Lieque (LU7) and Fengchi (GB20) are added; for wind heat involved, Quchi (LI11), Hegu (LI4) and Shaoshang (LU11) are added; for the liver *qi* stagnation, Taichong (LR3) and Yanglingquan (GB34) are added; for *yin* deficiency, Sanyinjiao (SP3), Taixi (KI3) and Zhaohai (KI6) are added. A reducing technique is applied for excess syndrome and reinforcing technique for deficiency syndrome. The treatments are applied based on such disease for acute and chronic laryngitis, strain of the vocal fold, vocal nodules and hysteric aphonia.

[CLINICAL EXPERIENCE]

1. CONVENTIONAL ACUPUNCTURE

(1) Puncturing Liyanxue

Point: Liyanxue (in the depression posterior to the middle of the ear lobe and angle of mandible)

Technique: The patient is in a sitting position with the eyes staring straight ahead. An 1.5-*cun* filiform needle is inserted toward the throat, 0.8 to 1.2-*cun* deep. Scraping needle technique is applied. The needle is retained for 30 to 60 minutes and scraped once every 10 to 20 minutes. The technique is for acute laryngitis. For fever, Dazhui (GV14) and Hegu (LI4) are punctured, and Shaoshang (LU11) is punctured to bleed. The treatment is given once daily.

(2) Puncturing Fengfu (GV16)

Points: Fengfu (GV16), Yemen (TE2) and Yuji (LU10)

Technique: Each point is punctured 0.3 to 0.5 *cun* deep and rotated for 2 minutes. This is for treating a sore throat with hoarse voice.

(3) Selecting the Points Along the Meridian

Points: Tianding (LI17) and Jianshi (PC5)

Technique: *Bai Zheng Fu* (*Fu on One Hundred Diseases*): "Tianding (LI17) and Jianshi (PC5) stop aphonia." Since the large intestine is related to the lung externally and internally, Tianding (LI17) is located beside the throat, good for promoting lung *qi* dispersal and benefiting the vocal chords following sudden loss of voice. Jianshi (PC5) can regulate heart functions. *Internal Classic* says: "The heart dominates speech and the liver dominates language." The speaking disorder is related to the heart and liver. The reducing needle technique is applied after the arrival of *qi*. Such a method is for treating hysteric aphonia.

(4) Puncturing Shenzhu (GV12)

Point: Shenzhu (GV12)

Technique: For hysteric aphonia, if there is no effect through treatment with Tiantu (CV22), Lianquan (CV23), Yamen (GV15), Yongquan (KI1), Hegu (LI4) and Baihui (GV20), Shenzhu (GV12) is punctured and good effect is achieved immediately.

(5) Puncturing Renzhong (GV26)

Point: Renzhong (GV26)

Technique: Renzhong (GV26) is punctured with a 1.5-*cun* fili-form needle with strong stimulation until the patient cries with tears running down the face. This had good effect for hysteric aphonia.

(6) Selecting the Nearby Points

Point: Lianquan (CV23)

Technique: Lianquan (CV23) is punctured with a No.30 filiform needle, 1.5 *cun* long, with the tip toward the tongue root obliquely about 1 *cun* deep. Reducing technique by lifting and thrusting the needle is applied to cause numbness radiating from the neck to the tongue.

(7) Selecting the Distal Points

Point: Yongquan (KI1)

Technique: Quick needling technique is applied on Yongquan (KI1) bilaterally with strong stimulation. The treatment is given once every two days, and is indicated for aphonia due to encephalitis B.

(8) Puncturing Luo-Connecting Points

Points: Neiguan (PC6) and Tongli (HT7)

Technique: One-*cun* filiform needles are applied to puncture the Luo-Connecting points of the heart meridian of Hand-Shaoyin and pericardium meridian of Hand-Yueyin with strong stimulation, and the needles are retained for 20 minutes. The method is for sudden loss of voice due to emotional disturbance.

2. BLEEDING METHOD

(1) Bleeding on Jing-Well Points

Points: Shaoshang (LU11), Guanchong (TE1) and Zuqiaoyin (GB41)

Technique: To prick Jing-well points with a thick needle to cause bleeding. The method is for aphonia due to heat syndromes.

(2) Bleeding Under the Tongue

Points: Jinjin (Ex-HN12) and Yuye (Ex-HN13)

Technique: The points are pricked with a syringe needle to get 0.5 ml blood. The method is for hysteric aphonia or aphonia due to cerebral vascular diseases.

3. ELECTRIC ACUPUNCTURE

Points: Renying (ST9), Tiantu (CV22) and Lianquan (CV23)

Technique: After routine acupuncture, two points are selected for electric stimulation for 15 minutes each time. The method is especially effective for inflammatory aphonia, strain of laryngeal muscles and functional aphonia.

4. AURICULAR THERAPY

Points: Lung, heart, throat, trachea and kidney

Technique: Two to three points are selected each time with moderate stimulation. Five treatments make one course. The treatment is given daily, and needles are retained for 20 minutes each time.

5. MEDICINAL APPLICATION ON ACU-POINTS

Point: Tiantu (CV22)

Technique: Tiantu (CV22) is compressed with a piece of medical plaster for pain relief (*Shang Shi Zhi Tong Gao*). The plaster is replaced once every three days. The treatment is effective for chronic laryngitis.

6. COMPREHENSIVE THERAPY

Points: Renying (ST9), Quchi (LI11) and Jianzhen (GB21)

Technique: Renying (ST9) is injected with berberine, 1-2 ml. At the same time, Quchi (LI11) and Jianzhen (GB21) are punctured and the needles are retained for 30 minutes after the arrival of *qi*. The method is for acute and chronic chorditis vocalis and vocal fold edema.

[REMARKS]

1. Acupuncture is especially good for acute and chronic laryngitis and congestion of the vocal fold.

2. Psychotherapy can improve the therapeutic effect for hysteric aphonia.

3. The patient should take light-taste food, and all kinds of spicy and fried food are avoided, such as peppers, garlic, spring onion and fried food.

17

EPIGASTRIC PAIN

[INTRODUCTION]

Although the diseased part involved in epigastric pain is the stomach, it is closely related with the liver and the spleen. This problem may be caused by invasion of exogenous pathogenic cold, overeating of raw and cold food, an attack on the stomach by liver *qi* or weakness of the spleen and stomach. Clinically, it is divided into excess type and deficiency type. In excess condition, the pain is very severe and aggravated by pressure, especially after a meal; in deficiency condition, the pain is dull, alleviated by warmth and pressure, and is aggravated by an empty stomach. The principle of treatment is to regulate the spleen and stomach, and promote the flow of *qi* to stop pain with Zhongwan (CV12), Pishu (BL20), Neiguan (PC6) and Zusanli (ST36) as the main points. For pathogenic cold, add moxibustion; for attack on the stomach by liver *qi*, add Ganshu (BL18), Taichong (LR3); and for weakness of the spleen and stomach, add Weishu (BL21), Zhangmen (LR13) and Sanyinjiao (SP6). Stomachache is more apparent in acute and chronic gastritis, gastric and duodenal ulcer, and stomach neurasthenia.

[CLINICAL EXPERIENCE]

1. CONVENTIONAL ACUPUNCTURE

(1) Puncturing Zhongshu (CV7)

Point: Zhongshu (CV7).

Technique: Puncturing a one-*cun* needle into the point as deep as 0.5 to 0.8 *cun* with even technique and retaining the needle for 5 to 10 minutes. This method is effective for acute stomachache.

(2) Puncturing Weile Point

Point: Weile [0.2 *cun* inferior and 4 *cun* lateral to Shuifen (CV9)].

Technique: Keep the patient in a supine position. Puncturing a 1.5 *cun* needle into the point 0.7 to 1 *cun* deep with strong stimulation and no retention of the needle. This method is indicated for stomachache due to gastric and duodenal ulcer and gastritis.

(3) Method of Promoting Qi by the Needle Tip

Point: Neiguan (PC6).

Technique: Puncture Neiguan (PC6) of the left side obliquely by a 1.5-*cun* needle with the needle tip toward the shoulder and arm, and manipulate the needle by rotating it to obtain *qi*, then forcefully insert the needle 0.1 *cun* deep obliquely upward five times, when the patient will be able to feel the needling sensation being conducted to the arm-pit.

(4) Puncturing the Tender Points Along the Vertebral Column

Technique: Ask the patient to keep a prone position, with the chest and abdomen kept higher to make the vertebral column curve like arch. The practitioner presses the points with even force from the first to the 12th thoracic vertebra, the tenderness indicating the points for needling. Puncture two or three points each time intermittently. Insert the needle slowly along the space of the spineous process 0.8 to 1 *cun* deep. It is forbidden to hurt the spinal cord when puncturing the thoracic vertebra region. Manipulating the needle by lifting and thrusting it slowly, scraping the needle until the pain is alleviated or disappears, and retaining the needle for 30 to 60 minutes. The method is indicated for gastric and duodenal ulcer.

(5) Puncturing Liangqiu (ST34) with Heavy Force

Technique: Puncture the point quickly by a No.28 needle, 1.5 *cun* long, and manipulate it by rotating, lifting and thrusting to send the needling sensation upward to the hip and abdomen. The needle is retained for 10 to 15 minutes. This method is effective for stomach spasms.

(6) Puncturing Banmen

Point: Banmen point [medial to Yuji (LU10), when locating the point, bend the thumb downward, the point is where the prominence is located on the thenar].

Technique: Puncture the point by a No.26 needle, 1.5 *cun* long, perpendicularly 0.5 to 1 *cun* deep to send the needling sensation through the whole hand or to the upper arm. This method is indicated for stomach spasm.

(7) Puncturing the Scapular Region

Point: The tenderness around Tianzong (SI11).

Technique: After confirming the tenderness around the point, apply massage first and acupuncture later to alleviate the pain. In case the pain refers to both sides of the costal region, puncture from Geshu (BL17) to Ganshu (BL18) with penetrating technique along the skin.

(8) Puncturing the Calcaneus Region

Point: The local region on the posterior aspect of the calcaneus tendon.

Technique: Let the patient remain in a prone or lateral recumbent position with the toes extended downward in a forceful way. The point is located in the depression in the middle of the calcaneus tendon. Insert a one-*cun* needle into the point 0.5 to 0.8 *cun* deep, and retain the needle for 5 to 15 minutes after the arrival of *qi*. The treatment is given once a day. This method has been used for 154 cases of acute and chronic epigastric pain, with a total effective rate of 98.1%.

2. MOXIBUSTON

(1) Moxibustion with Moxa Stick

Point: Gaohuang (BL43).

Technique: Let the patient remain in a prone position, applying moxibustion on the point bilaterally with a moxa stick for 30 to 40 minutes. This method is indicated for epigastric pain accompanied by hyperacidity.

(2) Moxibustion with Moxa Box

Point: On the local area with pain.

Technique: Let patient remain in a supine position, putting a moxa box on the abdomen in the area where the pain is detected. The treatment is given once a day, 30 minutes each time. This method is indicated for stomachache due to deficient cold.

(3) Moxibustion with Moxa Cone

Point: Yinbai (SP1).

Technique: Apply moxa cones on Yinbai (SP1) bilaterally. This method is indicated for epigastric pain accompanied by occult blood in the stool.

3. CUPPING

Points: Zhongwan (CV12) and Shenque (CV8).

Technique: Let the patient remain in a supine position. Applying cupping on these points with medium-sized cups. Retaining the cup on Zhongwan (CV12) for 10 to 15 minutes, and on Shenque (CV8) for five minutes. This method is indicated for gastrointestinal neurosis and ulcerative stomachache.

4. AURICULAR THERAPY

Points: Stomach, spleen, Shenmen, duodenum, Sanjiao, subcortex and sympathetic.

Technique: Puncture the ear points by needles with moderate stimulation. The treatment is given once a day or once every other day, and 10 times constitute one course of treatment. The seeds can be used instead.

5. HYDRO-ACUPUNCTURE

Point: Zusanli (ST36).

Technique: Let the patient remain in a supine position with two lower limbs flexed, while injecting 2 ml of painkiller into Zusanli (ST36). In 20 cases where the patients were treated with injection, pain stopped immediately in 16 cases, and within three minutes in another four cases. This method is indicated for severe pain due to ulcer.

6. ELECTRIC ACUPUNCTURE

Points: Zusanli (ST36), Zhongwan (CV12), Liangmen (ST21), Tianshu (ST25) and Neiguan (PC6).

Technique: After using the common method to obtain *qi*, apply strong stimulation, and then connect to the electric apparatus for one hour. The interval between two treatments is four hours. This method is used to treat acute perforation of the ulcer (acute stage), and abdominal pain will be significantly alleviated with the disappearance of the board-like abdomen and resumption of a gurgling sound after one or two treatments. Herbal medicine can be combined. At the same time, gastrointestinal decompression, common IV and a half-sitting position can be helpful for the patient, without using any painkiller. If the symptoms do not improve remarkably, an operation should be performed.

7. CATGUT-EMBEDDING METHOD ON ACUPOINT

Points: ① Weishu (BL21) to Pishu (BL20), and Zhongwan (CV12) to Shangwan (CV13). ② Liangmen (ST21) to Chengman (ST20), and Weicang (BL50) to Yishe (BL49).

Technique: First using the first group of points. If the first are not effective, use the second group of points. In the application, sterilize the point first, insert a big-curved triangular needle with No.1 catgut thread into the skin from a point 1 cm away from the acupoint and out from a point 1 cm away from another acupoint through the muscular membrane and muscular layer, cut away the end of the thread above the skin, lift the skin in order to embed the thread completely inside, and cover a piece of sterilized gauze on it for three to five days. Embedding again 20 to 30 days later.

8. MEDICINAL APPLICATION ON ACUPOINT

Points: Zhongwan (CV12), Pishu (BL20) and Weishu (BL21).

Technique: Grind Sichuan peppers 15 g, dried ginger 10 g, Fupian 10 g, sandalwood 10 g, Cangshu (the rhizome of Chinese atractylodes) 20 g into powder, sifting and mixing them with ginger juice into paste. During treatment, apply medicinal paste on the points, cover them with gauze, and fix them by the plaster. The dressing is given once or twice a day. The course of treatment is one month without stop. This method is indicated for gastric and duodenal ulcer.

[REMARKS]

1. Stomachache can be stopped immediately in most cases by acupuncture. There will be long-term satisfactory results in case of ulcer if the treatment is given persistently.

2. The patient with this problem should maintain a pleasant, balanced work routine with a good rest, pursue a regular daily life, and avoid eating spicy and hot food.

ABDOMINAL PAIN

[INTRODUCTION]

Abdominal pain refers to the pain happening in an area below the epigastria and above the transverse bone. This problem involves the dysfunction of the spleen, stomach, large intestine, small intestine, liver, and gall bladder. It can be caused by overeating cold and raw food, or by excessive attack of external cold to the umbilicus and abdomen, leading to accumulation of cold and obstruction of *qi*, or by overeating and overdrinking, or by emotional disturbance, resulting in stagnation of liver *qi*, or *yang qi* deficiency of zang-fu organs. Clinically, it can be divided into cold type, which is marked by acute and severe abdominal pain and is alleviated by warmth; secondly, by food retention, which is marked by distension, fullness and abdominal; thirdly, a type of stagnation of liver *qi*, which is marked by distending pain of the abdomen, especially, more severe degree of distension than that of pain, and unfixed pain; the fourth type is *yang* deficiency, which is marked by intermittent dull abdominal pain. To promote the flow of *qi* and stop pain, Zhongwan (CV12), Neiguan (PC6), Tianshu (ST25), Qihai (CV6) and Susanli (ST36) are used. In case of excessive cold, moxibustion is supplemented; in case of retention of food, Xiawan (CV10) and Lineiting (Extra) are selected; in case of stagnation of liver *qi*, Ganshu (BL18) and Taichong (LR3) are also selected; in case of *yang* deficiency, Pishu (BL20), Shenshu (BL23) and Guanyuan (CV4) are selected with moxibustion. Reducing technique is used for excess syndrome, and reinforcing technique is used for deficiency syndrome.

[CLINICAL EXPERIENCE]

1.   CONVENTIONAL ACUPUNCTURE

(1) Penetrating Technique

Points: From Neiguan (PC6) to Waiguan (TE5) with penetrating technique.

Technique: Puncture Neiguan (PC6) to Waiguan (TE5) unilaterally with penetrating technique, while encouraging the patient to breathe deeply. Retain the needle for 15 minutes after the arrival of *qi*, lift and thrust the needle with a sparrow-pecking method once every five minutes and apply massage gently on the patient's abdomen.

(2) Selection of Points According to the Affected Area

Points: In case of pain in the middle of the abdomen, Gongsun (SP4) and Diji (SP8) are selected; for pain around the umbilicus, Shuiquan (KI5), Yingu (KI10), Mingmen (GV4) are selected; for pain in the lower abdomen, Zhongdu (LR6) and Xingjian (LR2) are selected; and for pain on the lateral aspect of lower abdomen, Ligou (LR5) is selected.

Technique: Puncture the points with the common method and retain the needle for 20 minutes after the arrival of *qi*. Other points can also be used in terms of different etiology.

(3) Selection of Points According to the Nature of Pain

Points: For distending pain, Tianshu (ST25) and Yinlingquan (SP9) are selected; for pricking pain, Xuehai (SP10) and Quchi (LI11) are selected; for moving pain, Qihai (CV6) and Sanyinjiao (SP6) are selected; and for dull pain, Gongsun (SP4), Zhangmen (LR13) and Dabao (SP21) are selected.

Technique: Puncturing the points with the common method. Other points can also be used in terms of etiology and affected area.

(4) Puncturing Around the Umbilicus

Points: Four points around the umbilicus (one *cun* superior, inferior, left and right to the umbilicus respectively).

Technique: Both acupuncture and moxibustion can be applied on these points. It is indicated for all kinds of abdominal pain.

(5) Puncturing Jianli (CV11)

Points: Jianli (CV11).

Technique: Keep the patient in a supine position, and puncture the point perpendicularly one to two *cun* deep. When *qi* arrives, apply reinforcing or reducing technique in terms of deficiency or excessive syndrome, and retain the needle for 20 to 30 minutes.

(6) Selection of Points According the Time

Points: Dazhui (CV14) and Zusanli (ST36).

Technique: A patient had been feeling dull pain around the umbilicus for more than 10 years, the pain usually occurring between two and three o'clock in the afternoon and between seven and nine o'clock in the evening. These points were punctured at 2:00 p.m., and the pain disappeared completely after five treatments.

(7) Puncturing Along the Skin with the Penetrating Method

Points: Shangwan (CV13), Zhongwan (CV12), Jianli (CV11) and Xiawan (CV10).

Technique: Keep the patient in a supine position with both legs flexed upward slightly. The practitioner fixes and stretches the skin around Shangwan (CV13) with the left hand, and inserts a 3-*cun* needle into Shangwan (CV13) transversely along the skin to penetrate through Zhongwan (CV12), Jianli (CV11) and Xiawan (CV10), then rotates the needle repeatedly. After the arrival of *qi*, the needle should be retained for 20 to 30 minutes, while manipulating it intermittently until the pain is alleviated or disappears. Usually most cases of abdominal pain can be alleviated after 30 minutes of needle retention.

(8) Selection of Ah-shi Points on the Back

Points: Pressing the skin of the patient along the vertebral column 1.5 to 2 cm lateral to the mid-line up to down, the Ah-shi points are those tender spots.

Technique: Selecting one or two points every time and puncturing them with reducing technique. It is used for abdominal pain.

2. MOXIBUSTION

(1) Moxibustion with Moxa Box

Point: Painful area on the abdomen.

Technique: Keep the patient in a supine position, placing the moxa box on the area affected by pain and igniting the moxa stick. This method can alleviate abdominal pain due to various reasons, but it is especially good for pain caused by cold or *yang* deficiency.

(2) Moxibustion with Salt

Point: Shenque (CV8).

Technique: Cover Shenque (CV8) evenly by fried salt powder 0.3 cm thick and two or three cm in diameter, put big moxa cones as big as a yellow bean on it and ignite them. Three to five cones are applied successively, but be careful not to burn the skin.

(3) Moxibustion with Ginger

Points: Zhongwan (CV12), Shenque (CV8) and Guanyuan (CV4).

Technique: Place a big slice of ginger, 0.2 cm thick, on the points, then put some big moxa cones on top and ignite them. When the temperature becomes high, move the ginger slice. Apply moxa on one or two points with five to eight cones on each point.

3. CUPPING

Points: Zhongwan (CV12), Tianshu (ST25), Shenque (CV8) and Qihai (CV6).

Technique: Keep the patient in a supine position and apply cupping on the points with medium-sized cups. Do not put the cup on Shenque (CV8) heavily, but just leave it gently socked onto the skin. Retain the cup for 10 to 15 minutes once a day.

4. AURICULAR THERAPY

Points: Large Intestine, Stomach, Spleen, Shenmen and Sympathetic.

Technique: Puncture two to three points every time by filiform needles with moderate stimulation and retain the needles for 10 to 20 minutes. The treatment is given once a day or once every other day, with 10 treatments comprising one course.

5. HYDRO-ACUPUNCTURE

Point: Zusanli (ST36).

Technique: Mix Phenergan 50 mg with Atropine 0.5 mg and sterilize the skin with routine asepsis. Insert the needle into Zusanli (ST36) bilaterally, and inject the fluid when the patient feels sourness, numbness and distension on the point. Less dosage is used for weak patients and children. This method is much better than only using antispastic.

6. FINGER PUNCTURE

Point: Qishe (ST11).

Technique: The practitioner kneads Qishe (ST11) by the tip of middle finger for five to 10 minutes, after which the pain can be alleviated.

[REMARKS]

1. Acupuncture is effective for abdominal pain, but causes should be checked in order to make clear diagnosis. In case of severe abdominal pain, importance should be attached to nursing and clinical observation, and medicine and other methods can be supplemented if necessary.

2. The patient with abdominal pain is advised to take care of his diet. For example, one should eat more food of a sweet, warm nature for pain due to deficient cold; or control the intake of food for pain due to retention of food.

VOMITING

[INTRODUCTION]

The problem may be caused by upward perversion of stomach *qi* due to invasion of wind, cold, summer heat and damp, or retention of food, or interior retention of phlegm fluid, or attack of stomach by liver *qi*, or weakness of the spleen and stomach, or deficiency of stomach *yin*. The treatment is given to harmonize stomach and lower stomach *qi* by selecting the Front-Mu point and Lower He-Sea point of the stomach as the main points, such as Zhongwan (CV12), Neiguan (PC6), Zusanli (ST36) and other points as supplementary points. For example, for invasion of external wind and cold, Fengchi (GB20), Waiguan (TE5) and Hegu (LI4) are added; for invasion of summer heat and damp, Dazhui (CV14), Quchi (LI11), Weizhong (BL40) and Yinlingquan (SP9) are added; for retention of food,

Xiawan (CV10) and Fujie (SP14) are added; for internal retention of phlegm fluid, Zhongmen (LR13), Fenglong (ST40) and Gongsun (SP4) are added; for attack on the stomach by liver *qi*, Yanglingquan (GB34) and Taichong (LR3) are added; for weakness of the spleen and stomach, Pishu (BL20), Weishu (BL21) and Qihai (CV6) are added; for deficiency of stomach *yin*, Sanyinjiao (SP6) and Xiangu (ST43) are added. This disease is similar to neurotic vomiting, acute and chronic gastritis, pylorospasm or obstructive problems.

[CLINICAL EXPERIENCE]

1. CONVENTIONAL ACUPUNCTURE

(1) Puncturing Renying (ST9)

Point: Renying (ST9).

Technique: Keep the patient in a supine position with the head lowered. The practitioner seizes the patient by the throat, but it is not advisable to use this method if the patient feels any dizziness. In application, touch the artery on the point Renying (ST9) with the left hand to fix the artery, puncturing a 1.5-*cun* needle into the artery wall with the right hand. It is not allowed to puncture the point very deeply, as this may cause hematoma. It is enough to see the trembling of the needle handle, and then gently press deeper without manipulation. Normally, the needle should be removed after 10 seconds, and on no account must it remain more than two minutes.

(2) Selection of Zhiou Point

Point: Zhiou Point [0.5 *cun* distal to Daling (PC9) on the palm].

Technique: Insert a needle, 1 or 1.5 *cun* long, into the point forming an angle of 15° to 30° toward the tip of the middle finger, manipulating the needle with large amplitude to cause strong stimulation. The needle can be retained for about 10 minutes, but the needle may not be retained for children. One side can be punctured for mild cases, and both sides for severe cases. A total of 26 cases were observed, and all were effectively treated. Usually, one treatment is enough.

(3) Puncturing Yintang (Extra) to Ezhong (Extra) with Penetrating Technique as the Main Points

Points: Yintang (Extra) to Ezhong (1 *cun* above Yintang), Weizhong (BL40), Chengjiang (CV24) and Kunlun (BL60).

Technique: Puncture the points by reducing technique. This method is indicated for vomiting caused by invasion of external pathogenic factors.

(4) Selection of Points According to Time

Point: Neiguan (PC6).

Technique: The treatment starts before the onset of vomiting after the meal. Ask the patient to remain in a supine position. After sterilizing both sides of the points Neiguan (PC6) with routine asepsis, insert the needle rapidly 0.8 to 1 *cun* deep. After the arrival of *qi*, manipulate the needle on both sides of the points by the lifting and thrusting technique for 10 to 15 minutes. Meanwhile, ask the patient to breathe in and out deeply two to three times, and lift and thrust the needle once after 5, 10 and 15 minutes respectively. Retain the needle for 30 minutes. The treatment is given twice to three times a day.

2. MOXIBUSTION

(1) Mild-warming Moxibustion with Moxa Stick

Points: ① Zhongwan (CV12), Shangwan (CV13) and Zusanli (ST36). ② Pishu (BL20), Weishu (BL21) and Neiguan (PC6).

Technique: The two groups of points are used in turn and once a day. Apply moxa on each point for five to 10 minutes. This method is indicated for neurological vomiting.

(2) Moxibustion with Moxa Cone

Points: Zhongwan (CV12), Wangu (SI5), Zhongkui (located on the tip of the middle bone of middle finger on the back).

Technique: For regurgitation and vomiting, apply moxa cones on the above points, five to seven each.

3. CUPPING

Points: ① Dazhui (CV14), Ganshu (BL18) and Pishu (BL20); ② Shendao (CV11), Danshu (BL19) and Weishu (BL21).

Technique: Sterilize the points with routine asepsis, and then prick them with a three-edged needle, and apply cupping to cause bloodletting. Retain the cups for 10 to 15 minutes. Only one group of points is used once every other day.

4. BLEEDING

Point: Chengjiang (CV24).

Technique: Pinch up the point with the left hand and prick it with a three-edged needle in the right hand. Then, squeeze the point with both hands to cause bleeding. This method is indicated for heat type of vomiting.

5. ELECTRIC ACUPUNCTURE

Point: Penetrating from Juque (CV14) to Xiawan (CV10) and from Burong (ST19) to Taiyi (ST23).

Technique: Insert a 5-*cun* needle at an angle of 25° into the points. A G6805 Electric Apparatus is used with the negative lead connected to Juque (CV14) and the positive lead to Burong (ST19) for 20 to 30 minutes. The wave pattern is a dense-disperse wave and the current is limited based on the endurance of the patient. Ten treatments are considered as one course. This method is indicated for neurological vomiting.

6. AURICULAR THERAPY

Points: Stomach, Shenmen, Sympathetic Nerve, Occiput, Esophagus and Sub-cortex.

Technique: Two or 3 points are punctured each time with strong stimulation once daily. The needle are retained for 30 minutes. Needles and seeds can be embedded on the ear points instead.

7. HYDRO-ACUPUNCTURE

Points: Ear Shenmen (bilaterally).

Technique: After the routine asepsis, fix the helix with the thumb and middle finger of the left hand, and then support Shenmen with the index finger of the left hand while holding the syringe in the right hand. A No.4.5 needle is used to inject 0.1 ml of Vitamin B1 subcutaneously on the points to form white skin prominence. The needle is then withdrawn. Both sides of the points are injected. A total of 124 pregnant women of morning sickness being treated by this method were studied, and 64 cases were cured by one injection, 39 after two and 21 after three. Miscarriage or fetal deformity did not occur in any case.

8.   MEDICINAL APPLICATION ON ACU-POINT

Point: Neiguan (PC6).

Technique: Apply two pieces of fresh ginger on the points bilaterally, fixing them with plasters. This method is indicated for neurological vomiting.

9.   COMBINED TREATMENT

Points: Main point: Jianjing (GB21). Supplementary points: Dazhui (CV14), Zhongwan (CV12) and Zusanli (ST36).

Technique: Only both sides of points Jianjing (GB21) are used for neurological vomiting, post-operative vomiting, allergic vomiting, and vomiting due to stomach cancer and pregnancy. Zhongwan (CV12) is added for gastritis and ulcerative vomiting; Zusanli (ST36) for vomiting due to indigestion; and Dazhui (CV14) for vomiting due to encephalitis B. Only moxibustion is used for morning sickness or for a baby under one year old. But for other cases, needling is applied first and moxa later. The treatment is given once or twice a day. If there is no effect after four or six treatments, other methods may be adopted.

[REMARKS]

1.   Acupuncture can effectively treat vomiting, especially neurological and acute types. But cases of projectile vomiting and incessant vomiting should be treated by combining Western medicine to exclude the organic ailments.

2.   The patients with vomiting are advised not to eat cold, raw, greasy, spicy and fried food, but only food that can be easily digested and light food. It is good to eat small, frequent meals.

HICCUP

[INTRODUCTION]

Hiccup is marked mainly by short and frequent sounds over varying periods of time. In mild cases, it only lasts from a few minutes to a few hours. In the severe cases, however, it may occur intermittently for several days or even for several months. An upward adverse flow of stomach *qi* due to irregular food intake, emotional disturbances, or weakness of anti-pathogenic *qi* may cause this problem. Cold syndrome of stomach is manifested by deep and slow hiccups, alleviated by warmth, and with cold hands and feet. Heat syndrome is manifested by a loud and forceful sound and a strong preference for cold drinks. Stagnation of liver *qi* is manifested by its onset related to emotional disturbance accompanied by distention and fullness. Weakness of the spleen and stomach is manifested by a low and forceless sound, poor appetite and lassitude. Deficiency of stomach *yin* is marked by an abrupt and paroxysmal sound, accompanied by dry mouth and tongue, flushed face and nocturnal sweating. The principle of treatment is to harmonize the stomach and reduce the adverse flow of *qi*. The Back-Shu and Front-Mu points are selected as the main points, such as Zhongwan (CV12), Neiguan (PC6), Zusanli (ST36), Weishu (BL21), Geshu (BL17) and Tanzhong (CV17). Other points are selected as the supplementary points according to the differentiation of the syndrome. Reducing technique is used for excess syndrome, and reinforcing technique is used for deficiency syndrome with moxibustion. Some Western problems, like diaphragm spasms, gastrointestinal neurosis, esophagus cancer, and stomach cancer, can be treated by reference to these methods.

[CLINICAL EXPERIENCE]

1. CONVENTIONAL ACUPUNCTURE

(1) Regulate Diaphragm
Point: Geshu (BL17).

Technique: Puncture Geshu (BL17) bilaterally, and retain the needle for 20 minutes after the arrival of *qi*. This method has been used to treat five cases of hiccups continuing for four days after an operation. All of them were cured by one treatment without recurrence.

(2) Regulating Du Meridian

Point: Renzhong (GV26).

Technique: Puncture the point toward the nasal septum 0.5 *cun* deep with a one-*cun* needle. Manipulate the needle by lifting, thrusting and rotating it until hiccup stops, and retain the needle for 30 to 60 minutes. This method is indicated for intractable hiccups.

(3) Puncturing Eight Confluent Points

Points: Neiguan (PC6) and Gongsun (SP4).

Technique: Puncture Neiguan (PC6) one *cun* deep and Gongsun (SP4) 0.8 *cun* deep. Reducing technique is used on the points with lifting, thrusting and rotating of the needle. The treatment is given three times a week for hiatus hernia.

(4) Puncturing the Points with Shallow Insertion

Points: Zhongwan (CV12) and Taichong (LR3).

Technique: Puncture Zhongwan (CV12) and Taichong (LR3) shallowly with one-*cun* needles, and manipulate the needles by rotating them and keeping them in place for 20 minutes. This method is indicated for stagnation of liver *qi* and failure of stomach *qi* to descend.

(5) Penetrating Technique

Points: Puncturing from Jingqu (LU8) to Taiyuan (LU9), from Daling (PC7) to Neiguan (PC6), from Gongsun (SP4) to Taibai (SP3) and from Zusanli (ST36) to Shangjuxu (ST37).

Technique: Puncture the points with penetrating technique horizontally. Reinforcing technique is used, retaining the needles for 20 minutes. This treatment is given once a day. It is a method treating lung and stomach, spleen and stomach at same time.

(6) Selecting Ah-shi Points

Point: Tenderness on the border of the gastronemius lateral to Chengshan (BL57), and the point at end of medial end of the crease between the first and second digital joint of the middle finger with finger flexed.

Technique: When puncturing the joint of the middle finger, do so along the skin upward with strong stimulation. If the middle jiao is affected, Zhongwan (CV12) is added; if the lower jiao is affected, Yindu (KI19) and Guanyuan (CV4) are added.

(7) Selecting Experience Point

Point: New Futu [posterior to sternocleidomastoid muscle, at the junction between two third and one third, anterior and inferior to Futu (LI19)].

Technique: The patient is kept in a sitting position. Puncture the point perpendicularly toward the cervical vertebrae 0.5 to 1 *cun* deep. When the needling sensation like an electric shock travels to the upper limb, remove the needle immediately. This method was used to treat 15 cases of intractable hiccup, and the total effective rate was 93.3%.

(8) Puncturing Anding (Extra)

Point: Anding [0.5 *cun* directly above Suliao (GV25) and 0.3 *cun* lateral to the nose].

Technique: Puncture the point quickly and horizontally upward and rotate the needle gently for one minute. If the hiccup does not stop, continue rotating the needle for up to 15 or 20 minutes. The treatment is given once a day.

2. MOXIBUSTION

(1) Moxibustion with Moxa Cone

Point: Qimen (LR14).

Technique: Apply three to five moxa cones on Qimen (LR14) for hiccup after a woman gives birth to a child.

(2) Moxibustion on Zhongkui (Extra)

Point: Zhongkui (The midpoint of proximal digital joint of middle finger located by making a fist).

Technique: Apply a little Vaseline on the point, and place five to seven moxa cones as big as grain on it. Treatment may be given once or twice a day. If fluid appears on the scar, apply a little gentian violet on it and cover it with gauze. This method is indicated for hiccup in the later stage of lung cancer.

(3) Moxibustion with Moxa Stick

Points: Tanzhong (CV17) and Zhongwan (CV12).

Technique: Applying moxibustion with moxa stick above the two points or with a moxa box. This method is indicated for weakness of the spleen and stomach.

(4) Moxibustion with Dengxin

Point: Tiantu (CV22).

Technique: Burn Dengxincao with oil over the fire and burn the point Tiantu (CV22) rapidly. In mild case, only one treatment is given; in severe case, a second treatment may be carried out one week later.

3. CUPPING

Points: ① Dazhui (CV14), Geshu (BL17) and Ganshu (BL18); ② Tanzhong (CV17), Zhongwan (CV12) and Qihai (CV6).

Technique: The two groups of points are used in turn once a day. Cupping is used for deficiency syndrome, and bleeding technique for excess syndrome.

4. ELECTRIC ACUPUNCTURE

Points: Neiguan (PC6) and Hegu (LI4).

Technique: After inserting the needles into the points, rotate it with large amplitude. Retain the needles for 20 to 30 minutes after the arrival of *qi*, and then connect the points with the electric apparatus.

5. AURICULAR THERAPY

Points: Diaphragm, Shenmen and sub-cortex.

Technique: Puncture the points with filiform needles, and manipulate them with strong stimulation. The needles should be retained for one hour, or treatment given with an electric detector. In a mild condition, Geshu (CV17) is also pressed by a match head for a few minutes. Then the hiccup can be stopped.

6. PUNCTURING DIAPHRAGM NERVE

Point: Tiantu (CV22).

Technique: Puncture the point toward the cervical vertebrae 0.5 to 0.8 *cun* deep with a one-*cun* needle to make the fingers feel electric numbness. Lift and thrust the needle a few times, then withdraw it. Puncturing this point can directly inhibit excitation of the diaphragm nerve so as to reduce the adverse flow of *qi* and relieve the spasm.

7. FINGER PRESSING

(1) Pressing Tianding (LI17)
Point: Tianding (LI17).
Technique: The operator presses the point with the palm of the thumb or middle finger for one to three minutes. One side of points are used, once a day.

(2) Pressing Neiguan (PC6).
Point: Neiguan (PC6).
Technique: Press the points bilaterally with heavey pressure for three to five minutes. Mild cases can be cured by this method right away.

8. HYDRO-ACUPUNCTURE

Points: Ear Points: Diaphragm, Ear Middle and Shenmen; Body Points: Neiguan (PC6) and Zusanli (ST36).
Technique: Inject VB1 into the ear points Diaphragm, Ear Middle and Shenmen bilaterally with 0.05 ml in each point, and a prominence on the skin as big as a bean should appear on the points; then inject a mixture of 4 ml of VB1 and 4 ml of 2% of procaine into Neiguan (PC6) and Zusanli (ST36) bilaterally with 2 ml in each point. This method is used to treat intractable hiccupping.

9. MEDICINAL APPLICATION ON THE ACU-POINT

Points: Zhongwan (CV12), Yindu (KI19) and Weishu (BL21).
Technique: Mix equal amount of Wufuzi, Xiaohuixiang, Guang-muxiang, Qianghuo, Ganjiang, Mudingxiang, and salt together, grind the mixture into pieces and sift them. In treatment, place 15 g of the powder in the center of a plaster with an area of 5 square centimeters, making three plasters in all, and put them on three points and cover

with clean gauze. Fry wheat bran until it is hot, and then wrap it and compress the three points in turn. This method is used to treat hiccups due to deficient cold.

[REMARKS]

1.   Acupuncture is more effective for the treatment of hiccup of the excessive type, and not very effective for the deficient type.

2.   During the development of acute and chronic diseases, the onset of continuous hiccups belongs to the "exhaustion of stomach" and is a sign of aggravation of the condition.

3.   In case of mild hiccups, it can be stopped by sneezing induced by paper touching of the nose or shifting of attention.

DIFFICULTY IN SWALLOWING (*YEGE*)

[INTRODUCTION]

Ye refers to the difficulty of swallowing food, and *ge* refers to obstruction of food in the chest and diaphragm or vomiting after eating. *Ye* may happen separately, or may be a warning sign of *ge*, so they are termed together "*Yege.*" This problem may be caused by injury to the spleen by melancholy and mental agitation; stagnation of spleen *qi*, and failure of body fluid to be disseminated all over the body, bringing about production of phlegm; injury of the liver by depression, stagnation of liver *qi*, leading to poor blood circulation; stagnation of *qi* and blood; or by indulgence in pungent and hot food, leading to accumulation of heat, injury of *yin* leading to obstruction of *qi*, blood, phlegm and heat in the esophagus. The principle of treatment is to remove the obstruction, disperse the accumulation, regulate the flow of *qi*, resolve the phlegm, nourish *yin* and moisten the dryness. The points of Ren Meridian and Foot Yangming Meridian are selected as the main points, such as Tiantu (CV22), Tanzhong (CV17), Shangwan (CV13), Neiguan (PC6), Geshu (BL17) and Zusanli (ST36). For obstruction of phlegm and *qi*, add Fenglong

(ST40) and Pishu (BL20); for stagnation of liver *qi*, add Ganshu (BL18) and Taichong (LR3); for exhaustion of body fluid and stagnation of blood, add Xuehai (SP10), Sanyinjiao (SP6), Taixi (KI3) and Zhaohai (KI6). Reinforcing technique is more often used in needling. This disease is similar to cardiac spasm, inflammation of the esophagus, esophagus cancer, and esophagus diverticulum, as well as neurosis of esophagus in western.

[CLINICAL EXPERIENCE]

1. CONVENTIONAL ACUPUNCTURE

(1) Reducing Technique with Rotating the Needle

Points: Tiantu (CV22), Tanzhong (CV17), Juque (CV14) and Hegu (LI4).

Technique: A total of 35 cases of patients with esophagus cancer have been treated by reducing technique with rotating of the needle on the points, producing definite improvements in swallowing. Through the observation by X-ray, the movement of the esophagus is strengthened, the esophagus cavity is widened, so that the spasm is relieved, and food can quickly pass through.

(2) Even Reinforcing and Even Reducing Technique

Points: ① Geshu (BL17), Geguan (BL46), Weishu (BL21) and Neiguan (PC6). ② Tiantu (CV22), Zhongwan (CV12), Zusanli (ST36) and Gongsun (SP4).

Technique: The two groups of points are used in turn. For constipation, Dachangshu (BL25), Tianshu (ST25) and Fenglong (ST40) are added; for chest pain referring to the back, Xinshu (BL15) and Ah-shi points on the chest and back are added; and for fullness and belching, Daling (PC7) is added. An even technique is used on the points, the needle being retained for 30 minutes. This method can greatly ease the obstruction due to esophagus cancer.

(3) Puncturing Jiaji Points

Points: Jiaji points from C4 to C6.

Technique: Keep the patient in a sitting position. Insert the needle one *cun* deep, and leave it for 20 minutes after the arrival of *qi*.

Meanwhile, manipulate the needle twice. This method is used to treat swallowing pain due to inflammation of the esophagus.

(4) Puncturing Feishu (BL13)

Point: Feishu (BL13) bilaterally.

Technique: Keep the patient in a sitting position. Insert the needle 0.7 *cun* deep, and keep it in place for 20 minutes, manipulating it once every five minutes. This method is indicated for esophagus inflammation.

(5) Puncturing Futu (CV22)

Points: Futu (CV22) and Neiguan (PC6).

Technique: Puncture Futu (CV22), when a sensation of electric shock traveling to the fingers should be felt. Lift and thrust the needle a few times, and then remove it. One side of the point is often needled. Neiguan (PC6) is supplemented to relieve the chest and reduce the adverse flow of *qi*. This method is indicated for cardiac spasm due to the upward adverse of flow of stomach *qi*.

2. MOXIBUSTION

Point: Zhongkui (an extra point, located in the middle of back of middle finger on the digital joint).

Technique: Apply seven moxa cones each on both sides of the points to lower stomach *qi*. It has a certain effect in treating an inability to drink water and vomiting immediately after a meal.

3. BLEEDING

Points: Taiyang (extra) and Tiaokou (ST38).

Technique: Prick Taiyang (Extra) and Tiaokou (ST38) with a three-edged needle to cause a little bleeding. The treatment is given once every three days. It is good for cases of esophagus diverticulum because it can eliminate the stagnation and remove the obstruction. The condition usually can be alleviated through three treatments.

4. AURICULAR THERAPY

Points: Esophagus, Stomach, the end of the lower crus, Diaphragm, Spleen and Liver.

Technique: Every time, one or two points are selected, puncturing them with a short needle and applying moderate stimulation. The needle should be kept in place for one to two hours. The treatment is given once a day, and ten times is considered as one course. Or instead, seeds can be applied on five to six points each time on one ear, then change to the other ear every three to five days. The patients need to press the seeds a few times a day.

[REMARKS]

1. Acupuncture is effective for esophagus spasms, and can help improve the symptoms of esophagus cancer.

2. Patients with difficulty of swallowing are advised to keep pleasant, avoid excitation and not to eat cold and raw food.

DIARRHEA

[INTRODUCTION]

Diarrhea refers to a condition marked by frequent bowel movement, loose or watery feces, accompanied by abdominal pain and lassitude. It can be divided into acute and chronic types. Acute diarrhea is generally caused by invasion of cold-damp, or summer heat-damp or retention of food in the intestine and stomach, leading to dysfunction of transmission, mixture of water and food, or the failure of separation between the clear from the turbid. The principle of treatment is to eliminate the pathogenic factors, and regulate the intestine and stomach. The points of Hand and Foot Yangming Meridians are selected as the main points, such as Zhongwan (CV12), Tianshu (ST25), Hegu (LI4), Shangjuxu (ST37) and Yinlingquan (SP9), which are punctured with reducing technique. Moxibustion is added for cold-damp syndrome, and bleeding for heat syndrome. Chronic diarrhea is generally caused by dysfunction of zang-fu organs, weakness of the spleen and stomach, the decline of Mingmen fire and failure of the spleen to be warmed, counteraction of the liver on the spleen, leading to dysfunction of the latter in transportation and transformation, failure of separation of the clear from the turbid, which both move to the intestine together. The principle of treatment is to build up the spleen, sooth the liver and warm the kidney. The points of Ren Meridian, Foot Yangming Meridian and Back-Shu points are selected as the main points, such as Zhongwan (CV12), Tianshu (ST25), Zusanli (ST36), Pishu (BL20), Guanyuanshu (BL26), Ganshu (BL18) and Taichong (LR3), which are punctured with reinforcing technique, or plus moxibustion. Those Western diseases, like acute and chronic diarrhea, intestinal dysfunction, allergy of the colon, and tuberculosis of the intestine, can be treated by reference to this syndrome.

[CLINICAL EXPERIENCE]

1. CONVENTIONAL ACUPUNCTURE

(1) Four-Point Around the Umbilicus

Point: Four points around the umbilicus (located one *cun* lateral, left and right respectively to the umbilicus).

Technique: Use a No.28 or No.30 needle, 1.5 *cun* long. Puncture the four points in an order of upper, lower, left and right, the needle being inserted 0.5 to 1 *cun* deep in an adult, and 0.3 to 0.5 *cun* deep in children. For diarrhea due to deficient cold, insert the needle slowly and rotate for half a minute; and for diarrhea due to excess heat, puncture the points quickly and rotate the needle for 10 seconds, with no retention.

(2) Puncturing the Buttock with Deep Insertion

Point: Sensitive point on the buttock (located on the point three finger-widths below the midpoint between the superior anterior and superior posterior iliac spine, approximately on the upper border of piriformis).

Technique: The patient should be in a lateral position with the knees flexed. The practitioner presses the skin to find the tenderest point (there are sensitive points on each side, but more on the left side). After locating the point, insert a 3- or 3.5-*cun* needle into the point swiftly and straight to the bone membrane. Then lift the needle slightly away from the bone membrane and manipulate it with large amplitude for one or two minutes. Retain the needle for 20 minutes while lifting, thrusting and rotating it three times.

(3) Puncturing Tender Points

Points: The points are located 5 *cun* directly below Yinlingquan (SP9) and 1 *cun* posterior to the tibia, which will produce a different sensation or pain when pressed.

Technique: Insert a 1.5- or 2-*cun* needle straight into the point. Reducing technique is used for excess syndrome with acute onset; and reinforcing is used for deficient syndrome. The treatment is given once a day, retaining the needle for 30 minutes and manipulating the needle once every 10 minutes.

(4) Shallow Puncturing of the Points on the Four Limbs

Points: Taibai (SP3), Taixi (KI3), Quchi (LI11), Zusanli (ST36), Yinlingquan (SP9) and Quze (PC3).

Technique: Insert a one-*cun* needle straight into the points, 0.2 *cun* deep on Taixi (KI3), Yinlingquan (SP9), Quze (PC3) and 0.6 *cun* deep on Quchi (LI11) and Zusanli (ST36), retaining and rotating it for two minutes. This method is used for diarrhea due to summer heat-damp.

2. MOXIBUSTION

(1) Mild-Warming Technique with Moxa Stick

Point: Specific point for diarrhea (located directly below the highest point of external malleolus at the junction of red and white skin).

Technique: Apply moxibustion with a moxa stick on both sides of points for 10 to 15 minutes each, two or three times a day. A total of 120 cases of patients with diarrhea (32 with infantile simple indigestion and 88 cases with acute enteritis) were treated. Through one to four days of treatment, the curative rate was 98.3%.

(2) Moxibustion with Moxa Cone

Points: Guanyuan (CV4), Tianshu (ST25), Pishu (BL20) and Baihui (GV20).

Technique: Apply more than 10 moxa cones on each point. It is used to treat diarrhea due to weakness of spleen *qi* and is given once a day.

(3) Moxibustion with Salt

Point: Shenque (CV8).

Technique: Grind a certain amount of salt into fine powder, filling the umbilicus 0.5 to 1 cm above the surface. Put a 4-cm-diameter iron cover on the salt, and then moxa cones. Three to seven cones are used, and should be applied two or three times a day. A total of 748 cases with watery diarrhea were dealt with by a two-day course of treatment, with 680 cases cured (90.9%), 40 improved (5.3%), and 28 ineffective (3.8%).

(4) Moxibustion by Producing Pus

Points: Tianshu (ST25) and Guanyuan (CV4).

Technique: Make a moxa cone with fine moxa wool using a specially made model, each cone weighing 0.1 gm with a diameter of 0.7 cm at the bottom. Three to six cones are used on each point and pus should be formed. This method is indicated for chronic specific and ulcerative colitis.

(5) Moxibustion with Ginger

Points: ① Zhongwan (CV12) and Shenque (CV8). ② Guanyuan (CV4) and Tianshu (ST25).

Technique: The two groups of points are applied in turn with moxibustion, five to seven cones as big as yellow bean or date kernel being used on each point. The treatment is given once a day, and 10 times make up one course with intervals of five days. It is mainly used to treat chronic diarrhea due to *yang* deficiency of spleen and kidney.

3. MOVING CUPPING

Point: Back-shu points of zang-fu organs.

Technique: The patient should be in a prone position. Apply a little Vaseline along both sides of the Urinary Bladder Meridian, cupping with one cup, and then moving this cup along the running course of the Urinary Bladder Meridian two or three times until the skin is congested and red. It is given once a day, and 10 times are considered as one course with intervals of five days. This method is indicated for early morning diarrhea.

4. BLEEDING

(1) Applying Bleeding on He-Sea Point

Points: Chize (LU5) and Weizhong (BL40).

Technique: Prick the points with a three-edged needle to cause bloodletting to clear heat and damp, and harmonize the stomach. This method is used for acute gastroenteritis of the heat type.

(2) Applying Bleeding on the Tip of the Fingers

Point: Shixuan (Extra).

Technique: Prick Shixuan (extra) with a three-edged needle to cause bloodletting. This is indicated for acute gastroenteritis.

5. HOT-RED NEEDLING

Point: Changqiang (GV1).

Technique: Ask the patient to squat down. Use a No.26 needle, 1.5-*cun* long. Burn it over the fire until it is red, then insert it quickly into Changqiang (GV1) 1 *cun* deep, rotate the needle quickly a few times and withdraw it. This method can consolidate the prolapse and is effective for prolonged diarrhea.

6. AURICULAR THERAPY

Point: Shoulder joint.

Technique: Insert a 1.5-*cun* needle horizontally along the scapha upward about one *cun* deep, manipulating the needle for five minutes until the patient indicates the ear has become hot, and you can see it is red and feels hot. Retain the needle for 12 to 24 hours, or 36 hours at maximum. During the retention of the needle, whenever there is desire of defecation, rotate the needle for five minutes and this will disappear.

7. HYDRO-ACUPUNCTURE

Point: Zhixie point (2.5 *cun* below the umbilicus).

Technique: Inject Huangliansu fluid into the point, 2 to 4 ml for an adult and 1 to 2 ml for children under seven each time. The treatment is given once a day, or twice a day for severe cases. A study of 60 cases of acute enteritis that were treated four times confirmed a total effective rate of 85%.

8. CATGUT-EMBEDDING METHOD

Points: Chiyizhuxue (located on the upper border of the sixth thoracic vertebrae); and Chiyierxue (located on the upper border of the first lumbar vertebrae).

Technique: A No.16 puncturing needle for bone marrow is used. Grind the middle part of needle to flat to make it as long as the needle-tip. Insert two or three cm No.2 catgut thread into the front part of the needle. Hold the needle by the thumb and middle finger of right hand, insert it in the subcutaneous region with an angle of 45° on the middle line of the back. Puncture as deep as three to four cm, fixing the middle part of needle by the index finger of the right hand. Lift the needle tube by the thumb and middle finger of the right hand to the top of the middle part of the needle, and then withdraw, leaving the catgut thread in the subcutaneous region. This treatment is given once every two weeks, and two treatments are considered as one course. This method has been used to treat 64 cases of allergic colitis, of which 26 were cured, 19 were nearly cured, eight were remarkably improved, six improved and five failed.

9. MAGNETIC THERAPY

Points: Shenque (CV8), Tianshu (ST25), Zusanli (ST36), Guanyuan (CV4) and Zhongwan (CV12).

Technique: Apply 1500 g of magnetic iron on the points and fix them with a plaster. This method is indicated for allergic enteritis.

10. LASER THERAPY

Points: Yanglingquan (GB34), Zusanli (ST36) and Guanyuan (CV4).

Technique: He-Ne laser machine is used to radiate the points for 15 minutes on each point. The treatment is given once a day or every other day. Ten treatments are considered as one course. This method is used to treat chronic enteritis.

11. MEDICINAL APPLICATION ON ACU-POINT

Points: Yongquan (KI1), Shenque (CV8) and Zhixie point (2.5 *cun* below the umbilicus)

Technique: Grind 50 g of Kufan into fine powder, add 20 g of white flour and a proper amount of vinegar, and mix them into the paste. In the treatment, apply the medicinal paste on the points, covering them with gauze fixed in place with a plaster. Change the dressing three to five times a day. This method is used to treat prolonged diarrhea with sallow complexion, lassitude, shortness of breath and reluctance to speak.

[REMARKS]

1. The patients should follow an easily-digested diet and avoid cold, raw, spicy and greasy food.

2. Transfusion of fluids should be combined for acute diarrhea patients with severe dehydration.

3. Acupoint massage could be combined for chronic diarrhea on such points as Pishu (BL20), Weishu (BL21), Dachangshu (BL25), Zhongwan (CV12), Tianshu (ST25), and Zusanli (ST36), once daily, three or four points each time.

DYSENTERY

[INTRODUCTION]

Dysentery is a common intestinal infectious disease manifested as abdominal pain, tenesmus and diarrhea with pus and blood. Chinese medicine practice holds that the disease is due to eating cold, raw and unclean food, or through the invasion of external summer heat, damp and epidemic toxin. All of the factors may combine together to result in dysfunction of the larger intestine in transportation, accumulation of damp and heat and stagnation of *qi* and blood, further damaging the zang-fu organs and meridians and collaterals, resulting in dysentery. In clinical practice, acute and chronic dysentery are divided. Acute dysentery includes the damp heat type manifested as more blood lesser pus stool, while the cold damp type manifested itself as more pus and less blood, anorexia and nausea after eating. The treatment principle is to clear away heat, resolve damp, promote digestion and regulate *qi* and blood circulation. The points are selected from Hand-Yangming meridian mainly, i.e., Hegu (LI4), Tianshu (ST25), Shangjuxu (ST37) and Neiting (ST44). For severe heat syndromes, Quchi (LI11) is added; for severe damp, Yinlingquan (SP9); and for severe cold, moxibustion. Reducing needling technique is applied. Chronic dysentery refers to persistent dysentery, weakness of *qi* in the middle energizer and retention of pathogenic factors. In clinical practice, the main manifestation is intermittent dysentery. The treatment principle is to tonify the spleen and stomach, and eliminate cold and damp. The main points are selected from Foot-Yangming meridian and Back-Shu points, i.e., Tianshu (ST25), Qihai (CV6), Zusanli (ST36), Pishu (BL20) and Dashangshu (BL25). Acupuncture and moxibustion are applied together. The treatments are taken as reference for acute bacillary dysentery, toxic dysentery and amebic dysentery in modern medicine.

[CLINICAL EXPERIENCE]

1. CONVENTIONAL ACUPUNCTURE

Selecting the Tender Points in Spleen Meridian

Points: The tender points on about one finger width above Sanyinjiao (SP6), about 0.5 *cun* above or below Diji (SP5) and about 0.5 to 1 *cun* above and below Yinlingquan (SP9).

Technique: The patient lies in a supine position. Reducing needling is given once or twice a day for severe cases. The needles are retained for 30 to 60 minutes and reducing manipulation is applied once every 10 minutes. The method is effective for acute and chronic dysentery.

2. MOXIBUSTION

(1) Surrounding Moxibustion with Moxa Stick

Point: Shenque (CV8)

Technique: The patient is in a supine position. Surrounding moxibustion with a moxa stick is applied on Shenque (CV8) for 30 to 60 minutes until the patient feels warmth with the abdomen and the abdominal pain is reduced or disappears. The distance between the body and the ignited moxa stick is changeable depending on the patient's tolerance. The method is for bacillary dysentery.

(2) Direct Moxibustion with Moxa Cone

Points: Hegu (LI4), Guanyuan (CV4), Pishu (BL20) and Tianshu (ST25)

Technique: Twenty moxa cones are applied on Guanyuan (CV4), five cones on Tianshu (ST25) and Hegu (LI4), respectively, at first. Then, 20 cones are placed on Pishu (BL20). The method is for dysentery of the cold and damp type, manifested as a bloody and pus stool.

(3) Indirect Moxibustion with Garlic

Points: Qihai (CV6) and Ah-shi points (4 *cun* bilateral to CV6)

Technique: Three slices of garlic, 2.5 to 3 mm thick, are placed on the points and three to five moxa cones are required on each point. The fresh garlic slice is replaced when the previous one is burnt. The method is for acute dysentery.

3. ELECTRIC ACUPUNCTURE

Points: Shenshu (BL23) and Dashangshu (BL25)

Technique: The 2-*cun* filiform needles are inserted on the points bilaterally. The needles are retained for 30 minutes with electric stimulation. The treatment is given once a day.

4. HYDRO-ACUPUNCTURE

Points: Tianshu (ST25) and Zusanli (ST36)

Technique: The points are injected bilaterally with berberine 1 ml on each. The treatment is given once a day and continuously for two or three days.

5. MEDICINAL APPLICATION ON ACU-POINTS

Points: Shenque (CV8), Zhixiexue (Extra) and Pishu (BL20)

Technique: Grind three *Fanmubie* (Strychnotis, Semen) and 24 Mudingxiang (Flos Caryophylli) into powder and mixed the powder with 0.3 g *Yuancun*. The final herbal powder is stirred with water into a paste of pea-like size. The paste is placed on the points and fixed with plaster. The application is replaced once a day and two to three treatments are applicable. The method is for chronic dysentery.

6. COMBINED TREATMENT

(1) Puncturing and Bleeding

Points: Shixuan (Ex-UE11), Weizhong (BL40), Chize (LU5), Tianshu (ST25), Dachangshu (BL25), Zhongwan (CV12) and Zusanli (ST 36)

Technique: Shixuan (Ex-UE11), Weizhong (BL40) and Chize (LU5) are pricked with a three-edged needle to cause bleeding. The rest points are punctured with the filiform needle with rotating, thrusting and lifting technique. The needles are retained for 30 minutes and manipulated once every five to 10 minutes. The treatment is given once a day. The method is for bacillary dysentery.

(2) Pricking and Cupping

Points: Four points 1 *cun* around the umbilicus.

Technique: Pricking is given by a three-edged needle on the points and cupping is followed to get a little blood. The cup is retained for five to 10 minutes. The treatment is given once or twice a day. The proper treatment is applied for dehydrant acidosis and other complications.

[REMARKS]

1. Acupuncture can effectively control the symptoms and swiftly reduce fever with overall satisfactory effects.

2. The patient should be isolated and take liquid or semi-liquid food. Raw, cold, greasy and hard food should be avoided.

3. If acupuncture cannot control the symptoms rapidly for some severe cases, comprehensive treatment with Chinese and Western medicine is applied actively.

CONSTIPATION

[INTRODUCTION]

The onset of this disease is usually due to the transmission dysfunction of the large intestine that could be induced if there is a heat accumulation in the stomach and intestine, or liver *qi* stagnation, deficiency of *qi* and blood, or deficiency of kidney y*ang*. The treatment principle is to promote the smooth flow of *qi* in the large intestine. The main points selected should be the Back-Shu point, the Front-Mu point as well as the Lower He-Sea point of the large intestine such as Tianshu (ST25), Dachangshu (BL25), Shangjuxu (ST37) and Zhigou (TE6); the combination of points should be determined on a case-by-case basis. In the case of heat accumulation in the stomach and intestine, Quchi (LI11), Hegu (LI4), Neiting (ST44) and Fujie (SP14) should be combined; in the case of liver *qi* stagnation, Taichong (LR3), Yanglingquan (GB34) and Ganshu (BL18); in the case of the deficiency of *qi* and blood, Pishu (BL20), Zusanli (ST36), Qihai (CV6), Sanyinjiao (SP6) and Geshu (BL17); in the case of deficiency in kidney *yang*, Shenshu (BL23), Guanyuan (CV4) and Shenque (CV8). The treatment discussed in this section should be taken as a reference to the treatment of habitual constipation.

[CLINICAL EXPERIENCE]

1. CONVENTIONAL ACUPUNCTURE

(1) Needling Point Zhigou (TE6)

Technique: Needle the point Zhigou (TE6) bilaterally, and apply chiefly the reducing needling manipulation or the even needling manipulation. This method treats mostly constipation due to heat.

(2) Needling Unilateral Points

Points: Fenglong (ST40), Shuidao (ST28), Guilai (ST29) and points 2 *cun* lateral to Shuidao (ST28) and Guilai (ST29)

Technique: Needle each point 1.5 to 2 *cun* deep, apply the reducing needling manipulation achieved by rotation; keep manipulating the needles for 15 minutes, and retain them for 30 minutes. This treatment should be performed once a day to relieve intractable constipation.

(3) Needling Such Points as Changqiang (GV1)

Points: Changqiang (GV1), Dadun (LR1) and Yanglingquan (GB34)

Technique: The patient should lie prone. Needle Changqiang (GV1) first, rotate the needle five minutes after the arrival of *qi*, then needle Dadun (LR1) and Yanglingquan (GB34) bilaterally, using reducing needling manipulation. The method treats mostly constipation of the heat type.

(4) Needling Point Chengshan (BL57)

Technique: Take 1.5-*cun* filiform needles and puncture Chengshan (BL57) bilaterally. The method mainly relieves habitual constipation. The treatment should be performed once a day, 10 sessions in total.

(5) Needling Point Dubi (ST35)

Technique: Needle Dubi (ST35) unilaterally, either left or right, retaining the needle for 10 to 20 minutes. One session of treatment is performed a day and 10 sessions constitute one course.

2. INDIRECT MOXIBUSTION WITH CHINESE HERBS

Point: Shenque (CV8)

Technique: Take Gansui 3 g, Yuancun 0.3 g and salt 5 g (stir fried); mix the three herbs and grind them into fine powder (this is the amount for one time usage). Fill the point with the herbal powder. Rub the moxa leaves and shape into a moxa column. Place the moxa column on the herbs and ignite it. Usually after five to seven moxa columns are applied, bowel movement should be promoted. The method is applied to treat constipation due to heat, cold or deficiency.

3. AURICULAR THERAPY

Points: Lower portion of rectum, sympathetic nerve, sub-cortex, large intestine and small intestine

Technique: After the desensitizing plaster is used to stick the ear seeds on the ear points, the patient should press over 10 times the ear points where the ear seeds are located. Each time, the pressing should last five minutes. The patient should have a bowel movement at a regular time each day, and should also press the ear seeds while defecating.

4. NEEDLE-EMBEDDING METHOD

Points: Left Fujie (SP14)

Technique: After performing routine sterilization, embed one intradermal needle on the point. This method can promote the peristalsis of the sigmoid colon.

5. HYDRO-ACUPUNCTURE

Points: Jianweixue [about 2 *cun* below Zusanli (ST36)], Wenliu (LI7), Ah-shi point (abdominal pain point)

Technique: Take Vitamin B$_1$ injection fluid and inject 0.3 ml to 0.5 ml into each point, using points unilaterally in each treatment. One session is carried out once a day and seven sessions constitute one course.

6. MEDICINAL APPLICATION ON ACU-POINT

Point: Shenque (CV8)

Technique: Take 50 g of scallion stalks (the root is taken as well, but no washing is required, as it is enough just to clean away the mud), 30 g of ginger, 15 g of salt, 37 pieces of fermented soya beans, mixing, smashing and preparing them into a round cake. Before application, heat the round cake over the fire, and then place it on the point and fix it in place with an elastic bandage. Change the cake when it becomes cold. Usually, the *qi* will flow smoothly in 12 to 24 hours, and the constipation disappears. This method is applicable to constipation due to *yang* deficiency.

[REMARKS]

1. The patient should eat more vegetables and fruit than in usual times, and should follow a normal, regular lifestyle, paying attention to having a bowel movement at a regular time.

2. The patient should engage in physical exercise so that the peristalsis of the stomach and intestine can be improved.

3. The patient should not use purgatives, so as to prevent become reliant on the medicine.

4. The Chinese massage can be combined to improve the therapeutic effectiveness. The patient should lie supine; he or she should rub the abdomen in a clockwise direction for 10 minutes. The massage should be performed once a day and 10 sessions constitute one course.

HEMATOCHEZIA

[INTRODUCTION]

Hematochezia can be divided into deficient and excessive types. Hematochezia of the deficient type is caused by spleen *qi* deficiency and the failure of spleen *qi* in controlling blood. The main manifestations are stool tinged with dark black blood, discharge of stool prior to a discharge of blood, lassitude, sallow complexion, emaciation, pale tongue, thready and weak pulse. The treatment principle is to strengthen spleen to control blood. Moxibustion should be applied on Guanyuan (CV4), Zusanli (ST36), Pishu (BL20), Zhangman (LR13), Geshu (BL17) and Taibai (SP3). The excessive type of the hematochezia is due to the downward flow of damp heat to the large intestine causing blood extravasations. The main manifestations are stool tinged with fresh blood, discharge of blood prior to a discharge of stool, abdominal pain, fever, yellow sticky tongue coating, and a rolling, rapid pulse. The treatment principle is to clear the heat, resolve dampness and stop the hemorrhage. When acupuncture treatment is performed, the reducing needling technique should be used on Shangjuxu (ST37), Xiajuxu (ST39), Neiting (ST44), Yinlingquan (SP9), Dachangshu (BL25) and Tianshu (ST25). Those modern medical diseases like tumor or polyps in the duodenum and rectum, ulceration in the digestive tract, acute hemorrhagic necrotic enteritis and aplastic anemia all have manifestation of hematochezia.

The hematochezia caused by hemorrhoid and anal fissure does not belong to that discussed in this section.

[CLINICAL EXPERIENCE]

1. CONVENTIONAL ACUPUNCTURE

(1) Needling Point Liangqiu (ST34)

Technique: Use 1.5 *cun* filiform needles to puncture the point Liangqiu (ST34) bilaterally, keeping the needles for 30 minutes after the arrival of *qi*. The method is used in the case of gastric hemorrhage.

(2) Needling Points Chengshan (BL57) and Others

Points: Chengshan (BL57), Fuliu (KI7), Taichong (LR3), Taibai (SP3), Dachangshu (BL25), Changqiang (GV1) and Geshu (BL17)

Technique: Needle all these points bilaterally. The method treats bleeding from the distant part or local bleeding.

2. MOXIBUSTION

(1) Moxibustion with Moxa Cones on Spine

Point: On the spine at the same level of the center of the umbilicus.

Technique: Apply seven big moxa cones on the point. If the hematochezia cannot be relieved, another seven moxa cones can be used. The therapeutic result is better if this point on the spine is sore and painful when pressed.

(2) Moxibustion with Moxa Cones on Baihui (GV20)

Technique: Apply seven moxa cones as big as a soybean on Baihui (GV20). The method treats hematochezia without hemorrhoid.

(3) Moxibustion with Moxa Cones on Qihai (CV6) and Other Points

Points: Qihai (CV6), Zhongwan (CV12) and Zusanli (ST36)

Technique: Use seven to 10 moxa cones on each of the points above. The method treats abdominal pain and blood tinged diarrhea. The treatment can warm up the spleen and strengthen the stomach.

(4) Suspended Moxibustion with Moxa Stick

Points: Laogong (PC8), Taibai (SP3), Heyang (BL55) and Geshu (BL17)

Technique: Perform suspended moxibustion with moxa stick on these points bilaterally, applying five minutes of moxibustion on each point. The method relieves persistent hematochezia.

3. APPLYING BOTH ACUPUNCTURE AND MOXIBUSTION

Points: Pishu (BL20), Qihai (CV6), Tianshu (ST25), Zusanli (ST36) and Yinbai (SP1)

Technique: Needle Pishu (BL20) perpendicularly at a depth of 0.8 *cun*, and remove after one minute. The reinforcing needling manipulation is achieved by rotation. Puncture Qihai (CV6) and Tianshu (ST25) perpendicularly at a depth of 1 to 1.2 *cun*; puncture Zusanli (ST36) perpendicularly at a depth of 1.2 to 1.5 *cun*, applying the reinforcing needling manipulation achieved by lifting, thrusting and rotating. Needle Yinbai (SP1) perpendicularly at a depth of 0.2 *cun*, applying the reinforcing needling manipulation achieved by rotation. Retain needles on the last four points for 20 minutes. Ten to 15 minutes warm mild-moxibustion with moxa stick can also be applied on all the points. Moxibustion with three to seven moxa cones as big as wheat beans can be used on Yinbai (SP1). The method can be used in the case of spleen and stomach deficiency and dysfunction of *qi* in controlling blood in stool tinged with dark purple blood, sallow complexion, intolerance to cold, cold extremities, pale tongue body, thin and white tongue coating, and deep, thready and soft pulse.

[REMARKS]

1. It is better for the patient to take the food when it is at an appropriate temperature. The patient should eat neither hot nor boiling hot food. The patient should not take any food of a hot nature and of rough and hard properties such as spicy food, cigarettes, alcohol and fried food.

2. Principally, a patient with hematochezia should rest. In particular, a patient with repeated hematochezia that is hard to be relieved must calm down and take a rest. Patients with sever hemorrhage must stay in bed.

GASTROPTOSIS

[INTRODUCTION]

Gastroptosis refers to the condition when the lowest point of the lesser curvature of stomach is below the iliac crest line. The condition is clinically manifested by poor appetite, distended discomfort in the stomach, symptoms aggravated after meal, emaciation, lassitude, frequent epigastric and abdominal dull pain. The symptoms may also be accompanied by belching and acid regurgitation. This disease belongs to the scope of "abdominal distention" classified in traditional Chinese medicine, and it is mostly caused by weakness of the spleen and stomach and the sinking of *qi* of the middle Jiao (triple energizer). The treatment principle is to tonify *qi* of the middle Jiao (triple energizer), to strengthen the spleen and harmonize the stomach. Points chosen are mainly the Back-shu and Front-mu points of the stomach, and the points of the stomach meridian of Foot Yangming, such as Baihui (GV20), Zhongwan (CV12), Pishu (BL20), Weishu (BL21), Zusanli (ST36) and Qihai (CV6). Moxibustion is usually applied in the treatment.

[CLINICAL EXPERIENCE]

1. CONVENTIONAL ACUPUNCTURE

(1) Needling Back-shu Points

Points: Ganshu (BL18), Danshu (BL19), Pishu (BL20) and Weishu (BL21).

Technique: Ask the patient to lie prone. Use one-*cun* filiform needles to puncture the points bilaterally, choosing two pairs of points each time and using points from up to down repeatedly. The needle tip should point obliquely toward the intervertebral foramen, or the needles are inserted perpendicularly, the depth of the insertion determined by the size of the patient. After the arrival of *qi*, the reinforcing needling manipulation achieved by rotation should be applied until the patient feels his stomach is contracting upward. After that the needles are retained for 15 minutes. Ten sessions of treatment constitute one course, the interval between each course of treatment should be five to seven days. After one to two courses of treatment, improvement should have occurred. But the patient should be told not to stand too long.

(2) Penetrating Puncture from Tiweixue to Tianshu (ST25)

Points: Tiweixue [1.5 *cun* lateral to Shangwan (CV13) and Zusanli (ST36)].

Technique: Take six-*cun* needles and perform the penetrating puncture along the skin from Tiweixue to Tianshu (ST25), and put in three to five *cun* of the needle, giving strong stimulation and twisting the needles left and right simultaneously. The reinforcing needling technique is used on Zusanli (ST36), and needles should be retained for 30 minutes. The treatment should be given once a day, 10 sessions constituting one course. The patient should take a three-day rest after each course of treatment.

(3) Penetrating Puncture from Youmen (KI21) to Huangshu (KI16)

Technique: While the patient is supine, take an eight-*cun* filiform needle of size 28 and insert the needle through the skin from the right Youmen (KI21) from the upper abdomen. Apply rotating needle manipulation in small amplitude to make the needle pass the abdominal middle line under the skin. Stop the manipulation when the needle tip reaches the left Huangshu (KI16). After that, pull back the needle slowly at an even speed. While the practitioner is withdrawing the needle, he or she should feel the traction under it. When the needle has been withdrawn to the skin level, another penetrating puncture should be conducted. Such manipulation should be repeated several times. Needles should be retained for 20 minutes. Treatment is given once a day, 20 sessions being carried out successively. The effective rate of this method is 90%.

(4) Penetrating Puncture on Jianli (CV11)

Technique: With the patient lying supine, take two three-*cun* needles and insert them into the left and right Jianli (CV11) under the skin at a depth of two or three *cun*. After the arrival of *qi*, lift and thrust the two needles several times, then leave them in the place for

20 minutes. When the needles are removed, a cloth belt of 0.3 cm thick should be used to bind the waist, but it should be taken off before sleep. Ten days of acupuncture treatment constitute one course, with a break of two or three days between two courses.

(5) Penetrating Puncture on Weishangxue

Points: Penetrate puncture from Weishangxue [4 *cun* lateral to Xiawan (CV10)] to Qihai (CV6) or Guanyuan (CV4), and Zusanli (ST36)

Technique: With the patient lying supine, insert a five-*cun* needle of size 26 from Weishangxue, and penetrate the muscle layer. For a patient with a gastroptosis less than 6 cm, the needle tip should point toward Qihai (CV6); for a patient with a gastroptosis more than 6 cm, the needle tip should point toward Guanyuan (CV4). When the penetrating puncture is completed, the "supporting stomach" manipulation should be performed to assist the lifting of the stomach. During the treatment, Zusanli (ST36) should be needled bilaterally. The treatment is conducted once every other day, and strong stimulation should be given. Ten to 20 sessions constitute one course.

2. ELECTRIC ACUPUNCTURE

Points: Zhongwan (CV12), Tiweixue [1.5 *cun* lateral to Shangwan (CV13)], Weishangxue [4 *cun* lateral to Xiawan (CV10)]

Technique: Let the patient to lie supine, use two-*cun* filiform needles, needle points other than Qihai (CV6) obliquely downward at a 45° angle to a depth of 1 to 1.5 *cun*, and puncture Qihai (CV6) perpendicularly to a depth of 1.5 *cun*. The dense-disperse pattern of the electric stimulation should be used. The negative wire should be connected to the needle in Zhongwan (CV12) while the positive wire should be split into five and then be connected to the needles in bilateral Tiweixue, as well as to the needles in bilateral Weishangxue and Qihai (CV6). The amount of the electric stimulation should be determined upon the contraction of the abdominal muscles and the tolerance of patient. In each treatment, the electric stimulation should be applied 20 to 30 minutes, and the treatment is given once a day. Twelve sessions of the treatment make up one course, with a break of three days between two courses. The total effective rate of three courses of treatment is 77.8%.

3. CATGUT-EMBEDDING METHOD

Points: From Pishu (BL20) to Weishu (BL21) and from Zhong-wan (CV12) to Shangwan (13)

Technique: Thread the triangular suture needle with the complex catgut of size 2 to 4, insert the suture needle into the muscle layer from Pishu (BL20), penetrate the suture needle out from Weishu (BL20) and cut the catgut to embed it in the muscle layer. The same method is used to embed the catgut between points Zhongwan (CV12) and Shangwan (CV13). After the operation, the site operated should be covered with the gauge and tape to fix it. Another treatment should be conducted 15 to 20 days later.

4. HYDRO-ACUPUNCTURE

Points: Zusanli (ST36), Weishu (BL21) and Pishu (BL20)

Technique: Take Huangqi injection fluid, and inject 3 ml fluid into each point. Each hydro-acupuncture treatment should be conducted on one pair of bilateral points. The treatment is performed once a day. The patient should take a three-day break after receiving six sessions of treatment. The above points should be used alternately. After one month of this treatment had been carried out in 142 patients with gastroptosis, the total effective rate was found to be 96.7%.

5. AURICULAR THERAPY

Points: Stomach, Liver, Ear-Shenmen, Sympathetic Nerve and Sub-cortex

Technique: After locating points accurately, the vaccaria seeds should be put on points on both ears. The seeds should be changed every three to five days, and the treatment should be performed one to two months in succession.

6. MEDICINAL APPLICATION ON ACU-POINT

Point: Baihui (GV20)

Technique: Prepare 9.8 g of castor beans, 2 g of gallnuts. Clean the shell of gallnuts first, grind them into powder and then filter the powder. Add the plump and the white castor beans into the powder and pound them into paste, preparing the paste into a medicinal cake that is 3 cm in diameter, 1 cm in thickness and 10 g in weight. This is one dose for the adult. When it is applied on Baihui (GV20) on the patient, the hair of the hairy area as big as the medicinal cake over Baihui (GV20) should be shaved. Place the medicinal cake on Baihui (GV20), put on a hard paper ring that is 3 cm in diameter around the cake, and fix the cake with the gauge and the elastic bandage. Fill the saline bottle with boiling water and then put it on top of the medicinal cake, performing the treatment once in the morning, once at moon, and once in the evening and carrying out 15 minutes application each time. The temperature should be regulated to the extend that the skin would not be burnt. The medicinal cake should be changed once every two days. Six days successive application make up one course. One day's break should be taken between two treatment courses.

[REMARKS]

1.　The patient should take a good rest, and avoid standing over a long time. What is particularly helpful to the recovery of the disease is that the patient should lie in bed an hour after meal.

2.　The food should be those easy to be digested. The patient should not eat too much each meal. It is beneficial for the patient to eat less at each meal but to take more numbers of meal. For the patient with a severe gastroptosis, the "stomach supporter" can be used to correct the location of the stomach.

PROCTOPTOSIS

[INTRODUCTION]

The disease tends to occur in aged people and in people having a weak constitution due to chronic disease. In mild cases, the rectum protrudes after bowel movement, but the protrusion corrects itself; in severe cases, the rectum protrudes after coughing, sneezing or even slight exertion to defecate, and the rectum cannot move back and has to be supported to return to its correct location. The disease is mainly due to the deficiency of primary *qi*, the sinking of *qi* of the middle Jiao (triple energizer) and weakness in contraction. To solve the problem, it is beneficial to tonify *qi* of the middle Jiao (triple energizer), lifting up *qi* and promoting contraction. The points of the Governor Vessel and the Back-shu point of the large intestine are intended to be the main points. Examples are Baihui (GV20), Dachangshu (BL25), Changqiang (GV1) and Chengshan (BL57). The reinforcing needling technique should be used. If acupuncture can be applied together with moxibustion, the result tends to be more satisfactory.

[CLINICAL EXPERIENCE]

1. CONVENTIONAL ACUPUNCTURE

(1) Needling Points Baihui (GV20) and Qihai (CV6)

Technique: Needle Baihui (GV20) obliquely to a depth of 0.3 *cun* at first, retaining the needle for five minutes. Then Qihai (CV6) is needled perpendicularly to a depth of 0.8 to 1 *cun*. When the needle is at a certain depth, it should be rotated along with forward movement of the thumb so that soreness and distention are felt on the point. The needle should be taken out when the soreness and distention reach the perineum. Treatment is conducted once every other day.

(2) Needling Points Changqiang (GV1), and Erbai (4 cun below the mid-Point of the wrist crease, between the two tendons)

Technique: Puncture Erbai perpendicularly to a depth of 0.8 *cun*, giving a mild stimulation and then retaining the needle for 10 minutes. Changqiang (GV1) is punctured obliquely upwards to a depth of 1.5 *cun*, the needle being rotated gently with a mild stimulation until the patient feels contraction around the anus. The treatment is performed once a day, 10 sessions constituting one course. A five-day break should be taken between the courses of treatment.

(3) Needling Point Xiazhibian

Technique: The patient should lie on the side with lower leg straight and upper leg flexed, keeping the popliteal fossa of the upper leg bent at an angle of 130° and the body trunk turned inward slightly. A correct posture should be kept in which the anterior superior iliac spine and the mid-point of the great trochanter form sides of an isosceles triangle. The crossing point of the other sides of the triangle is this point. When the treatment is performed, a 3.5 to 5 *cun* needle of size 28 is inserted perpendicularly through the skin. The needle body is then turned obliquely backward (dorsal gluteal side) at an angle of 10°. Through this insertion the needling sensation can reach the anal intestinal area. After the needling sensation reaches the affected area, the needle can be retained one to two minutes and then taken out.

2. MOXIBUSTION

(1) Mild Warm Moxibustion with Moxa Stick
Point: Baihui (GV20)

Technique: The patient should sit upright. The practitioner parts the patient's hair with his left hand to expose the point, then holds the moxa stick with his right hand and performs the mild warm moxibustion for five minutes. Afterwards, a 15-minute sparrow pecking moxibustion is carried out. The treatment is performed once daily or every other day.

(2) Indirect Moxibustion with Salt
Point: Shenque (CV8)

Technique: The patient lies in a supine position. Take an appropriate amount of the fine salt to fill the whole umbilicus. Place the moxa cone on the salt. Five to 10 moxa cones should be used each time, each moxa cone being as big as a soybean. The treatment is carried out once daily or every other day, five to seven sessions being one course. When the moxibustion treatment is performed, great attention should be paid to preventing the patient from being burnt.

(3) Indirect Moxibustion with Ginger
Points: ① Baihui (GV20), Weishu (BL21), Changqiang (GV1)

and Chengshan (BL57). ② Shenque (CV8), Qihai (CV6), Henggu (KI11) and Zusanli (ST36)

Technique: Use the two groups of points alternately. Apply moxibustion once a day, placing five to seven moxa cones on ginger on each point each time. The moxa cone is in the size of a soybean or a date pit. Three sessions of treatment constitute one course.

3. PRICKING METHOD

Point: Lumbosacral region

Technique: Locate the vertical line from the third lumbar vertebrae to the second sacral vertebrae and 1 to 1.5 *cun* lateral to the midline of the spine, and choose any point on the line to prick. After the point is located accurately, a three-edged needle is used to prick the point. Two points should be pricked each time, cupping then applied. The treatment is performed once every three days.

4. AURICULAR THERAPY

Points: Lower portion of rectum, large intestine, subcortex and spleen

Technique: Apply acupuncture with the filiform needle, give a medium amount of stimulation and retain the needles for 30 minutes. The treatment is performed once daily and 12 sessions of the treatment represent one course.

[REMARKS]

1. This disease can often be secondary to chronic dysentery, chronic diarrhea, postpartum weakness of women, constipation and a chronic cough, hence attention should be paid to preventing the diseases mentioned above.

2. The patient should pay attention to rest, not undertake too much strain or stress, keep a regular life style and ensure good hygiene of the anus.

3. Better results are gained if the treatment is given in the early stage of this disease. Results are less satisfactory if the disease is chronic, and also if the patient is elderly.

INSOMNIA

[INTRODUCTION]

This disease occurs mainly because of the excessive mental activity, overstrain and stress, heart blood deficiency, and malnourishment of the heart and mind. It can also occur because of damage to the kidney by sexual indulgence, *yin* deficiency with hyperactive deficient fire, disharmony between the heart and kidney; emotional depression, upward disturbance of liver fire, irritability; improper food intake, disharmony of the stomach and the retention and accumulation of phlegm damp. The treatment principle is to calm down the heart and mind. Points on the Hand Shaoyin and three *yin* meridians of Foot should be used as the main ones, such as Baihui (GV20), Anmian (Extra 13), Taiyang (Ex-HN5), Yintang (Ex-HN3), Neiguan (PC6), Shenmen (HT7), Sanyinjiao (SP6) and Taichong (LR3). In case of heart blood deficiency, points like Xinshu (BL15), Geshu (BL17) and Zusanli (ST36) should be added. In case of disharmony between the heart and kidney, points like Xinshu (BL15), Shenshu (BL23) and Taixi (KI3) should be combined. In case of upward disturbance of liver fire, points like Yanglingquan (GB34), Xingjian (LR2) and Ganshu (BL18) should be added. In case of retention of phlegm damp in the interior, points like Pishu (BL20), Weishu (BL21), Yinlingquan (SP9) and Fenglong (ST40) should be combined. Insomnia can be found in such Western medical diseases as neurasthenia and neurosis.

[CLINICAL EXPERIENCE]

1. CONVENTIONAL ACUPUNCTURE

(1) Needling Head Triangle Points

Points: Locate the cross points of the line straight up from the inner canthus of the eyes with the anterior hairline and locate the other point on the mid-line of the nose forming an isosceles triangle with the previous two points (that is also the projection of the cerebral frontal lobe on the scalp). The three apexes are known as head triangle points.

Technique: Use a filiform needle (Size: No.32), insert it between the scalp and the bone membrane obliquely at an angle of 150° quickly to a depth of 1 cm and rotate it slightly. The needle should be retained for one hour. Two or three times of further stimulation can be conducted during the treatment. The treatment is performed once a day, 10 sessions being one course.

(2) Needling Point Shuimianxue

Point: It is midway between Hegu (LI4) and Sanjian (LI3).

Technique: Apply the rotating needling insertion technique, and needle the point to a depth of 0.5 to 1 *cun*. A constant rotation should be carried out for two to three minutes, and the needle is retained for 20 minutes.

(3) Needling Positive Reaction Point on the Back

Technique: With the patient sitting upright, look for nodules on the two sides of the upper thoracic vertebrae that are shapes like cords. Soreness and distention should be felt distinctively when pressure is exerted on the nodules. The needling is carried out right on the positive reaction point. Two to three reaction points are chosen for each treatment.

(4) Needling Shimianxue

Point: Shimianxue (right in the center of the heel)

Technique: Puncture it perpendicularly to a depth of 0.2 *cun*, without retention. The treatment should be conducted two to three hours before sleep. This is good for treating insomnia due to various reasons.

(5) Needling Point Zanzhu (BL2)

Technique: Use the filiform needle to puncture the point along the skin to a depth of 0.5 *cun*, retaining the needle for 20 minutes. The method has a soporific function.

2. MOXIBUSTION

Point: Baihui (GV20)

Technique: Apply suspended moxibustion with moxa stick over Baihui (GV20) for 10 to 15 minutes every night before sleep. Usually, the patient will fall asleep within five to 15 minutes after moxibustion is performed. After one to four sessions of moxibustion, the patient should sleep eight to 12 hours. The treatment had been carried out with satisfactory results in 21 cases.

3. CUTANEOUS PUNCTURE

Points: Baihui (GV20), Fengchi (GB20), Taiyang (Ex-HN5), Frontal areas, Jiaji (Ex-B2) of the neck and chest sections, the palm of the hands and the sole of the feet

Technique: Use the plum blossom needle to tap the above points and regions from up to down, and keep tapping until the skin in the localized area turns slightly red. The treatment is performed once daily, 10 sessions being one course.

4. NEEDLE-EMBEDDING METHOD

(1) Anmianxue [midway between Fengchi (GB20) and Yifeng (TE17)]

Technique: Use the thumb tags, and embed the needles on the points bilaterally. Fix the needles with adhesive plaster. The tags should be taken out after two to three days.

(2) Sanyinjiao (SP6) (bilaterally)

Technique: After sterilizing the local skin, use the needle holder to hold the handle of the cutaneous needle. For the needle on the right side, turn the tip up; for the needle on the left side, turn the tip down. Put the needle quickly under the skin, shaking the needle holder slightly. Fix the needle with a small piece of adhesive plaster as long as the patient feels no discomfort. The needle should be retained for three days.

5. AURICULAR THERAPY

(1) Medicinal Application

Points: Brain, Heart, Kidney, Spleen, Intertragic Region, Ear-Shenmen and Sub-cortex

Technique: After locating the points accurately, put vaccaria seeds or magnetic balls onto the ear points of both ears. Tell the patient not only to press the seeds several times a day, but also stimulate the points a couple of minutes before sleep. The vaccaria seeds should be taken off five days after they are put on. One to two days after the previous treatment, the next treatment may begin.

(2) Needle-embedding on Auricular Points

Points: Heart, Ear-Shenmen, Kidney and Sub-cortex

Technique: After locating the points correctly, perform strict sterilization. Use forceps to hold the handle of the cutaneous needle, inserting it into the points gently. Usually, two thirds of the needle body is inserted. Then fix the needle in place with adhesive plaster. Each time, two to three points are selected. The treatment is conducted on the unilateral points. The needles should be retained three to five days each time.

(3) Bleeding Ear Root

Point: Use the ear point detector to find the sensitive points on the ear root.

Technique: After sterilizing the skin, use a spring needle or a three-edged needle to prick the sensitive points quickly, letting out one drop of blood as big as a mung bean. The treatment is given once a day or once every other day. Only the sensitive points on one side are pricked each time.

6. ELECTRO-STIMULATION THERAPY

Points: Taiyang (Ex-HN5), Waiguan (TE5), Yangbai (GB14), Fengchi (GV20), Touwei (ST8) and Neiguan (PC6)

Technique: The induced direct current electric apparatus of the buzzer type should be used, the electrode board of the apparatus being larger than 3 cm in diameter. First, apply low current (two to three volts) stimulation on Taiyang (Ex-HN5) on both sides, then move the two electrodes to Yangbai (GB14) on both sides. Afterwards, move the electrodes from Yangbai (GB14) to Touwei (ST8). This process should be repeated three times. Use a stronger current (4 to 6 volts) to stimulate Fengchi (GB20), Waiguan (TE5) and Neiguan (PC6) bilaterally. In general, the treatment is better performed in the morning. To a few patients whose inhibition can be induced quickly, the treatment may be conducted at 4 o'clock in the afternoon. Each treatment lasts 10 minutes once a day. Seven to 10 sessions make up one course.

7. HYDRO-ACUPUNCTURE

Points: Xinshu (BL15), Jueyinshu (BL14), Pishu (BL20), Shenshu (BL23) and Zusanli (ST36)

Technique: Choose one to two pairs of points each time and inject 0.5 to 1 ml Huangqi (the root of membranous milk vetch) injection fluid into each point. The treatment is performed once daily, and 30 sessions represent one course.

8. MEDICINAL APPLICATION ON ACU-POINTS

Point: Shenque (CV8)

Technique: Take an equal amount of pearl powder, powder of the root of red-rooted salvia, salphur powder and borneol, mix them up and store them in a bottle for use. When the treatment is conducted, a certain amount of the above medicinal powder is taken to fill up the whole umbilicus and then sealed with adhesive plaster. The medicinal powder should be changed once every five to seven days.

[REMARKS]

1. Acupuncture can achieve good results in treating insomnia.

2. Insomnia relates closely to the emotions, hence psychotherapy should be combined as well. The relief of such unstable emotional factors as worry, excessive mental activity, fear, fright and anxiety are vitally important to the therapeutic effect of the treatment.

3. The patient should pay attention to physical exercise, and do appropriate labor work that is beneficial to recovery.

LETHARGY

[INTRODUCTION]

Lethargy refers to a condition whereby a person feels sleepy all the time no matter whether day or night. The disease can appear when the patient is caught in the rain or he walks through water, sits or lies in wet places, or when the patient has constitutional excessive endogenous dampness. Other causes include deficiency of both the heart and spleen when he suffers from excessive mental activity and improper food intake; or in case the patient has declined kidney *yang* after just recovering from a disease, or due to old age. The treatment principle is mainly to activate the *yang qi*. Chosen points include Baihui (GV20), Xinshu (BL15), Shenshu (BL23), Neiguan (PC6), Tongli (HT5), Guanyuan (CV4), Mingmen (GV4), Zusanli (ST36) and Taixi (KI3). Acupuncture and heavy moxibustion should be used together. The disease is commonly seen in Western medical treatises as "paroxysmal sleep" and "neurasthenia."

[CLINICAL EXPERIENCE]

1. CONVENTIONAL ACUPUNCTURE

(1) Reinforcing Shenmai (BL62) While Reducing Zhaohai (KI6)

Points: Shenmai (BL62), Zhaohai (KI6), Baihui (GV20) and Sanyinjiao (SP6)

Technique: Take Shenmai (BL62) first, and use the reinforcing needling technique achieved by rotation. When the patient experiences local warmth and a distending sensation, Baihui (GV20) is needled. The needles on these two points should be twisted alternately so as to achieve a matching needling sensation. Further needling manipulation should be performed every five minutes while the needles are retained for 30 minutes. The reducing needling technique achieved by rotation should be used on Zhaohai (KI6). When the needling sensation reaches Sanyinjiao (SP6), the quick needling technique should be used on Sanyinjiao (SP6). The needle should be inserted to a depth of 1.5 *cun*. Strong lifting and thrusting of the needle should be carried out three to five times, and the needle can be removed with the arrival of *qi*. The treatment is given once a day.

(2) Needling Bijiaoxue (on the midline of the nose, in the intranasal suture superior to the base of the nasal bone)

Technique: Take a one-*cun* filiform needle, and insert it towards the nose tip to a depth of 0.2 to 0.3 *cun*, with slight rotation. The needle is retained for 60 minutes after the arrival of *qi*. Other points like Shenmen (HT7) and Sanyinjiao (SP6) can be used, too. The treatment is given once a day and five sessions constitute one course. The interval between the courses of treatment should be two days. The method is applied to treat paroxysmal sleep.

(3) Needling Shenmen (HT7)

Technique: Needle Shenmen (HT7) bilaterally with one-*cun* filiform needles, applying the reducing needling techniques. The needles are retained for 30 minutes after the arrival of *qi*. Other manipulations of needles should be carried out every five minutes. The treatment is performed daily and it treats lethargy.

2. MOXIBUSTION

(1) Moxibustion with Moxa Stick

Points: Ganshu (BL18), Genshu (BL17), Baihui (GV20), Erjian (LI2), Sanjian (LI3), Taixi (KI3), Zhaohai (KI6) and Lidui (ST45)

Technique: One moxa cone is applied on each of Erjian (LI2) and Sanjian (LI3); three to five moxa cones should be applied on each of the remaining points. The method treats mainly hypo-activity of spleen *yang*, manifesting in being sleepy the whole day, with a deficient and slow pulse.

(2) Moxibustion Applied on Proximal Interphalangeal Joint of Ring Finger

Technique: Hold the moxa stick to perform the suspended moxibustion over the proximal interphalangeal joint of ring finger until the skin turns red. The treatment is given once daily.

[REMARKS]

1. Treatment with medicines may be combined with the acupuncture.

2. Attention should be paid to the amount of mental and labor work, and the patient should not get too tired or stressed.

PALPITATION

[INTRODUCTION]

Palpitation is a symptom when a patient feels subjectively the palpitation, uneasiness, liability to be scared or frightened and inability to sit or stand still. The disease occurs when a patient who usually has a diffident and timid character receives sudden stimulation, in which case the heart and mind are not at ease. The disease may also be due to insufficiency of heart blood leading to malnourishment of the heart; disturbance of the heart and mind by hyperactive heart fire where the kidney *yin* is deficient and water fails to check fire; hypo-activity of heart *yang* and the upward perversion of pathogenic fluid. The treatment should be to calm down the heart and mind. The points of Hand Shaoyin and Jueyin meridians are the main ones, such as Xinshu (BL15), Jueyinshu (BL14), Neiguan (PC6), Shenmen (HT7) and Daling (PC7). If a patient has *qi* deficiency of the heart and gallbladder, Danshu (BL19), Juque (CV14), Tongli (HT5) and Qihai (CV6) should be added. If the patient has heart blood deficiency, Pishu (BL20), Geshu (BL17) and Zusanli (ST36) should be added. If the patient has hypo-activity of heart *yang*, Tanzhong (CV17), Guan-yuan (CV4) and Zusanli (ST36) should be combined. The treatment discussed here can be taken as reference when the palpitation caused by various heart diseases and neurosis diagnosed by Western medical theory is treated.

[CLINICAL EXPERIENCE]

1. CONVENTIONAL ACUPUNCTURE

(1) *Penetrating Puncture of the Interior-exteriorly Related Meridians*

Point: Penetrating from Yanglao (SI6) to Tongli (HT5)

Technique: Tell the patient to sit straight with palms down. The practitioner uses the left thumb to press the ulnar head posterior to the wrist, and the index finger to locate the spot where Tongli (HT5) is located. The needle is inserted in Yanglao (SI6) to a depth of 0.5 *cun*. After the arrival of *qi*, the needle is pushed toward Tongli (HT5), the needling sensation traveling along the wrist. Points are needled bilaterally and needles are retained for 20 minutes. The technique treats palpitation due to the restlessness of the heart and mind caused by the emotional injury.

(2) Needling Such Points as Suliao (GV25)

Points: Suliao (GV25), Neiguan (PC6) and Anmian (Extra)

Technique: It is enough to insert the needle in Suliao (GV25) just under the skin. Use the finger to scrape the needle handle for one minute, scraping once a second. Other points are needled with a 1.5-*cun* filiform needle, after the arrival of *qi*. The reinforcing manipulation achieved by rapid and slow insertion and withdrawal of the needle is performed. Needles are retained for five minutes. The treatment has been applied in 54 cases of sinus bradycardia, with an effective rate of 88%.

(3) Needling Zanzhu (BL2) Only

Technique: Insert a one-*cun* filiform needle obliquely through the skin to a depth of 0.3 to 0.5 *cun*. After the arrival of *qi*, the needles are retained for 15 minutes. Other rotations of the needle are performed once every three minutes.

(4) Needling Points of Lower Limb

Points: Zusanli (ST36), Sanyinjiao (SP6), Tiaokou (ST38) and Chengshan (BL57)

Technique: Perform routine acupuncture technique, retaining needles for 20 minutes after the arrival of *qi*. The method has been used to treat 112 cases of organic heart disease complicated by ventricular bigemina, with an effective rate of 72.6%.

(5) Needling Mainly Extra Points

Points: Xinshu[1] (between the 2nd and 3rd thoracic vertebrae), Xinshu[2] (between the 4th and 5th thoracic vertebrae), the point beside cervical vertebra (between the 5th and 6th cervical vertebrae, 0.5 *cun* lateral to the midline), the heart point [3 *cun* below Shaohai (HT3)], Jianshi (PC5) and Yanglingquan (GB34)

Technique: Apply strong stimulation in acupuncture treatment, and manipulate the needle until the arrival of *qi*. The needles may not be retained or retained 5 to 10 minutes. Twelve daily sessions of treatment constitute one course, and three-day break should be taken between courses.

2. MOXIBUSTION

(1) Moxibustion with Moxa Stick

Points: Zhongwan (CV12), Tanzhong (CV17) and Shenmen (HT7)

Technique: Use the moxa stick to perform suspended moxibustion, 10 minutes on each point. The method treats patients with *qi* and blood deficiency.

(2) Indirect Moxibustion with Ginger

Points: Shenque (CV8) and Guanyuan (CV4)

Technique: Prepare big pieces of ginger, place them on the points and put five to eight moxa cones onto two slices of ginger on each point. The method treats patients with hypo-activity of heart *yang*.

3. ELECTRIC ACUPUNCTURE

Points: Main points: Neiguan (PC6), Jianshi (PC5), Ximen (PC4) and Sanyinjiao (SP6). Supplementary points: Zusanli (ST36) and Diji (SP8) in the case of dysfunction of stomach and weak constitution; Xinshu (BL15) and Jueyinshu (BL14) in the case of bradycardia; Shenshu (BL23) and Yiming (Extra) in the case of restlessness, penetrating technique from Tanzhong (CV17) to Jiuwei (CV15) in the case of pressure in the chest.

Technique: With the arrival of *qi* after the acupuncture technique has been performed, the electric stimulator is connected. The frequency of the stimulation is 0.3 Hz, and the stimulation should last 15 to 30 minutes. The intensity should be regulated to the extent that the patient can tolerate. The method is used to treat arrhythmia.

4. AURICULAR ACUPUNCTURE.

Points: Heart, sympathetic nerve, Ear-Shenmen, Sub-cortex, Small Intestine and Jiaodian (midway between the urinary bladder points and the brain point)

Technique: Give mild stimulation with filiform needles for 30 to 60 minutes. While the needles are in place, they can be rotated two or three times. The treatment is conducted once a day. For patients with a short duration of disease, one to three treatments should work. For patients with a long duration of disease, 10 sessions of treatment make up one course. Vaccaria seeds can be used for stimulation.

5. HYDRO-ACUPUNCTURE

Points: Neiguan (PC6), Ximen (PC4), Jianshi (PC5), Shaohai (HT3), Xinshu (BL15), Zusanli (ST36) and Sanyinjiao (SP6)

Technique: Use the compound Danshen injection fluid, choose two or three points each time, and inject 0.5 to 1ml fluid into each point. The injection is given once every other day, 10 sessions being one course.

6. WRIST-ANKLE ACUPUNCTURE

Points: Neiguan (PC6) and Shenmen (HT7)

Technique: Use the 2 to 6-*cun* filiform needle of size 28, insert them quickly through the skin, and keep the needle body and the skin at an angle of 30°. When the needle is under the skin, every effort should be made to insert the needle close to the dermis rather than too deep. The first insertion should be quick and accurate, but further insertions should be slow. No rotation should be made while the needle is inserted to a depth of 2 to 6 *cun*. The needles are retained for 20 to 30 minutes, and the treatment is given once daily or once every other day. Ten sessions make up one course. The interval between two courses should be 10 days. The treatment was applied in 90 cases of arrhythmia, with a remarkably effective rate of 58.2%, an effective rate of 28.5% and failure rate of 13.3%.

[REMARKS]

1. Emotional changes have a great impact on this disease. The practitioner should do more psychological work so that the patient has a sound emotional balance, and can regulate the body calmly. All of these are favorable to recovery.

2. A modern medical examination should be performed. If it is necessary, combined traditional Chinese and Western medicine may be adopted.

CHEST BI SYNDROME

[INTRODUCTION]

The syndrome refers to pectoral pain with stuffiness. In mild cases, the patient feels chest suffocation and in severe cases, experiences colic pain, shortness of breath and asthmatic breathing. The factors causing it are mostly the accumulation of *yin* cold and obstruction in the meridians and collaterals occurring in the aged with *qi* deficiency of the heart and lung and the hypo-activity of chest *yang*, invaded by exogenous pathogenic cold; or chest *yang* is blocked by phlegm. Other factors are obstruction of *qi* activities, which happens when the dampness, produced by the spleen deficiency due to the improper food intake or over-intake of greasy and high flavored food, has accumulated and turned into phlegm; or prolonged stagnation of liver *qi* has impaired the smooth flow of blood and produced stagnation of *qi* and blood. The treatment principle is to regulate *qi* activities. Points of the conception vessel, Jueyin meridians and Back-shu points are selected, such as: Xinshu (BL15), Jueyinshu (BL14), Tanzhong (CV17), Juque (CV14) and Neiguan (PC6). In the case of hypo-activity of chest *yang*, Feishu (BL13), Qihai (CV6), Guanyuan (CV4) and Ximen (PC4) are combined, and the moxibustion is also used in the treatment. In the case of the retention of phlegm damp, Pishu (BL20), Zhongwan (CV12), Zusanli (ST36) and Fenglong (ST40) are used; for stagnation of *qi* and blood, Geshu (BL17), Yinxi (HT6) and Taichong (LR3) are adopted. The reducing technique is used to treat the excess syndrome, while the reinforcing technique is used to treat the deficiency syndrome. Chest pain can be found in some Western medical diseases, including the coronary arteriosclerosis, cardiopathy and other acute and chronic cardiopulmonary diseases.

[CLINICAL EXPERIENCE]

1. CONVENTIONAL ACUPUNCTURE

(1) Needling Mainly Tanzhong (CV17)

Points: Penetrating technique from Tanzhong (CV17) to Jiuwei

(CV15), Neiguan (PC6), Zusanli (ST36), Tongli (HT5), Shenmen (HT7), Rugen (ST18), Jianshi (PC5) and Ximen (PC4)

Technique: Apply the penetrating technique from Tanzhong (CV17) to Jiuwei (CV15) under the skin, then insert the needle transversely to a depth of 2.5 to 2.8 *cun*. Other points are needled with regular acupuncture technique. The treatment was carried out on 621 cases of coronary heart disease and angina pectoris, with a total effective rate of 89.2%.

(2) Choosing Separate Groups of **Points**

Points: ① Jiaji (Ex-B2) point lateral to the spinous process of the 5th thoracic vertebrae, Juque (CV14), Xinping [3 *cun* below Shaohai (HT3)]. ② Jiaji (Ex-B2) point lateral to the spinous process of the 4th thoracic vertebrae, Tanzhong (CV17) and Neiguan (PC6)

Technique: Use the two groups of points alternately, needle the back points with the needle tip pointing toward the vertebrae, and puncture points of the four extremities perpendicularly. A soreness, numbness, distention or traveling sensation should be gained. The needles on the back should be removed after their handles are scraped for two minutes. The needles on the points of four extremities should be retained for 20 minutes. The treatment is given once a day or once every other day, 10 sessions being one course. This treatment was applied in 130 cases of coronary heart disease and angina pectoris, and remarkable effect was found in 32 cases (24.62%), improvement in 73 cases (60%) and no improvement in 20 cases (15.38%). The total effective rate was 84.62%.

(3) Penetrating **Technique** *from Qiuxu (GB40) to Zhaohai (KI6)*

Points: Qiuxu (GB40) and Zhaohai (KI6)

Technique: The acupuncture treatment should be applied with strong stimulation. The method is used for coronary heart disease and angina pectoris.

2. MOXIBUSTION

(1) Mild Moxibustion with Moxa Stick

Points: Tanzhong (CV17) and Tianjing (TE10)

Technique: Apply moxibustion for 15 to 30 minutes on each point each time, until the skin turns slightly red. Treatment is given once a day, 10 sessions being one course.

(2) Indirect Moxibustion with Ginger

Point: Shenque (CV8)

Technique: With the patient lying supine, place a fresh ginger slice on Shenque (CV8), then perform moxibustion with moxa cones. Each time, five to seven moxa cones can be used. Once the moxa cone gets too hot, the ginger slice can be moved a bit until the patient can tolerate the heat.

3. CUPPING

Points: Dazhui (GV14), Xinshu (BL15), Tanzhong (CV17), Shendao (GV11), Juque (CV14) and Jueyinshu (BL14)

Technique: Apply cupping only or apply bleeding and cupping, using the chest and back points alternately. The method can promote circulation in the meridians and collaterals and remove the stagnation from the heart meridian.

4. ELECTRIC ACUPUNCTURE

Points: Feishu (BL13), Jueyinshu (BL14), Xinshu (BL15) and Dushu (BL16)

Technique: After the arrival of *qi*, the electric stimulator is connected. Stimulation with an electric impulse at low frequency should be applied. The output amount is by what the patient can tolerate. A treatment lasts 10 minutes, once a day, 12 sessions making up one course. There should be an interval of four days between two courses. The above method was used in 110 cases of coronary heart disease, and ECG results showed a total effective rate of 72.2%, while the total effective rate of the relief of angina pectoris was 92.3%.

5. AURICULAR THERAPY

Points: Heart, Small Intestine, Sympathetic Nerve, Sub-cortex, Lung, Chest, Excitation Point and Occiput

Technique: Choose three to five points each time and insert two needles in the heart region. The electric stimulator is connected. The needles are retained for one hour, and the treatment is conducted once every other day. Vaccaria seeds can be embedded on other points.

6. WRIST-ANKLE ACUPUNCTURE

Point: Bilateral Shang[1]

Technique: Use a two-*cun* filiform needle, insert to a depth of 1.5 *cun* under the skin and retain the needle for 20 to 30 minutes.

7. MAGNETIC THERAPY

Points: Neiguan (PC6), Tanzhong (CV17), Xinshu (BL15) and Ah-shi points in cardiac region.

Technique: Put the small magnetic pads of 300 to 2,000 GAOSI on the points and apply the medium or big magnetic pads on the Ah-shi points in the cardiac region.

8. LASER THERAPY

Point: Neiguan (PC6)

Technique: Use a helium-neon laser to irradiate the point bilaterally and apply 15 minutes of irradiation on each point. When the treatment is applied to patients with coronary heart disease, in most cases the function of the left ventricle is improved.

9. HYDRO-ACUPUNCTURE

(1) Compound Danshen Injection

Points: Xinshu (BL15), Jueyinshu (BL14), Neiguan (PC6) and Ximen (PC4)

Technique: Choose one to two points each time, and inject 0.5 to 1 ml of injection fluid in each point, performing the injection treatment once a day or once every other day. The treatment is indicated for coronary heart disease.

(2) Dolantin Injection

Point: Neiguan (PC6)

Technique: Prepare 10 mg dolantin, and dilute it with injection water to prepare 5 ml injection fluid. Insert the syringe needle perpendicularly into Neiguan (PC6) bilaterally, perform strong stimulation after the arrival of *qi*, and inject 2.5 ml fluid into each point. When this treatment was used in seven recorded cases of acute cardiac infarction, the pain disappeared in five to 10 minutes in six of them. In the other case, the pain eased but did not go away completely. Thirty minutes after the first injection, 5 mg dolantin was injected into Jianshi (PC5) of both sides, and the pain was completely gone within five minutes.

10. MEDICINAL APPLICATION ON ACU-POINT

Points: Tanzhong (CV17) and Neiguan (PC6)

Technique: Prepare 3 g Chuanxiong (the rhizome of chuanxiong), 1 g borneol and 1 pill nitroglycerin, and grind them into powder to make pills as big as a soybean for use. When the application treatment is given, one pill should be put on each point on Tanzhong (CV17) and Neiguan (PC6), then use adhesive plaster to fix the pills on the points. The medicinal application on the acu-point can be performed once daily, five sessions of treatment being one course. The method treats coronary heart disease. In general, the treatment works in three to 15 minutes.

11. FINGER ACU-PRESSURE

Point: Lingdao (HT4)

Technique: Rub the left Lingdao (HT4) gently for 1.5 minutes with the thumb, massage the point heavily for two minutes, and gently rub the point again for 1.5 minutes. The treatment is given once daily. Fifteen sessions constitute one course. The interval between two courses of treatment should be three days.

[REMARKS]

1. Acupuncture can achieve a good effect in treating coronary heart disease. But for a patient whose disease is severe and one who has cardiac infarction and is in a critical condition, comprehensive treating measurements should be taken in time.

2. For a patient with hidden coronary heart disease, even if there are no subjective symptoms, routine acupuncture treatment should be

conducted to dilate the blood vessels, improve blood circulation and slow down the narrowing of the lumen of the coronary artery.

3. Keeping a sound and smooth emotion, not getting worried or anxious and being optimistic are vital to recovery. Striking a proper balance between work and rest, and avoiding strenuous exercises are also helpful.

MANIC AND DEPRESSIVE MENTAL DISORDERS

[INTRODUCTION]

Manic and depressive mental disorders belong to the disease category of mental abnormalities. The clinical manifestations such as hyper-activity, dementia, depression, incoherent speech, and crying or laughing without reason usually signify a depressive mental disorder. While clinical manifestations of violent movement, lots of anger, climbing to a high point to sing songs, running around without clothes on, shouting, beating others, even desiring to kill people are related to manic mental disorder. Depressive mental disorder is mainly caused by emotional injury. Emotional injuries lead to liver *qi* stagnation, cause failure of spleen *qi* in transportation and transformation, which, in turn, means the body fluid would accumulate and become phlegm. Once the turbid phlegm goes upward and mists the heart and mind, the disease occurs. The proper treatment should be to regulate the flow of *qi* and remove stagnation, calm the heart and resolve the phlegm. The points of Hand Shaoyin, Jueyin and Foot Jueyin meridians are taken as the main points. The examples are Baihui (GV20), Sishencong (Ex-HN1), Shenmen (HT7), Neiguan (PC6), Daling (PC7), Taichong (LR3) and Sanyinjiao (SP6). Acupuncture and moxibustion should be used together, and both the reinforcing and reducing techniques should be applied. As for manic mental disorder, it is mostly due to emotional depression, which leads to excessive fire in the liver and stomach. Once the fire brings up phlegm to disturb the mind, it becomes misted and the heart fails to house the mind, so disease occurs. The treatment should be to reduce liver fire, clear heart fire and break up the phlegm. Points of the Conception Vessel and Governor Vessel, points of the Hand Jueyin and Foot Shaoyin meridians are taken as the main points, such as Renzhong (GV26), Laogong (PC8), Shaofu (HT8), Fenglong (ST40), Dazhong (KI4) and Xingjian (LR2). The reducing needling technique is applied. The treatment discussed in this section can be taken as reference for the treatment of schizophrenia, manic and depressive psychosis and involutional psychosis diagnosed in Western medicine.

[CLINICAL EXPERIENCE]

1.   CONVENTIONAL ACUPUNCTURE

(1) Needling Thirteen Ghost Points

Points: Renzhong (GV26), Shaoshang (LU9), Yinbai (SP1), Daling (PC7), Shenmai (BL62), Fengfu (GV16), Jiache (ST6), Chengjiang (CV24), Jianshi (PC5), Shangxing (GV23), Yumentou (Extra), Quchi (LI11) and Shexiazhongfeng (Extra)

Technique: Perform acupuncture treatment on the above points in the order listed, applying the reducing needling technique and retaining the needles for 40 to 60 minutes. The treatment is given once a day. Ten sessions make up one course.

(2) Penetrating Puncture

Points: Penetration from Hegu (LI4) to Laogong (PC8), from Quchi (LI11) to Shaohai (HT3), from Yanglingquan (GB34) to Yinlingquan (SP9), and from Taichong (LR3) to Yongquan (KI1)

Technique: Perform the penetrating puncture on the above points with a 1.5-*cun* filiform needle, and give strong stimulation, retenting for 30 minutes following the arrival of *qi*. After the needles are removed, the quick needling technique is applied on Huantiao (GB30). The treatment is carried out once daily, and seven sessions make up one course.

(3) Needling Mainly Points of Governor Vessel

Points: Fengfu (GV16), Dazhui (GV14), Shenzhu (GV12), Taodao (GV13), Renzhong (GV26), Daling (PC7) and Taichong (LR3)

Technique: The patient is in a sitting position, with the head slightly lowered. Needle Fengfu (GV16) to a depth of 2 *cun*, the needle tip pointing downwards. Dazhui (GV14), Shenzhu (GV12) and Taodao (GV13) are all needled when the patient is in a sitting posture, but the needles are not retained on these points. Daling (PC7) and Taichong (LR3) should also be punctured deeply to clear the brain and wake up the mind. The treatment is performed once daily, and 10 sessions constitute one course. This treatment is applied for manic mental disorder.

2. MOXIBUSTION

(1) Moxibustion with a Moxa Cone

Points: Baihui (GV20), Shaoshang (LU11), Yinbai (SP1) and Dadun (LR1)

Technique: Use the moxa cone to do moxibustion on the above points, applying three moxa cones on each point. Moxibustion is performed from the upper points to the lower points and once daily. Usually, two or three hours after moxibustion, the manic behavior will be relieved and consciousness become clearer.

(2) Moxibustion with Moxa Stick

Point: Zhongwan (CV12), Zusanli (ST36) and Neiguan (PC6)

Technique: Apply warm moxibustion with a moxa stick on the above points for 10 minutes each. The treatment is carried out once daily and successively for one month. The treatment is applicable for depressive mental disorder caused by spleen deficiency and liver stagnation that lead to the obstruction of phlegm and *qi*.

3. ELECTRIC ACUPUNCTURE

Points: Baihui (GV20) and Yintang (Ex-HN3)

Technique: Use a one-*cun* filiform needle to puncture the points along the skin and apply electric stimulation. Use dense and disperse wave stimulation for one hour. The treatment is conducted once daily, and 30 sessions make up one course. This method can achieve certain effects in treating depression.

4. BLEEDING METHOD

Points: Taiyang (Ex-HN5) and Weizhong (BL40)

Technique: Use a three-edged needle to prick the points bilaterally, letting out a small amount of blood. The bleeding treatment is performed once every other day, and should be carried out successively three to five times. The method can be used to treat both the excessive and heat types of schizophrenia.

5. AURICULAR THERAPY

Points: Heart, Ear-shenmen, Sub-cortex, Brain Point, Kidney, Endocrine and Adrenal

Technique: Choose three points each time and needle the points bilaterally, totaling six points. Use filiform needles to puncture the points. Electric stimulation is applied, the frequency being 3 times/second. Each treatment lasts 30 minutes. The treatment is given once daily and 10 sessions make up one course. The method can achieve good results in treating auditory hallucination and visual hallucination accompanying mental disorders, and the involutional depression. Or the compound Dongmianling is injected into the Ear-shenmen of both ears, 0.1 to 0.2 ml injection fluid being injected into each point. This treatment can deal with the manic type of mental disorders.

6. HYDRO-ACUPUNCTURE

Points: Xinshu (BL15), Ximen (PC4), Sanyinjiao (SP6) and Fenglong (ST40)

Technique: Divide points into two groups, use each alternately, and inject 25 to 50 mg of chlorpromazine injection fluid into each point. The injection is given once daily, sessions determined by the condition of the disease.

7. LASER THERAPY

Point: Yamen (GV15)

Technique: Apply helium neon irradiation of 5.9 to 25 mw on Yamen (GV15), one treatment a day, 15 minutes each time. Six weeks of treatment make up one course. During the treatment, no medicine for psychosis should be taken. The clinical remarkable effective rate was 78%.

8. COMBINED TREATMENT

Points: Penetration from left Fengchi (GB20) to right Fengchi (GB20), from the point 1 *cun* above the anterior end of axillary fold to the posterior end of axillary fold, from Quchi (LI20) to Shaohai (HT3), from Hegu (LI4) to Houxi (SI3), from Yanglingquan (GB34) to Yinlingquan (SP9), from Kunlun (BL60) to Taixi (KI3), from the point one *cun* or so above the medial end of the femoral crease to its lateral end (locating the line when the knee is flexed at a right angle).

Technique: Apply the lifting, thrusting and rotating needling manipulation on all the points, giving quick needle manipulation or retaining the needles. The treatment is performed once daily and is combined with Chinese herbal medical treatment. Take 30 to 120 g of Jiujun, 9 g of the root-tuber of aromatic turmeric, 30 g of calamus, and decoct the herbs. The patient should take the decoction once on an empty stomach in the morning. Thirty minutes after the herbal decoction is taken, the patient will feel a slight abdominal pain and then have diarrhea, passing a loose stool with mucous. The method is applicable for the manic type of psychosis, in which case the pulse manifestation is surging, wiry and excessive. In general, after the medicine is taken, the patient becomes quieter, but this kind of herbal medicine is contraindicated for patients with ulceration and intestinal tuberculosis.

[REMARKS]

1. The course of acupuncture treatment will be longer.

2. For patients with manic type of mental disorder, it is better to apply the comprehensive treatment. Measures should be taken to prevent a patient from committing suicide, hurting others or destroying things.

3. While the acupuncture treatment is applied to treat the disease, attention should be paid to psychological treatment as well. It is better to comfort the patient, trying to straighten him or her out. These measures are favorable to the recovery of the disease.

EPILEPSY

[INTRODUCTION]

It is believed in traditional Chinese medicine that the disease originates in the fetus, when the pregnant women is suddenly frightened, the fear interrupting the development of fetus, or that fear, fright and repressed anger cause the stagnation of liver *qi*, which further induces the dysfunction of the spleen in transportation and transformation, ultimately producing phlegm damp from the interior, so that *qi* and fire bring up the phlegm and travel in the meridians collaterals and mist up the clear orifice. Clinically, it can be divided into deficient and excessive types. The excessive type manifests itself as sudden falling in a faint, loss of consciousness, locked jaw, frothy mouth, opisthotonus, severe convulsion, making roaring sounds, incontinence of urine and stool. The deficient type manifests itself as chronic epilepsy with repeated attacks, decreased severity of convulsion, low spirits, lassitude, weakness, soreness and weakness in the lower back and knees. The treatment for the excessive type is to calm the interior part of the body, relieve epilepsy, tranquilize the heart and resolve the phlegm. Points selected include Baihui (GV20), Fengfu (GV16), Neiguan (PC6), Taichong (LR3), Shenzhu (GV12), Benshen (GB13) and Jiuwei (CV15). The treatment to the deficient type is to tonify the heart and spleen, resolve phlegm and calm down the mind. Points selected are Tongli (HT5), Yanglingquan (GB34), Fenglong (ST40), Sanyinjiao (SP6), Jinsuo (GV8) and Shenshu (BL23). The reinforcing needling technique can be used, and moxibustion can be combined.

[CLINICAL EXPERIENCE]

1. CONVENTIONAL ACUPUNCTURE

(1) Needling Fengfu (GV16) Deeply

Points: Fengfu (GV16), Dazhui (GV14), Shenzhu (GV12), Taichong (LR3) and Fenglong (ST40)

Technique: Place the patient in a sitting position with the head flexing slightly, or ask the patient to lie down on the side or lie prone in case sitting is not feasible. Turn the needle tip slightly downwards, inserting it to a depth of 2 to 2.5 *cun*. When the needling sensation comes, the patient should feel numbness traveling up and down or radiating to the left and right shoulders. The needle is removed after the arrival of *qi*. The treatment is performed once a day and it is indicated for epilepsy.

(2) Penetrating Puncture

Points: Penetrating from Baihui (GV20) to Qianding (GV21), Fengchi (GB20), Fengfu (GV16) and Mingmen (GV4)

Technique: With the patient in a prone position, use a two-*cun* filiform needle to perform the penetrating puncture, inserting the needle to a depth of 1.5 *cun*. The needle on Mingmen (GV4) should be inserted to a depth of 1.2 *cun*. The reducing technique achieved by lifting, thrusting and rotating should be applied. The needles are retained for 20 minutes; other needles should be rotated once every five minutes.

(3) Needling Dazhui (GV14)

Technique: Tell the patient to sit down. Take a 1.5-*cun* filiform needle to puncture Dazhui (GV14) to a depth of 0.8 to 1 *cun*. Repeated lifting and thrusting of the needle is prohibited. The treatment is given once daily and the therapeutic effect can be increased if anti-epileptic medicines are taken.

(4) Surrounding Puncture of Changqiang (GV1)

Point: Changqiang (GV1)

Technique: Ask the patient to rest on chest and knees. After sterilizing the point, pinch up the local tissues of the point with the left hand, and take thicker filiform needles to puncture Changqiang (GV1) and other points to the front, back, left and right of Changqiang (GV1). The needles are inserted to a depth of 0.3 to 0.5 *cun* and distributed like a plum blossom. The four points around Changqiang (GV1) should be 0.5 *cun* lateral to Changqiang (GV1). The needles are retained two or three minutes. After they are removed, blood should be let out. The treatment is conducted two or three times a week, 10 sessions being one course. The short-term effect of this treatment is good.

(5) Needling Renzhong (GV26) and Other Points

Points: Renzhong (GV26), Yamen (GV15), Fengchi (GB20), Houxi (SI3), Neiguan (PC6) and Yaoqi (2 *cun* above the tip of coccyx, about where the sacral hiatus is)

Technique: During the attack, Renzhong (GV26) and Neiguan (PC6) should be needled; during the intermission, other points should be needled too. A filiform needle is of 2.5 to 3 *cun* used to puncture Yaoqi (extra) with the needle tip pointing upward. The treatment is performed once daily. No needle retention is applied on Yamen (GV/5), while 20 to 30 minutes of needle retention is applied on other points.

(6) Needling Shangchi (Extra), Yaoqi (Extra) and Other Points

Points: Shangchi (Extra) (on the hand dorsum, between the second and third matacarpal bones, 2 *cun* above the wrist crease) and Yaoqi (Extra)

Technique: Take one-*cun* filiform needles to puncture Shangchi bilaterally to control the epileptic attack. In the usual time, the treatment on Shangchi and Yaoqi can prevent an attack. The treatment is performed once daily and the needles are retained for 30 minutes each time.

2. MOXIBUSTION

(1) Scarring Moxibustion

Points: Shenzhu (GV12), Shentang (BL44) and Geshu (BL17)

Technique: Use one point, or use all the three points, in each moxibustion treatment. The moxa cones are prepared as big as a soybean. Three to five moxa cones are applied on each point every time. It is better to have the moxa scar become purulent. The moxibustion treatment is given once every 20 to 30 days.

(2) Burning Rush Moxibustion

Points: Baihui (GV20), Chonggu (below the spinous process of the 6th cervical vertebrae) and Huiyin (CV1)

Technique: Apply the burning rush moxibustion on the above points, using one burning rush moxibustion on each point every time.

According to the disease condition, this should be done once every 10 days.

3. SCALP ACUPUNCTURE

Points: Xiongqiangqu and Yuntingqu

Technique: Use 1.5 to 2 *cun* filiform needles to puncture the scalp areas bilaterally, applying the reducing manipulation achieved by rapid and slow insertion and withdrawal of the needle. Three sessions of treatment should be performed every week. When the treatment is done, the intra-dermal needles should be embedded on the Xiongqiangqu (thoracic cavity area) and Yuntingqu on both sides. If the above treatment is given successively for two or three months, the onset of attacks can be controlled.

4. AURICULAR ACUPUNCTURE

Points: Stomach, Sub-cortex, Ear-shenmen, Heart, Occiput and Brain Point

Technique: Use one-*cun* filiform needles to puncture the points of both ears, retaining the needles for 20 minutes. The treatment is given once a day. Vaccaria seeds can also be embedded on the above points, but the seeds should be changed every four to five days. This method is applicable in the intermission of epilepsy.

5. CATGUT-EMBEDDING METHOD

Points: Dazhui (GV14), Yamen (GV15), Xinshu (BL15), Ganshu (BL18) and Sanyinjiao (SP6)

Technique: Choose two or three points each time, using the suture needle to embed two or three cm catgut into the points. This is done once every 20 days.

6. PRICKING METHOD

Points: Three points in total that are 0.5 *cun*, 1 *cun* and 1.5 *cun* above Changqiang (GV1), respectively

Technique: After performing routine sterilization, pinch up the subcutaneous tissues with the left hand, and hold a three-edged needle or syringe needle with the right hand, pricking the subcutaneous tissues to let out some blood. The pricking method is used once a week, three sessions being one course.

7.   MEDICINAL APPLICATION ON ACU-POINT

Point: Shenque (CV8)

Technique: Take 0.25 g phenytoin sodium, 1 g powder of the root of red-rooted salvia, 1 g borax, a certain amount of borneol, and grind them into powder. Store the mixed powder in a sealed bottle for use. Upon application, the powder fills the whole of the umbilicus, and adhesive plaster is used to cover it. The powder is changed once every three days.

8.   COMBINED TREATMENT

(1) Cutting and Cupping Therapy

Points: ① Dazhui (GV14), Yaoqi and Dianxian [midway between Dazhui (GV14) and the tip of coccyx, about the spinous process of the 11th thoracic vertebrae]. ② Taodao (GV13), Geshu (BL17) and Mingmen (GV4). ③ Ganshu (BL18), Shenzhu (GV12) and Yaoyangguan (GV3)

Technique: Apply one group of points each time, changing groups alternately. A lancet is used first to make a cut on the point 0.5 cm long, then the subcutaneous fiber tissues are pricked completely. Afterwards, cupping is applied over the pricked points five to 10 minutes, so that some blood is sucked out. After the cup is removed, sterilized gauze is applied over the point. The pricking treatment is performed once every week, and three sessions constitute one course.

[REMARKS]

1.   Acupuncture treatment can achieve certain effect in treating epilepsy. Its effect can be increased if the oral administration of Chinese herbal and Western medication is combined.

2.   When the treatment is given while the patient is in the severe attack, the limbs are twitching. So great care should be paid to prevent bending of the needles.

MELANCHOLIA

[INTRODUCTION]

Melancholia manifests itself as emotional depression, emotional anxiety, distending pain in the hypochondrium, excessive mental activity, worry, liability to anger or crying, foreign body sensation choking in the throat and insomnia. The disease is mainly caused by suppressed anger damaging the liver leading to liver *qi* stagnation and a traverse attack on the spleen by the liver. Alternatively, it is caused by liver stagnation transformed into fire that brings up liver fire attacking stomach; when excessive mental activity damages the spleen, causing its failure in transportation and transformation which in turn generates phlegm and damp in the interior, leading to phlegm and *qi* accumulating above the diaphragm in the chest; when overstrain, stress and excessive thinking damage both the heart and spleen and lead to deficiency of *qi* and blood; or when there is the dysfunction of *yin, yang, qi* and blood of zangfu organs. The treatment principle is to sooth the liver, remove liver stagnation, strengthen the spleen, resolve phlegm and tonify *qi* and blood. The points of the Hand and Foot Jueyin, Foot Taiyin and points of Conception Vessel are taken as the main ones, such as Tanzhong (CV17), Neiguan (PC6), Shenmen (HT7), Xinshu (BL15), Fenglong (ST40), Sanyinjiao (SP6) and Taichong (LR3). Neurasthenia, hysteria and menopausal syndrome as diagnosed by Western medicine can be classified into this disease category.

[CLINICAL EXPERIENCE]

1. CONVENTIONAL ACUPUNCTURE

(1) Selecting Separate Groups of Points

Points: ① Kunlun (BL60) and Houxi (SI3). ② Renzhong (GV26), penetration from Hegu (LI4) to Laogong (PC8). ③ Baihui (GV20), penetration from Neiguan (PC6) to Waiguan (TE5)

Technique: Perform the acupuncture treatment once a day, choosing one group of points in each treatment. Apply reducing manipulation achieved by lifting, thrusting and rotating. The method is used to treat hysteria.

(2) Needling Tiantu (CV22)

Points: Tiantu (CV22) and Shangchi (on dorsum of hand, between the second and third metacarpal bones, 1.5 *cun* posterior to the metacarpophalangeal joint).

Technique: Needle Tiantu (CV22) with the needle tip pointing downward. Needle Shangchi perpendicularly, apply rotating and scrap manipulation on all needles, giving strong stimulation and combining psychological suggestion to treat globus hystericus. According to clinical observation of 440 cases, a total recovery rate came to 88%.

(3) Needling Yinbao (LR9) Deeply

Point: Yinbao (LR8)

Technique: Tell the patient to sit (Someone should assist the patient). Use the thicker needle, inserting it deeply to a depth of 3 to 4 *cun*. When something like a cord is felt under the needle, one should try to avoid puncturing it. The method is indicated for hysteria.

(4) Choosing Mainly the Eight Confluent Points

Point: Houxi (SI3), Shenmai (BL62), Neiguan (PC6), Taichong (LR3) and Fenglong (ST40)

Technique: Apply reducing needling technique to treat once a day and retain the needles for 30 minutes. The treatment is good for mental derangement, liability to cry, protruding/staring eyes and inability to sleep the whole night.

(5) Selecting the Yuan-primary Point of Pericardium Meridian

Point: Daling (PC7)

Technique: Needle Daling (PC7) of both sides, retaining the needles for 20 minutes. This method is mainly to treat globus hystericus.

2. MOXIBUSTION

(1) Using Moxibustion over the Epigastrium

Point: Zhongwan (CV12)

Technique: It is written in *Bian Que's Comprehension Book* that "symptoms of being unaware of one's behavior and looking like a dead person are caused by worry, excessive thinking, fear and fright, and the symptoms are found more in women. Fifty moxa cones should be applied on Zhongwan (CV12)."

(2) Moxibustion on Points like Tanzhong (CV17)

Points: Tanzhong (CV17), Neiguan (PC6), Shenmen (HT7), Zusanli (ST36) and Taichong (LR3)

Technique: Apply moxibustion with three moxa cones on each point. The treatment is given once daily for treating depression.

3. BLEEDING METHOD

Point: Taiyang (Ex-HN5)

Technique: Use a three-edged needle to prick Taiyang (Ex-HN5) of one side, letting out some blood. Taiyang (Ex-HN5) of the other side should be pricked three days later. The treatment is good for globus hystericus.

4. PRICKING METHOD

Points: Ah-shi points of throat, Feishu (BL13), Ganshu (BL18) and Jiaji (Ex-B2) points from the 3rd to 6th cervical vertebrae

Technique: Select two or three points to prick each time, applying mainly the tendon pricking method. Conduct treatment once a day or once every other day. Five sessions constitute one course. This method has good effect in relieving the foreign body sensation, choking in the throat.

5. ELECTRIC ACUPUNCTURE

(1) Selecting Head Points

Points: Baihui (GV20) and Yintang (Ex-HN3)

Technique: With the arrival of *qi* after the acupuncture treatment is performed, the electric stimulator is connected to the needles. The treatment is given once a day, and it takes one hour each time. Thirty sessions constitute one course. The method can achieve a certain effect in relieving melancholia.

(2) Selecting Points on Lower Extremities

Points: Sanyinjiao (SP6) and Yongquan (KI1)

Technique: Needle points bilaterally, applying electric stimulation and connecting one pair of points on the same side of the body. The treatment is performed once daily, and 10 sessions make up one course. The method is applicable to melancholia.

6. CUTANEOUS PUNCTURE

Points: Neck region, and the Governor Vessel and Bladder Meridian on the nape and back

Technique: Use a cutaneous needle to tap the regions gently until the skin turns slightly red. The treatment is performed once a day or once every other day, 10 sessions making up one course.

7. MEDICINAL APPLICATION ON ACU-POINT

Points: Tiantu (CV22) and Quchi (LI11) (unilaterally)

Technique: Prepare 3 g of Chinese blister beetles, 1 g centipedes, 1 g scorpions, 0.5 g borneol, grind them into fine powder and prepare the medicament into a paste with some Vaseline. Medicinal paste, as much as a match tip, is taken out with a small bamboo spatula, and the paste is put in the middle of an adhesive plaster to be applied on the point. The medicinal application should be kept three days. There will be local foaming, so measures should be taken to prevent infection. The treatment is used to treat globus hystericus.

[REMARKS]

1. Acupuncture has a certain effect in relieving melancholia.

2. When acupuncture and psychological treatment are combined, the therapeutic effect can be improved. Before the acupuncture treatment is conducted, careful observation should be made on the emotions and mental condition of the patient. The patient should be encouraged to keep him/her vigorous and build up confidence in curing the disease.

WIND STROKE

[INTRODUCTION]

This disease is mainly characterized by sudden falling down in a fit, loss of consciousness, deviation of the corner of the eye and mouth, speech debility and hemiplegia. Before the onset of the disease, the patient usually has such preliminary symptoms as dizziness and numbness of limbs. The disease occurs when the patient is obese and overeats greasy and sweet food that cause too much dampness generating an accumulation of phlegm, turning into heat. The disease also occurs when the patient has overindulged in sexual activities, or has been subject to overstrain and stress, leading to deficiency of kidney *yin* that further generates hyperactive liver *yang*. It can also occur when there are dysfunctions of zangfu organs, the preponderance of *yin* and *yang* and the derangement of *qi* and blood that are induced by worry, excessive thinking, anger and alcoholic indulgence. The disease is mild if it is due to the up-stirring of liver wind, the obstruction of the turbid phlegm and blood stagnation in the meridians and collaterals when the location of the disease is shallow. In this case, the manifestations are those symptoms of meridians and collaterals like numbness and paralysis of limbs. The type of disease is therefore termed "attack on meridians and collaterals." The treatment is to open and regulate meridians and collaterals, to harmonize *qi* and blood. The points chosen are Jianyu (LI15), Qichi (LI11), Waiguan (TE5), Hegu (LI4), Huantiao (GB30), Yanglingquan (GB34), Zusanli (ST36), Taixi (KI3), Chongyang (ST42) and Taichong (LR3). The disease is severe if it is due to the sudden uprising of liver *yang* that is mixed with phlegm and fire, creating rising of *qi* and blood; when the *yin-yang* balance has been damaged badly and phlegm and heat are misting the heart orifice, the location of the disease is deep. In this case, the manifestations are those symptoms of zangfu organs, such as the paralysis of limbs, unconsciousness and aphasia. This type of the disease is thus termed the "attack on zangfu organs." The attack on zangfu organs can be divided into tense and flaccid types. The treatment for the tense type is to calm down the liver and eliminate wind, clear fire and break phlegm and open the orifice. The points selected are Shuigou (GV26), 12 Jing-well points, Taichong (LR3), Fenglong (ST40) and Laogong (PC8). Treatment for the flaccid type is to restore *yang* to rescue the patient from collapse. Moxibustion with big moxa cones should be used on Guanyuan (CV4) and Shenque (CV8). Cerebrovascular diseases including cerebral hemorrhage, cerebral embolism and cerebral thrombosis belong to the disease discussed in this section.

[CLINICAL EXPERIENCE]

1. CONVENTIONAL ACUPUNCTURE

(1) Two Steps Opposing Needling

Points: Binao (LI14), Quchi (LI11), Sidu (TE9), Hegu (LI4), Huantiao (GB30), Yanglingquan (GB34), Tiaokou (ST38) and Fengshi (GB31)

Technique: The treatment to the sequelae of wind stroke is divided into two steps. The first step is to use points mainly on the healthy side. According to the diseased area, the points of the upper or lower extremities are needled with the reducing needling technique. After the needling manipulation has been carried out for a few minutes, the patient is told to try to exercise the affected limb. If the treatment is not effective, the needle manipulation is repeated every five minutes. When the patient is able to move the affected limb slightly, the points of the affected side are needled. The needles should be retained for 20 minutes after the arrival of *qi*. This treatment should be performed daily, 10 sessions making up one course. One to two courses of treatment can be given in the way described above. Once the movements of the patient's limb have improved greatly, the second step of treatment is carried out, namely, to needle the points of the affected side with the reinforcing needling technique first, then one to two points on the healthy side should be punctured with the reducing needling technique.

(2) Needling Points of Governor Vessels

Point: Dazhui (GV14), inter-vertebral spaces between the 4th and 5th cervical vertebraes, Zhiyang (GV9), Yaoyangguan (GV3), Mingmen (GV4) and Jinsuo (GV8)

Technique: Use 1 to 1.5-*cun* needles to puncture the above points, retaining the needles for 15 minutes. The patient is prohibited from moving while the needles are retained so as to prevent accidents such as bending of the needles.

(3) Needling Points of Conception Vessels

Points: Chengjiang (CV24), Lianquan (CV23), Tiantu (CV22), Tanzhong (CV17), Jiuwei (CV15), Zhongwan (CV12), Qihai (CV6), Guanyuan (CV4) and Zhongji (CV3)

Technique: When the points on the chest are needled, the tip of the needle should point downward. The points on the abdomen should be needled perpendicularly to a depth of one to two *cun*. The method is indicated in hemiplegia caused by the disharmony of the spleen and stomach that leads to accumulation of dampness, which, in turn, is producing phlegm that finally induces an accumulation of excessive phlegm fluid or the lingering of phlegm damp.

(4) Needling Back-shu Points of Six Fu Organs

Points: Danshu (BL19), Weishu (BL21), Sanjiaoshu (BL22), Dachangshu (BL25), Xiaochangshu (BL27) and Pangguangshu (BL28)

Technique: With the patient lying prone, needle the Back-shu points bilaterally. The method is indicated for a patient with hemiplegia who has not recovered over a long period of time so that there is also dysfunction of the stomach and intestine and the dysfunction in urination and defecation.

(5) Needling Back-shu Points of Five Zang Organs

Points: Xinshu (BL15), Feishu (BL13), Ganshu (BL18), Pishu (BL20), Shenshu (BL23) and Geshu (BL17)

Technique: Use one-*cun* needles and insert the needles to a depth of 1 *cun* for heavy patients or 0.5 to 0.6 *cun* for thin patients. Needle manipulation is performed until the arrival of *qi*. The method is applicable for a patient with wind stroke, hemiplegia of long duration, where the five zang organs are deficient and along with weak yin and *yang*.

(6) Needling Renying (ST9)

Points: Renying (ST9) is taken as the main point, and Hegu (LI4) and Shenmen (HT7) of the upper limbs are combined in addition to Yongquan (KI1) and Chongyang (ST42) on the lower limb.

Technique: A one-*cun* needle is taken to puncture Renying (ST9) to a depth of 0.5 to 0.8 *cun*. The needle is removed with the arrival of *qi*. When the needle is taken out, a dry cotton ball is used to close the needle hole. The treatment is given once everyday. The point on the different sides should be needled alternately, while the supplementary points are punctured everyday only on the affected side. Seven to 10 sessions make up one course. This method is applied in the case of the sequelae of wind stroke.

(7) Needling Sympathetic Nerve

Points: Points 1.5 cm lateral to the thyroid cartilage.

Technique: Tell the patient to sit. Use 1.5-*cun* needles to puncture points on both sides perpendicularly to a depth of 1 to 1.2 *cun*, retaining them for five minutes. Attention should be paid to avoiding puncturing the carotid artery. Lifting and thrusting manipulation is prohibited. The method is applicable for aphasia caused by cerebrovascular diseases.

(8) Penetrating Puncture on Head Points

Point: Penetration from Baihui (GV20) to Qubin (GB7)

Technique: Insert a 1.5 to 2 *cun* needle of size 28 under the scalp from Baihui (GV20) to Qubin (GB7). Quick rotation of the needle is performed once the patient feels distention and numbness. Rotation is carried out about 200 times per minute. After five minutes of continuous rotation, there should be a five-minute break. This kind of manipulation should be repeated three times. The treatment is conducted daily and is given successively over 15 sessions. In the case of left hemiplegia, the penetration is made from Baihui (GV20) to right Qubin (GB7). In the case of right hemiplegia, the penetration is made from Baihui (GV20) to left Qubin (GB7).

(9) Penetrating Puncture on Four Extremities' Points

Points: Penetration from Jianyu (LI15) to Binao (LI14), from Quchi (LI11) to Shaohai (HT3), Waiguan (TE5) to Neiguan (PC6), Hegu (LI4) to Laogong (PC8), Yangchi (TE4) to Daling (PC7), Huantiao (GB30) to Fengshi (GB31), Yangguan (GB33) to Ququan (LR8), Yanglingquan (GB34) to Yinlingquan (SP9), Juegu (GB39) to Sanyinjiao (SP6), Qiuxu (GB40) to Shenmai (BL62), Taichong (LR3) to Yongquan (KI1)

Technique: The above points are needled to 1.5 to 2 *cun*. When the penetration is made and the needle reaches the other point, manipulation is performed to achieve the arrival of *qi*. This travels along with the direction that the needle points, therefore the arrival of *qi* can reach the diseased area. The method is applicable for a patient with hemiplegia who has had the disease over a long period and whose improvement in limb function has been slow.

(10) Needling Xinshe and Other Points

Points: Xinshe (straight down from Fengchi (GB20) on the nape, 1.5 *cun* below the posterior hairline, leveled with the transverse process of the 4th cervical vertebrae), and Yinlingquan (SP9)

Technique: Tell the patient to lie on the side first. Use a 2-*cun* needle to puncture Xinshe on the affected side, pointing the needle tip toward the transverse process of the 4th cervical vertebrae. Insert the needle to a depth of 1 to 1.5 *cun*, asking the patient to move the affected limb after the arrival of *qi*. The needle should be removed once the functions of limb have been restored. Then ask the patient to lie supine, and needle Yinlingquan (SP9) on the healthy side, giving a strong stimulation. In this case, the needling sensation should travel to the sole of foot. The patient should be told to exercise the affected limb after the arrival of *qi*. Once the functions of the affected limb have been restored, the needle can be retained for 30 minutes. During the needle retention, the lifting, thrusting and rotating manipulation can be performed three times, and the patient should be told to move the affected limb each time.

(11) Needling Lower Surface of Tongue

Points: Shegen (in the depression of the root of sublingual ligaments), Yepang (medial to the left and right sublingual veins, 1/3 proximal to the root of tongue), and Zhimai (to the left and right of sublingual veins, 2/3 proximal to the root of tongue)

Technique: Use thicker needles to prick the above points, inserting the needles 0.5 *cun* deep and applying the lifting and thrusting manipulation several times. The needle can be taken out when the numbness and distention felt under the root of the tongue travels to the throat. The method is applicable for a patient with hemiplegia and speech debility.

2. MOXIBUSTION

(1) Moxibustion with Moxa Stick

Points: Tianchuang (SI16) and Baihui (GV20)

Technique: In the case of left hemiplegia, apply moxibustion on the right Tianchuang (SI16), and in the case of right hemiplegia, apply moxibustion on left Tianchuang (SI16). In the case of simple aphasia, perform moxibustion on Baihui (GV20), keeping the moxa stick 3 to 4 cm away from the skin. Each moxibustion treatment should last 15 minutes, and it is carried out daily.

(2) Indirection Moxibustion on Salt with Moxa Cone

Point: Shenque (CV8)

Technique: Tell the patient to lie supine. Fill the whole umbilicus with salt, applying dozens of big moxa cones on the point. The method is indicated for the flaccid syndrome of wind stroke and has the function of restoring *yang* to rescue the patient from collapse.

3. SCALP ACUPUNCTURE

Points: Choosing the contra lateral motor area for the motor dysfunction; selecting the speech area I and II for the speech debility; using the contra lateral sensory area for the sensory dysfunction.

Technique: Needle the treatment area with a thick filiform needle, and apply rotating needling manipulation. The needle is rotated 180 to 200 times per minute and the rotation should last three to five minutes each time. The needles are retained for 30 minutes, and another three cycles of rotation should be conducted during this time. The method is applicable to the sequelae of wind stroke.

4. ORBITAL ACUPUNCTURE

Points: Bilateral upper triple energizer area and bilateral lower triple energizer area in the eye region around the orbit.

Technique: Use a 0.5-*cun* filiform needle of size 30 to puncture the points transversely and respectively in the introduced order from the point 0.2 *cun* to the lateral border of the orbit, retaining the needle for five to 10 minutes. When the needles are removed, a cotton ball is used to press the needle hole to prevent bleeding. The treatment is performed once a day, 10 treatments being one course. The interval between courses of treatment is three to five days. After two courses of treatment, however, treatment will be given every other day.

5. AURICULAR THERAPY

Points: Points relevant to the paralyzed regions, sub-cortex, liver, Sanjiao and middle border. Heart and liver are combined for aphasia; mouth and throat are added for swallowing debility.

Technique: The above-mentioned points should be needled with filiform needles. The points on one side of the ear are punctured in each treatment. A strong stimulation is applied and the needles are retained for 30 minutes to one hour. The treatment is carried out once a day, and points on different ears are used alternately. Semen Vaccaria seeds can be used in the treatment. These are put on points of both ears and changed once every five days.

6. HYDRO-ACUPUNCTURE

Points: Ganshu (BL18), Shenshu (BL23), Quchi (LI11), Yanglingquan (GB34), Zusanli (ST36) and Lanquan (CV23)

Technique: Take 5% *danggui* (Chinese angelica) injection fluid and inject 1 ml fluid into each point, choosing three to four points each time, and performing the treatment once every other day.

7. MAGNETIC THERAPY

Points: Jianyu (LI15), Quchi (LI11), Hegu (LI4), Waiguan (TE5), Zhongzhu (TE3), Huantiao (GB30), Fengshi (GB31), Yanglingquan (GB34) Xuanzhong (GB39), Zusanli (ST36), Kunlun (BL60) and Taichong (LR3)

Technique: According to the different conditions of the upper and lower extremities, two to four points are chosen each time. The spiral magnetic machine is used for 20 minutes, and then the magnetic pad of 500 to 1,500 gauss is applied topically on the points on the affected side. Other points are used 10 days later. This method has a certain effect for the patient who has hemiplegia accompanied with pain in the limb.

8.   COMPREHENSIVE TREATMENT

(1) Acupuncture and Bleeding Method

Points: Renzhong (GV26), 12 Jing-well points, Fengfu (GV16), Fengchi (GB20), Baihui (GV20), Neiguan (PC6), Daling (PC7), Hegu (LI4), Laogong (PC8), Zusanli (ST36), Yongquan (KI1) and Taichong (LR3)

Technique: At first, the filiform needles are taken to puncture Renzhong (GV26), Neiguan (PC6) and Yongquan (KI1), then the three-edged needle is used to prick the Jing-well points to let out blood. If the effect is not remarkable, other points should be needled. This method is applicable for the tense syndrome of wind stroke.

(2) Electric Acupuncture Combined with Moxibustion

Points: Baihui (GV20), Jianyu (LI15), Quchi (LI11), Shousanli (LI10), Hegu (LI4), Ganshu (BL18), Yanglingquan (GB34), Zusanli (ST36), Juegu (GB39), Taixi (KI3), Sanyinjiao (SP6) and Taichong (LR3)

Technique: At the beginning, three to five moxa cones are applied respectively on Baihui (GV20), Ganshu (BL18), then the points on the affected side are punctured with filiform needles. The electric stimulator is connected to the filiform needles and the continuous wave used. Each treatment lasts 30 minutes and one course consists of 10 sessions.

[REMARKS]

1.   Acupuncture and moxibustion do achieve good results in treating wind stroke. If the treatment is given earlier, the therapeutic results can be improved. Patients with sequelae of wind stroke usually recover faster, within the first six months. But even patients with lengthy illness can gain some therapeutic effect if they can keep up the treatment.

2.   The patient who has hemiplegia should pay more attention to functional exercises of the limbs, maintaining pleasant emotions and regular bowel movements, all of which are favorable to recovery.

3.   To the patient with hemiplegia as well as hypertension, attention should be paid to stabilizing the blood pressure. Treatment with Chinese and Western medication should be combined. When the

blood pressure is too high, measures should be taken to prevent the aggravation of the disease and the relapse of wind stroke.

HYPERTENSION

[INTRODUCTION]

Hypertension is a chronic general vascular disease manifested clinically as an increase of arterial pressure, especially the constant increase of diastolic pressure. In the early stages, there is dizziness, headaches, palpitations, insomnia, tinnitus, restlessness, lassitude, hypomonesis, and even numbness of limbs. In the later stages, diseases of the brain, heart and kidney can be found. Hypertension can be divided into primary and secondary categories. This disease is commonly seen in people over 40 or who are engaged in work requiring high concentration for a long time. It is believed in traditional Chinese medicine that the causative factors of this disease are related to the constitutional excess and deficiency of *yin* and *yang*. It can be due to long-term depression and anger leading to prolonged *qi* stagnation turning into fire, which then consumes the liver *yin* and generates hyperactivity of the liver *yang*. It can also be caused by constitutional kidney *yin* deficiency depriving the liver of nourishment, which means the liver and kidney *yin* becomes deficient and liver *yang* becomes hyperactive. Equally, it can be caused by improper food intake such as excessive intake of greasy and highly flavored food generating endogenous turbid dampness, which then turns into phlegm and causes the excess retention of phlegm and dampness. The treatment principles are to pacify the liver and subdue liver *yang*, to nourish the kidney and soften the liver, and to eliminate dampness and resolve phlegm. It is supposed to choose points mainly from the Foot Jueyin meridian, Foot Shaoyin meridian, Yangming meridians of the Hand and Foot and Governor Vessel. Some examples are Baihui (GV20), Fengchi (GB20), Quchi (LI11), Hegu (LI4), Fenglong (ST40), Sanyinjiao (SP6), Taichong (LR3) and Taixi (KI3).

[CLINICAL EXPERIENCE]

1. CONVENTIONAL ACUPUNCTURE

(1) Pointing Technique

Points: Juegu (GB39) and Sanyinjiao (SP6)

Technique: Use 1.5-*cun* filiform needles to puncture Juegu (GB39) and Sanyinjiao (SP6) with the needles pointing toward each other, using points bilaterally in each treatment. Apply reinforcing needling technique for the deficiency syndrome and reducing needling technique for the excess syndrome. It is required to get the needling sensation spread around. The needles are retained for 15 minutes, with rotating manipulation every five minutes during needle retention. The treatment is conducted once a day and 10 sessions constitute one course. After the treatment is carried out, the blood pressure will be lowered and the subjective symptoms will disappear or improve.

(2) Needling Blood Pressure Regulation Line

Point: Blood pressure regulation line (on the horizontal line leveled with the ear lobe, at the junction of the anterior 1/3 and the middle 1/2 of the sternocleidomastoid muscle)

Technique: The perpendicular puncturing method is applied, the depth of insertion for adults usually being two or three cm. The rotating needling technique is applied in small amplitude two or three times. The needle rotation is performed once every five minutes, and the needling sensation should radiate to the same side of the head. The needles are removed after remaining in place for one to two hours. The treatment is conducted once a day, 10 sessions being one course. The acupuncture treatment is stopped for three to five days between courses of treatment.

(3) Needling Artery at Taiyuan (LU9)

Point: Taiyuan (LU9)

Technique: Use points bilaterally, inserting a one-*cun* filiform needle at the Cunkou region of the radial artery. No manipulation is required. It is enough when the needle handle is vibrating. If the needle handle does not shake, some adjustments can be made by lifting up the needle slightly. The needle is punctured on the wall of the radial artery, so it should not be pushed too deep. The needle is retained for five to 10 minutes. The blood pressure should decrease after the treatment is performed.

(4) Reducing Taichong (LR3)

Point: Taichong (LR3) (bilateral)

Technique: Apply the reducing needling technique achieved by lifting and thrusting. The method is applicable for hypertension accompanied by severe dizziness due to hyperactivity of liver *yang*.

(5) Reinforcing Zusanli (ST36)

Point: Zusanli (ST36) (bilateral)

Technique: The reinforcing needling technique achieved by lifting and thrusting is applied. The method is used for the patient with a weak constitution or a patient who has gastrointestinal diseases and hypertension.

(6) Renying (ST9) Puncture

Point: Renying (ST9)

Technique: Tell the patient to lie supine and keep the head low. First, the hand is used to grasp the neck. If the patient feels dizzy, it means that this method is not appropriate. The doctor uses the left hand to palpate and fix the artery at Renying (ST9) and uses the right hand to insert a 1.5-*cun* needle on the wall of the artery. The insertion should not be made too deep otherwise the artery might be pierced, causing a large hematoma. After the needle insertion is made, it is better to see that the needle handle is shaking, after which no other needling manipulation should be applied. The needle is removed 10 seconds afterwards, and retention should never exceed two minutes.

(7) Lowering Blood Pressure with Shimen (CV5)

Point: Shimen (CV5)

Technique: A 2-*cun* filiform needle is used to puncture Shimen (CV5). The method is applicable for the patient who has the excess of the Conception Vessel, chest and abdominal fullness and distention, or for the female patient who has amenorrhea and leukorrhea.

(8) Using Mainly Fengchi (GB20) and Quchi (LI11)

Points: Fengchi (GB20), Quchi (LI11), Baihui (GV20), Shangxing (GV23), Touwei (ST8), Tianzhu (BL10) and Taiyang (Ex-HN5)

Technique: After the above points are needled, the needling sensation should be obtained before the needles are retained for one hour. Other further needle manipulations are performed once every 10 minutes. The treatment is conducted once a day, but can be given twice a day for a patient whose condition is severe. Seven to 10 days of treatment will be one course, with a two to three day interval between courses. To most of the patients, after two or three treatments, their subjective symptoms, such as dizziness and headache, should be relieved. After one to two courses of treatment, some patients' blood pressure can be reduced to normal.

2. MOXIBUSTION

(1) Moxibustion with Moxa Cone
Point: Baihui (GV20)

Technique: Shave the hair in the area where Baihui (GV20) is located, and apply three moxa cones as big as grain on Baihui (GV20) one after the other. The moxibustion is carried out once a day and three times successively. If a blister forms, infection should be avoided. After the moxibustion treatment is performed, the dizziness will be relieved and the blood pressure will decrease.

(2) Scaring Moxibustion with Moxa Cone
Point: Zusanli (ST36) and Juegu (GB39)

Technique: Tell the patient to lie on the side or in a supine position. Sterilize points on one side with 75% alcohol, and before the alcohol evaporates, put the moxa cones (as big as grain) on the points and light them. Apply three to seven moxa cones on each point each time. The moxibustion is carried out until there are small blisters on the points. When the moxibustion is done, 2 cm^2 elastic plasters are applied topically on each point. The next visit is made one day later. If there are no sores, another moxibustion is applied on the same points until sores are formed. If there are already sores, the patient should be told to come back for more moxibustion after the sores have healed. This method was used in 20 patients with hypertension. The highest number of the moxibustion treatments was seven and the lowest was one, when the symptoms disappeared and the blood pressure became stable.

(3) *Warm Moxibustion with Moxa Stick*

Points: Qihai (CV6), Guanyuan (CV4) and Zusanli (ST36)

Technique: Light the moxa stick, applying the moxibustion on each point five to 10 minutes until the skin turns slightly red. This method is applicable for a patient whose hypertension is caused by *yang* deficiency.

3. CUPPING

Points: Points on the first lateral line of urinary bladder meridian on the back

Technique: Choose big and medium cups, applying 10 cups each time and leaving them on for 10 to 15 minutes.

4. BLEEDING THERAPY

Points: Taiyang (Ex-HN5) and Yangjiao (GB35)

Technique: Use a three-edged needle to prick Taiyang (Ex-HN5) and Yangjiao (GB35) bilaterally, letting out 5 to 6 drops of blood from each point. Up to 10 drops of blood can be let out to the patient who has a strong constitution and a severe headache. The treatment is conducted once a day and can achieve a quick effect in lowering the blood pressure.

5. CUTANEOUS PUNCTURE

Point: Jiaji (Ex-B2) points lateral to the spine (mainly the ones on the lumbosacral region), forehead, after-brain, superciliary arch, ends of four extremities, sole of palm and sole of foot

Technique: Tap the points lateral to the spine from up to down first, then tap points on the head and four extremities. A mild stimulation is given. The treatment is performed once every other day and 10 sessions form one course.

6. INTRA-DERMAL NEEDLING

Point: Geshu (BL17)

Technique: Embed two intra-dermal needles on Geshu (BL17) with one on each point. The needles are taken out after five to seven days of needle retention. One to two days rest is taken before the start of a new needle embedding treatment.

7. SCALP ACUPUNCTURE

Point: Yunting line, the upper 1/5 of the ganjue line the zuyungan line or the lower 2/5 of the yundong line. Combining the lower 2/5 of the ganjue line for migraine, and combining the xueguanshusuo line for cortical edema. Lines are used bilaterally.

Technique: Insert 1.5-*cun* filiform needles between the skin and the bone membrane to a depth of 1 *cun*, retaining the needles one to two hours. Usually, the treatment is carried out once every other day, seven sessions forming one course, with three to five days rest usually between two courses.

8. AURICULAR THERAPY

(1) Ear Acu-Pressure with Seeds

Points: Heart, Ear-shenmen, Adrenal, Endocrine, Liver, Kidney and Forehead

Technique: Put the vaccaria seeds on the points above, and press them three times a day. Seeds should be changed after five days.

(2) Bleeding the Groove for Lowering Blood Pressure

Technique: On the upper 1/3 of the back of the ear, there are veins visible. A three-edged needle is taken to prick the veins and the blood as big as a bean is let out.

9. HYDRO-ACUPUNCTURE

Points: Quchi (LI11), Zusanli (ST36) and Taichong (LR3)

Technique: Take 0.2 ml reserpine and 0.5% procaine adding up to 2 ml; inject the medicine into one point, changing the point alternately. The injection is conducted twice a week or once every other day.

10. MAGNETIC THERAPY

Points: Baihui (GV20), Fengchi (GB20), Taiyang (Ex-HN5), Quchi (LI11), Shenmen (HT7) and Taichong (LR3)

Technique: Take small magnetic pad of 500 to 2,000 gauss, putting the magnetic pads on two to four points each time. The treatment should last 20 to 30 minutes daily, and 10 sessions form one course. This method works well for the I and II stages of primary hypertension.

11. LASER THERAPY

Points: Renying (ST9), Quchi (LI11), and the groove to lower the blood pressure on the back of the ear

Technique: Apply laser irradiation emitted from a 6 watt helium neon laser irradiator on the points bilaterally, giving five minutes irradiation on each point. The treatment is performed once a day or once every other day, 10 to 15 sessions making up one course.

12. MEDICINAL APPLICATION ON ACU-POINT

Point: Yongquan (KI1)

Technique: Take 12 g peach kernels, 12 g apricot hernels, 3 g Cape jasmine, seven pieces of peppers, 14 pieces of sticky rice, pound the above medicine, and add egg white to prepare the medicine in a paste used for three applications. Every night, the medicine should be applied on Yongquan (KI1) before the patient goes to bed and should be removed next morning. The medicinal application is performed once a day and the application is performed on one foot each time. The medicine application should be conducted alternately on two feet and six applications form one course. This method can achieve a short-term remarkable effect in relieving hypertension.

[REMARKS]

1. Acupuncture and moxibustion can achieve a satisfactory result in treating hypertension. However, in some patients, the long-term effect is not stable. When the clinical symptoms are relieved or disappear, and the blood pressure is lowered, the treatment can be given once every three to five days. A satisfactory long-term effect will be obtained.

2. To a patient who has hypertension for a long time, when the acupuncture and moxibustion treatment is not satisfactory, a small

amount of hypo tensor can be combined in the treatment to improve the therapeutic result.

3.   This disease relates closely to the emotions and diet. At usual times, attention should be paid to keeping a good mood and the patient should take food low in salt and fat and containing low cholesterol.

WEI SYNDROME

[INTRODUCTION]

Wei syndrome refers to the disease manifesting itself as the flaccidity and weakness of limbs, muscular atrophy and the inability to move freely. The disease can be found in all four extremities, especially the lower ones. The disease is usually due to the lung being burnt by heat leading to the consumption of body fluids; or it is caused by the invasion of meridians and collaterals by pathogenic damp heat; or it is induced by the liver and kidney deficiency. It can happen after a traumatic injury that deprives the tendons and meridians of nourishment, which then leads to muscular flaccidity. The treatment principles are to soothe the meridians and collaterals and to nourish the tendons and vessels. The points are selected according to the location of the disease and the points are also chosen according to the differentiation. To treat the diseases of the upper extremities, Jianyu (LI15), Jianliao (TE14), Binao (LI14), Waiguan (TE5), Zhongzhu (TE3), Quchi (LI11) and Hegu (LI4) should be used. To treat diseases of the lower extremities, Huantiao (GB30), Zhibian (BL54), Fengshi (GB30), Yanglingquan (GB34), Weizhong (BL40), Zusanli (ST36) and Jiexi (ST41) should be applied. In the case of the consumption of body fluid by the heat in the lung, Feishu (BL13) and Chize (LR5) should be selected; in the case of the invasion of pathogenic damp heat, Pishu (BL20), Yinlingquan (SP9) and Neiting (ST41) are combined; in the case of the deficiency of the liver and kidney, Ganshu (BL18), Shenshu (BL23), Sanyinjiao (SP6) and Taixi (KI3) should be added. This disease can be found in acute myelitis, progressive myatrophy, myasthenia gravis, multiple neuritis, hysterical paralysis or traumatic paraplegia.

[CLINICAL EXPERIENCE]

1. CONVENTIONAL ACUPUNCTURE

(1) Selecting Points of Governor Vessel

Points: Baihui (GV20), Fengfu (GV16), Dazhui (GV14), Taodao (GV13), Shenzhu (GV12), Shendao (GV11), Zhiyang (GV9), Jinsuo (GV8), Jizhong (GV6), Xuanshu (GV5), Mingmen (GV4), Yangguan (GV3) and Changqiang (GV1)

Technique: Tell the patient to lie supine. Use 1 to 1.5 *cun* needles to puncture the above points, manipulating the needle until the arrival of *qi*, and retaining them for 30 minutes. This method can open the governor vessel and regulate the flow of *qi* in it. It can nourish the marrow and strengthen the brain and is applicable for paraplegia.

(2) Mainly Choosing Points of Conception Vessel

Points: Juque (CV14), Zhongwan (CV12), Xiawan (CV10), Qihai (CV6), Guanyuan (GV4), Zhongji (CV3), Liangmen (ST21), Tianshu (ST25), Shuidao (ST28) and Zhangmen (LR14)

Technique: With the patient lying supine, perform the standard needling manipulation, retaining the needles for 30 minutes after the arrival of *qi*. This method is mainly used to nourish *yin* and foster the foundation of the body. When paraplegia is treated, these points are used alternately with the points of the governor vessels. The treatment is given once a day and 20 sessions form one course.

(3) Selecting Jiaji (Ex-B2) Points

Points: Starting from the second thoracic vertebrae to the fourth lumbar vertebrae, 0.5 *cun* lateral to the lower border of each vertebrae. There are altogether 16 points on the left and right sides.

Technique: With the patient lying prone, needle the points perpendicularly, and turn the needle tip slightly toward to vertebra. Insert the needle to a depth of 1 *cun* when the points located above the 2nd lumbar vertebra are punctured, or 1.5 to 2 *cun* when the points located below the 2nd lumbar vertebra are punctured. The method activates blood flow and removes stagnation. It is mostly applied for traumatic paraplegia.

(4) Selecting Back-shu Points

Points: Xinshu (BL15), Feishu (BL13), Ganshu (BL18), Pishu (BL20), Shenshu (BL23) and Geshu (BL17)

Technique: Ask the patient to adopt a sitting posture. Use one-*cun* needles to puncture the points perpendicularly to a depth of 0.5 *cun*. The method can regulate the functions of the zangfu organs and promote the recovery of paraplegic limbs. The method is applied in the later stage of the disease, and is combined with the local points. The treatment is given once a day.

(5) Choosing Points of Stomach Meridian as the Main Points

Points: Qichong (ST30), Biguan (ST31), Futu (ST32), Dubi (ST35), Zusanli (ST36), Shangjuxu (ST37), Xiajuxu (ST39), Jiexi (ST41), Xiangu (ST43), Sanyinjiao (SP6) and Neiting (ST44)

Technique: With the patient in a supine position, needle the points according to the routine method, retaining the needles for 30 minutes after the arrival of *qi*. This method is used mainly to regulate the stomach meridian of Foot Yangming, and it helps nourish the blood and tendons. The method is used to treat any types of paraplegia.

(6) Choosing Nine Points on Cross-section

Points: Point of the governor vessel as well as Jiaji (Ex-B2) points that are level with the spinous process right above the plane of the injured spinal cord; point of the governor vessel and Jiaji (Ex-B2) points level with the spinous process of the 5th lumbar vertebra; and points of the governor vessel and Jiaji (Ex-B2) points level with the mid-point of the damaged vertebra and the 5th lumbar vertebra. There are all together nine points in the upper and lower parts.

Technique: Use 1 or 1.5 *cun* filiform needles to puncture the points to a depth of 1 *cun*. The needling sensation is expected to go downward. The treatment is given once a day, 10 sessions to one course. Points on the affected limbs can also be combined.

2. THICK-NEEDLE PUNCTURE

Points: Penetrating from Dazhui (GV14) to Shenzhu (GV12) and from Shendao (GV11) to Zhiyang (GV9). In the case of diseases of the upper extremity, Shousanli (LI10), Neiguan (PC6) and Hegu (LI4) are combined; in the case of diseases of the lower extremity, Huantiao (GB30), Yinmen (BL37) and Chengshan (BL57) are combined.

Technique: Use the specially prepared thick needle with a diameter of 0.8 mm to penetrate from Dazhui (GV14) to Shenzhu (GV12) and from Shendao (GV11) to Zhiyang (GV9), retaining the needle for two hours. The rest points are punctured with the thick needle whose diameter is 0.45 mm. Strong stimulation is applied and no needle retention is required. This method is applicable in the case of gelinbali syndrome.

3. ELECTRIC ACUPUNCTURE

Points: Main points: Points located at one or two spinous processes above and below the plane of the affected spinal cord. Combination of points: ① Guanyuan (CV4), Zhongji (CV3) and Tianshu (ST25). ② Shenshu (BL23), Dachangshu (BL25), Yinmen (BL37), Weizhong (BL40) and Qunlun (BL60) ③ Biguan (ST31), Futu (ST32), Chongyang (ST42), Zusanli (ST36), Juegu (GB39) and Yanglingquan (GB34)

Technique: The main points must be used each time. The combined points can be applied according to the condition of the disease. Points in group ① are applicable in the case of the dysfunction in defecation and urination. Points in group ② and points in group ③ can be used alternately. In each treatment, electric stimulation can be applied on four to six points, on either the main points or the combined points. A continuous wave of low frequency is used. The treatment is given once a day or once every other day. Twenty sessions make up one course. This method is applied to treat traumatic paraplegia.

4. HYDRO-ACUPUNCTURE

(1) Danshen Injection Fluid

Points: Shenshu (BL23), Xuehai (SP10), Zusanli (ST36), Yanglingquan (GB34), Chengshan (BL57) and Sanyinjiao (SP6)

Technique: Take the *danshen* (the root of red-rooted salvia) injection fluid, choose three points each time, and inject 0.5 to 1 ml injection fluid into each point once every other day.

(2) Vitamin B Injection Fluid

Points: Mingmen (GV4), Yaoyangguan (GV3), Jiaji (Ex-B2) points on the lumbar region, Huantiao (GB30), Yinmen (BL37), Weizhong (BL40), Zusanli (ST36), Yanglingquan (GB34) and Juegu (GB39)

Technique: Inject 4 ml vitamin B_1 as well as 4 ml vitamin B_{12} injection fluid into Mingmen (GV4), Yaoyangguan (GV3) and Jiaji (Ex-B2) points on the lumbar region, injecting 0.5 to 1 ml into each point. On other points, the filiform needles are used in the treatment. Strong stimulation is used and no retention of the needle is required. The treatment is conducted once a day and 10 sessions form one course. This method is used to treat transverse myelitis.

(3) Galanthamine Injection Fluid

Points: Zusanli (ST36), Yanglingquan (GB34), Xuanzhong (GB39) and Yangfu (GB38)

Technique: Choose two points each time, taking 1 g galanthamine and injecting it into the point slowly. This treatment is conducted once every other day and 10 sessions form one course. The interval between the courses of the treatment is one week. This method treats the paralysis of the common peroneal nerve.

5. POINT CATGUT-EMBEDDING AND LIGATURE

Points: Shenshu (BL23) and local atrophic muscle

Technique: Use 0.5 cm catgut, thread the catgut through the sewing needle, and perform the embedding by rectilinear puncture or perform triangular or circular ligature. The treatment is conducted once every 15 days, and one to two points are used each time. It is applicable to treat poliomyelitis.

6. PLUM-BLOSSOM THERAPY

Points: Jiaji (Ex-B2) points and points of Governor Vessel located below the affected area, points of Hand and Foot Yangming meridians.

Technique: Tap the points once a day, tapping each meridian for 10 minutes each time. Ten sessions of treatment form one course.

7. ACUPUNCTURE COMBINED WITH PYSCHOLOGICAL TREATMENT

Point: Yongquan (KI1)

Technique: Psychological work should precede the acupuncture treatment. When the patient has the confidence to cure his disease, the doctor should take the thick needle of Size 26 and insert it quickly into the right and the left Yongquan (KI1). Needle manipulation achieved by rotating, lifting and thrusting is applied. After the arrival of *qi*, the patient should be told to move the limbs, and during this period, verbal suggestions are given to the patient. This method is applicable for hysteric paraplegia.

[REMARKS]
1. The increase of the functional exercises can promote recovery.
2. To the patient who has been in bed for a long time, massage of the muscles performed with the application of 5% safflower oil can improve the *qi* and blood circulation and can prevent the occurrence of bed sores.

BI SYNDROME

[INTRODUCTION]
When *yin* and *yang* of the body are in imbalance, and the striae of skin and muscles are deficient, the pathogenic wind, cold and damp will invade the meridians and collaterals, Then, *qi* and blood circulation are blocked and cannot flow freely. It results in pain, numbness and motor impairment in the limbs and joints, with perhaps swelling and deformity of the joints. The condition described above is known as Bi syndrome. In clinical practice, when the pathogenic wind is predominant, the condition is known as the wandering Bi syndrome and

is characterized by migrating pain in joints. When the pathogenic cold is predominant, the condition is known as painful Bi syndrome and is characterized by a severe pain alleviated by warmth but aggravated by cold. When the pathogenic damp is predominant, the condition is termed as fixed Bi syndrome, and is characterized by localized pain, heaviness of limbs and numbness of the skin. Apart from these symptoms, to one with a constitutionally excessive *yang qi*, after the pathogenic wind cold damp invades, the pathogens follow the heat transformation. If heat is accumulating in the meridians and collaterals, there is heat Bi syndrome characterized by redness, swelling, hotness and joint pain. The treatment principles are to eliminate wind and dampness, and warm up the meridians to dispel cold, or the principles are to clear away heat and damp and open the meridians and collaterals. It is supposed to combine points selected locally, points chosen along the running course of the meridian and points selected on the basis of differentiation. The local points applied may be Jianyu (LI15), Jianliao (TE14), Quchi (LI11), Chize (LU5), Waiguan (TE5), Hegu (LI4), Huantiao (GB30), Yanglingquan (GB34), Dubi (ST35), Xiyangguan (GB33), Shenmai (BL62), Jiexi (ST41) and Taixi (KI3). In the case of the wandering Bi syndrome, Geshu (BL17) and Xuehai (SP10) are added; in the case of the painful Bi syndrome, Shenshu (BL23) and Guanyuan (CV4) are added; in the case of the heat Bi syndrome, Dazhui (GV14) and Quchi (LI11) are added. The reducing needling technique should be used more in the treatment. Moxibustion should be combined in the cases of painful and fixed Bi syndromes. This syndrome is similar to the rheumatic arthritis, the rheumatic myelitis, rheumatoid arthritis and osteoarthrosis deformans endemica.

[CLINICAL EXPERIENCE]

1. CONVENTIONAL ACUPUNCTURE

(1) Using Five Needles on the Knee

Points: Heding, Neixiyan, Waixiyan, Liangqiu (ST34) and Xuehai (SP10)

Technique: Use 1.5-*cun* filiform needles to puncture the points, retaining the needles for 30 minutes after the arrival of *qi*. This method treats various types of the knee pain. The warming needling technique is combined to relieve cold damp Bi syndrome.

(2) Using Four Elbow Points

Points: Zhouliao (LI12), Quchi (LI11), Shousanli (LI10) and Zhoujian

Technique: Use 1.5-*cun* filiform needles, retaining them for 30 minutes after the arrival of *qi*. The treatment is indicated by pain in the elbow joint. Moxibustion is used in the condition caused by cold damp.

(3) Selecting Points of Governor Vessels on Vertex

Points: Qianding (GV21) and Houding (GV19)

Technique: Use Qianding (GV21) for the pain in the upper extremities, and Houding (GV19) for that in the lower extremities. Tell the patient to take either a sitting or prone posture. Insert a 1.5-*cun* needle into the points along the skin obliquely toward the back, performing rotating needling manipulation after the arrival of *qi*. Massage the head of the patient with the left thumb while pressing the needle body with other fingers, and asking the patient to move the affected limbs. Usually after the needles are retained and rotated for 20 minutes, most of the pain can be relieved.

(4) Selecting Points Along Meridians from the Two Ends

Points: Tongziliao (GB1) and Zuqiaoyin (GB44)

Technique: Needle the above points with one-*cun* filiform needles. Apply the reducing needling technique achieved by rotation. The method treats mainly pain along the mid-line of the lateral side of the unilateral leg below the knee.

(5) Selecting Knee Disorder Points

Point: Xiji [medial Xiji point is 1 *cun* superior and 0.5 *cun* posterior to Xuehai (SP10); lateral Xiji point is 1 *cun* superior and 0.5 *cun* posterior to Liangqiu (ST34)]

Technique: Tenderness points can be found on the medial and lateral Xiji points, and both points are treated. This method is applied mainly for knee pain.

(6) Choosing Lower Points for Upper Disorder

Point: Fengchi (GB20)

Technique: The treatment is used mainly for pain in the heel, including calcaneeous spur, calcaneeous bursitis, Achilles tendonitis, fracture of the calcaneus and symptomatic painful heels. Choose the unilateral Fengchi (GB20), and use a 1.5-*cun* filiform needle of Size 28 to puncture the point. Needle the point to a depth of 0.5 to 1 *cun* with the needle tip pointing toward the contra lateral mouth corner, rotating the needle five to 10 times after the arrival of *qi*. The needle is retained for 50 minutes, and manipulation should be repeated once every 10 minutes. This treatment was performed on 216 patients, with an effective rate of 92.1%.

(7) Combining Distal and Local Points

Points: Tianzhu (BL10), Daling (PC7) and Houxi (SI3)

Technique: It is indicated in painful heels. First of all, use Tianzhu (BL10) on the back of the neck bilaterally, and insert the needle to a depth of 0.8 to 1 *cun* to obtain the arrival of *qi*, before applying the reinforcing technique achieved by lifting and thrusting. Afterwards, needle Houxi (Si3) bilaterally, and puncture points with a quick needle insertion to a depth of 1 *cun*, gain the arrival of *qi* before applying the reducing technique achieved by lifting and thrusting. Finally, needle Daling (PC7) bilaterally to a depth of 0.3 to 0.5 *cun*, gain the arrival of *qi* and then perform the even needling technique achieved by rotation. The patient is told to move the affected limb once every five minutes. The needles are retained for 40 to 60 minutes. This treatment is given once every other day while 10 sessions constitute one course.

(8) Technique of Setting Mountain on Fire

Points: Jianyu (LI15), Quchi (LI11), Zusanli (ST36) and Sanyinjiao (SP6)

Technique: The technique of setting the mountain on fire is applied to needle Jianyu (LI15) and Quchi (LI11). Quchi (LI11) of the diseased side should be needled first. When the heat sensation gained in the point reaches the shoulder, other points can be needled. This method is used in the case of pain in the shoulder and arm that is classified as fixed Bi syndrome.

2. MOXIBUSTION

(1) Warming Needling Technique

Points: Local points on the painful area

Technique: Based on the size of the pain area, three to five points should be needled first, then the moxa stick as long as 1 *cun* is put on the needle handle. Two pieces of the moxa stick are applied on each point.

(2) Moxibustion with Moxa Box

Points: Ah-shi points

Technique: The wooden moxa box is placed over the pain area, and two pieces of moxa stick are put inside. Moxibustion can be carried out when the moxa sticks are lit. This treatment is carried out once a day.

(3) Indirect Moxibustion with Ginger

Point: Pain area

Technique: Cut fresh ginger into slices to a thickness of 0.3 to 0.5 cm. Use the needle to puncture several holes in the middle of the slices, shape the moxa wool into a cone and put the moxa cone on the ginger slice. Five to eight moxa cones are applied each time. When the moxibustion is over, the ginger slices are used to rub the affected region. The treatment is conducted one to two times a day.

(4) Moxibustion with Jingfang Steaming

Point: Local affected region

Technique: Put 30 g Jingjie (*Schizonepeta tenuifolia*), 30 g Fangfeng (*Saposhikovia divaricata*), 30 g Aiye (*folium artemisiae argyi*) and 30 g garlic (without peel) into a basin, add water and boil the mixture. The patient is told to steam the affected region over the basin for one to two hours. When the steaming is finished, a dry towel is used to wipe and clean the affected region and the towel is also used to prevent the affected region from being affected by cold. This steaming is conducted once daily and five sessions form one course. The interval between the courses is three days.

(5) Indirect Moxibustion with Salt

Point: Shenque (CV8)

Technique: Fill the entire umbilicus with fine salt and place a moxa cone as big as a soybean on it. Five to eight moxa cones are applied each time. Moxibustion is carried out once every other day. Five sessions make up one course. The interval between two courses is three to five days. This treatment is indicated for cold, damp Bi syndrome. It can also be combined with acupuncture treatment performed on some local points.

(6) Long Snake Moxibustion

Point: The midline of the spine

Technique: The patient lies prone with the back exposed. Perform standard sterilization of the spine and apply the garlic juice. Spread 1.5 g Banshe powder on the midline of the spine (the powder is composed of 50% musk, 20% Chinese blister beetle powder and 15% lilac powder and 15% Chinese cassia tree), and put the garlic smash in 2 *cun* width, 0.5 *cun* thickness on the governor vessel from Dazhui (GV14) to Yaoshu (GV2). Afterwards, apply moxa cones tracing the shape of the spine on the garlic smash, and light up the head, body and tail of line, letting it burn naturally. When the moxa cones are burnt out, another long snake moxibustion is applied. It is better to use two or three lines of cones in general. When the moxibustion is done, the garlic smash can be removed. If blisters occur, take measures to prevent infection. Three days later, a sterilized needle is used to drain out the fluid from the blister, which is then wiped off with medicinal cotton. Gentian violet is then used; a sterilized gauze is taken to cover the blister and an elastic bandage is used to fix the gauze in place until the scab scales off. This method is applicable for rheumatoid arthritis, spinal hyperosteogeny and overstrain of the lumbar muscles.

3. CUPPING

Points: Affected region and points of the diseased meridians

Technique: Moving cupping is applied for joint pain in the spine and back. Flash cupping is used for acute joint pain. Bleeding or cupping is applicable for a local sprain with blood stasis.

4. ELECTRIC ACUPUNCTURE

Points: ① Xiyan, Heding, Yangguan (GB33), Ququan (LR8) and Weizhong (BL40) ② Liangqiu (ST34), Xuehai (SP10), Yinlingquan

(SP9) and Yanglingquan (GB34) ③ Zusanli (ST36), Sanyinjiao (SP6), Kunlun (BL60) and Zhaohai (KI6)

Technique: Choose one to three points from each group each time, and conduct treatment once every other day, using points alternately. Using a size 28 filiform needle to needle the point to a depth of 1 to 1.5 *cun*, with strong stimulation. The electric stimulator is connected to the needles. Dense and dispersed waves are used in the treatment, which should last 20 to 30 minutes. The intensity of the stimulation should be adjusted to the patient's level of tolerance.

5. ELECTRO-STIMULATION THERAPY

Points: Tenderness points symmetrical to the diseased area

Technique: Each pair of electrodes should be connected to the symmetrical tenderness points, and fairly strong electric stimulation applied. Each stimulation should last 10 to 20 seconds, this intermittent treatment lasting 20 minutes.

6. INTRA-DERMAL NEEDLING

Points: Ah-shi points

Technique: Based on the pain area, two to five intra-dermal needles are embedded each time. These needles are fixed with elastic tape and should be changed every three to five days.

7. PRICKING THERAPY

Points: ① Local points ② Distal points (searching for the distal tenderness points from the affected meridians)

Technique: To the patient whose condition is acute, or whose symptoms are obvious, the treatment is given once daily and one to four points are pricked each time. This should relieve the pain. If the patient's condition is chronic, or the diseased area is large, two to four points are pricked every day or every other day, 10 sessions making up one course.

8. HYDRO-ACUPUNCTURE

(1) Danggui Injection

Points: Tenderness points or the starting and the ending parts of the painful muscle

Technique: Inject 0.5 to 1 ml Danggui injection fluid into each point, choosing two or three points each time. The injection is performed once every other day, and 10 sessions constitute one course.

(2) Weilingxian Injection

Points: Fengchi (GB20), Geshu (BL17), Quchi (LI11), Xuehai (SP10) and Zusanli (ST36)

Technique: Four ml of Weilingxian injection fluid is injected into the above points every day or once every other day. Ten sessions form one course, the second course of treatment starting after a break of three to five days. This method treats rheumatoid arthritis.

9. LASER THERAPY

Point: Hegu (LI4), Quchi (LI11) and Jianyu (LI15) are applied for pain in the upper limb; and Shenshu (BL23) and Mingmen (GV4) are applied for pain in the lumbar region. For pain in the lower limb, Huantiao (GB30), Zhibian (BL54), Xiyan, Dubi (ST35) and other local points can be combined as well.

Technique: Two or three points are selected in general, and 10-minute laser irradiation is applied on each point each time. The treatment is performed once a day using a helium-neon laser. Ten sessions form one course and the interval between courses should be seven to 10 days.

10. COMBINED TREATMENT

(1) Bleeding and Cupping Therapy

Point: Affected region

Technique: A three-edged needle is used to prick the swollen joint to cause bleeding, followed by cupping. The method can eliminate heat, relieve swelling and pain, and is good for rheumatoid arthritis.

(2) Acupuncture Combined with Medicinal Steaming and Washing

Points: Dazhui (GV14), Dazhu (BL11), Yanglingquan (GB34), Shenshu (BL23) and points on the affected area.

Technique: Both acupuncture and moxibustion should be used on the affected region, other points are only punctured with filiform needles. The even needling technique should be applied and the needles should be retained for 30 minutes. This treatment can be performed once daily. Fupian, Rougui (Chinese cassia tree), Danggui (Chinese angelica), Qianghuo (notopterygium), Duhuo, Xixin (the root of Chinese wild ginger), Jixueteng (reticulate millettia), Tougucao, Honghua (safflower), Ruxiang (frankincense), Aiye (Chinese mugwort) are decocted, and the medicinal water is used to wash and steam the painful joints.

[REMARKS]

1. Acupuncture can achieve a remarkable effect to relieve pain occurring in Bi syndrome. A patient with a chronic Bi syndrome should keep receiving the treatment.

2. A patient with cold damp Bi syndrome should be careful to stay away from wind cold. The patient should live in a dry and warm place, keep the affected area warm, a cotton or medicinal cushion used to wrap the affected region.

FACIAL PARALYSIS

[INTRODUCTION]

This disease refers to peripheral facial paralysis. The chief clinical manifestations are the deviation of the mouth and eye, paralysis of the facial mimetic muscle of the affected side, incomplete closure of the eye, lacrimation, disappearance of the nasolabial sulcus, ptosis of the labial angle, salivation, inability to raise the eyebrow, frown, show the teeth or to whistle, and hold food in the mouth. Some patients feel pain below the ear or in the mastoid process. This disease occurs suddenly, and the paralysis appears mostly on one side. It can be found in patients of any age, but more in patients between the ages of 20 to 40. Traditional Chinese medicine believes that the disease appears mostly because the pathogenic wind cold taking advantage of the weakness of the meridians and collaterals to invade the facial meridians and collaterals. The pathogens obstruct the meridian *qi*, deprive the meridians and collaterals of nourishment so that muscles can no longer contract. The treatment principles are to warm the meridians and dispel cold, eliminate wind and promote circulation in the collaterals. The points are mainly taken from the Hand and Foot Yangming meridians, while points of the Hand and Foot Taiyang (Ex-HN5) and Shaoyang meridians are taken as the supplementary ones. Examples are Fengchi (GB20), Yangbai (GB14), Zanzhu (BL2), Sibai (ST2), Dicang (ST4), Jiache (ST6), Yifeng (TE17), Xiaguan (ST7), Hegu (LI4) and Zusanli (ST36). Both acupuncture and moxibustion are used and the penetrating puncture is applied more in acupuncture treatment.

[CLINICAL EXPERIENCE]

1. CONVENTIONAL ACUPUNCTURE

(1) Contralateral Puncture

Points: Yangbai (GB14), Sibai (ST2), Dicang (ST4), Hegu (LI4) and Neiting (ST44)

Technique: On the basis of the disease's location, use the right points for the left disease and the left points for the right disease. Take a 1.5-*cun* filiform needle to puncture Sibai (ST2), or needle the point transversely from up to down, performing the penetration from Yangbai (GB14) to Yuyao, and from Dicang (ST4) to Jiache (ST6). It is better to apply even needling technique with a moderate stimulation, conducting the treatment once a day or once every other day, retaining the needles for 30 minutes each time. Ten sessions form one course, while the interval between courses of treatment is two to four days. This method is applied mainly in the middle or later stages of the disease.

(2) Puncturing More Points But Shallowly

Points: Zanzhu (BL2), Yangbai (GB14), Sizhukong (TE23), Yuyao, Taiyang (Ex-HN5), Sibai (ST2), Shangyingxiang, Juliao (ST3), Renzhong (GV26), Heliao (LI19), Dicang (ST4), Jiachengjiang, Jiache (ST6), Xiaguan (ST7), Touwei (ST8), Fengchi (GB20) (all on the affected side), Hegu (LI4) and Zusanli (ST36) (on both sides)

Technique: Use one-*cun* filiform needles (Size No.30) to puncture points shallowly to a depth of 0.2 to 0.3 *cun*. Use a one-*cun* filiform needle to puncture Fengchi (GB20) 0.5 to 0.6 *cun* deep with the needle tip pointing to the opposite eye corner. Puncture Hegu (LI4), Zusanli (ST36) perpendicularly about 1 *cun* deep, and perform the reinforcing needling technique after obtaining the arrival of *qi*, retaining the needles for 30 minutes. Ten sessions of treatment form one course.

(3) Puncturing Less Points But Deeply

Points: Jiuzheng (at the ulnar end of the metacarpophalangeal crease of the small finger, at the margin of the red and white skin), and Zusanli (ST36)

Technique: Use a two-*cun* filiform needle to puncture Jiuzheng (Ex) of the affected side deeply to Hegu (LI4). Use two-*cun* filiform needles to puncture Zusanli (ST36) deeply and bilaterally. The treatment is conducted once a day and 10 sessions make up one course.

(4) Selecting Miantan Point

Points: Shangmiantan [0.5 *cun* lateral to Taiyang (Ex-HN5)], Xiamiantan [0.5 *cun* below the middle point of the line connecting Dicang (ST4) and Jiache (ST6)]

Technique: Use a two-*cun* filiform needle to puncture Shangmiantan to a depth of 1.8 *cun*, with the needle tip pointing to Xiamiantan, when using a two-*cun* filiform needle to puncture Xiamiantan, pointing the needle toward Shangmiantan. Point needles toward each other, and manipulate them simultaneously, retaining them for 30 minutes. This method is quite effective to relieve facial paralysis.

2. MOXIBUSTION

(1) Warming Needling Technique

Points: Fengchi (GB20), Yangbai (GB14), Taiyang (Ex-HN5), Quanliao (SI18), Yifeng (TE17), Xiaguan (ST7), Dicang (ST4) and Jiache (ST6)

Technique: When the arrival of *qi* is obtained after needling, the warming needling technique is applied on Xiaguan (ST7), Yifeng (TE17) and Fengchi (GB20). Moxibustion is performed 20 minutes each time. The treatment is conducted once daily and 10 sessions form one course.

(2) Moxibustion with Reed Tube

Point: External auditory canal of the affected side

Technique: Take a piece of reed tube whose two ends are open (as thick as the shaft of a writing brush), and put one end into the ear. Prepare a semicircular metal pad and insert it into the other end of the reed tube. Place the big moxa cone on the reed tube, and light the moxa cone to make smoke and allow the hot air to enter the ear. Three to five moxa cones are applied each time and the treatment is performed once daily.

3. FLASH CUPPING

Point: Affected face

Technique: Use a medium-sized glass cup to perform flash cupping on the affected face until the skin in the area turns lightly red. Make sure the skin is not burnt. The treatment is conducted once daily, 10 minutes each time, and 10 sessions form one course.

4. BLEEDING THERAPY

Points: Taiyang (Ex-HN5), Xiaguan (ST7), Yangbai (GB14), Dicang (ST4) and all of the affected side

Technique: Prick the points with a three edged needle to let out a small amount of blood, using 2 points each time. Give the treatment once a day or once every other day.

5. ORAL CAVITY BLEEDING THERAPY

Point: Mouth mucous membrane

Technique: Perform regular sterilization, then take a three-edged needle to puncture the mouth mucous membrane of the affected side to cause bleeding. Let the blood flow out by itself. The mouth should not be rinsed to prevent infection. The bleeding therapy can be performed once a week.

6. CUTANEOUS PUNCTURE

Points: Affected forehead, cheek, Yifeng (TE17), Fengchi (GB20) and regions around the eye

Technique: Tap the above points gently to cause a slight bleeding, or apply cupping with small cups 5 to 10 minutes. Give the treatment once every other day. This method is applicable to patient who has such facial sequelae as the facial stiffness.

7. HYDRO-ACUPUNCTURE

Points: Fengchi (GB20), Qianzheng, Zusanli (ST36) and Shangjuxu (ST37)

Technique: Take 100 mg Vitamin B_1 and 0.1 mg Vitamin B_{12}, or use Danggui (Chinese angelica) injection fluid at the same time, injecting the injection fluid into the above points, one to two ml for each point. The injection treatment is conducted once a day or once every other day, the points being used alternately.

8. CATGUT–EMBEDDING METHOD

Points: Point 0.5 *cun* below the ear lobe to Jiache (ST6), Sibai (ST4) to Quanliao (SI18), Dicang (ST4) to Sanxiao (lateral inferior to Yingxiang (LI20), at the middle point of the nasal labial groove), Yangbai (GB14) to Touguangming (0.3 *cun* right above Yuyao). Other distal points can be combined, such as Hegu (LI4), Lieque (LU7), Xuehai (SP10) and Zusanli (ST36).

Technique: According to the location of the paralysis, choose one pair of points close to the diseased region alternately. Embed the thin catgut in the point, using one to two distal points each time. This treatment is applied to the patient whose disease has lasted a long time.

9. LASER THERAPY

Points: Yangbai (GB14), Sibai (ST2), Xiaguan (ST7), Jiache (ST6), Dicang (ST4) of the affected side and Hegu (LI4) of the healthy side

Technique: Use a Helium Neon Laser Stimulator of low power to radiate the above points, keeping the laser beam 0.2 to 0.5 cm away from the points. The size of the light spot is 0.1 to 0.2 cm^2 and the laser light should penetrate the tissue as deep as 10 to 15 mm. Laser irradiation is applied on each point for five minutes, each irradiation treatment lasting 30 minutes. The treatment is given once every other day and 12 sessions form one course.

10. MEDICINAL APPLICATION AND MOXIBUSTION ON ACU-POINT

(1) Steaming with Badou

Point: Laogong (PC8)

Technique: Take four to eight pieces of peeled Badou, dip them into 250 g of 50° white spirit, and then boil the mixture over a fire. Pour the white spirit into a small-mouthed bottle. Steam Laogong (PC8) of the healthy and affected side for 20 minutes while the white spirit is hot. The treatment is carried out once daily and 10 sessions make up one course. During the treatment, there will be slight diarrhea or local desquamation.

(2) Moxibustion with Maqianzi Application

Points: Points on the affected face

Technique: Grind certain amount of Maqianzi into fine powder and store it in a bottle for use. When moxibustion is applied, 0.2 g of the medicinal powder (the amount of powder applied on each point) is taken. Spread the powder in the middle of Xiaoyanzhentong Paste (plaster for diminishing inflammation and relieving pain), and apply the paste on the points of the affected side. Each application is kept for five days. Another application is performed two days after the previous application is removed.

11. COMBINED TREATMENT

Points: Fengchi (GB20), Yifeng (TE17), Yangbai (GB14), Taiyang (Ex-HN5), Yingxiang (LI20), Quanliao (SI18), Dicang (ST4), Jiache (ST6) and Hegu (LI4)

Technique: The disease is divided into three stages according to its course. At the initial stage (first one to two weeks of the disease), heavy moxibustion treatment is applied on the affected face and either the warming needle technique or reed tube moxibustion is applied for 40 minutes each time every day. In the middle stages (from the 3rd to the 7th week), penetrating puncture is mainly applied on the affected side, moxibustion is combined as well, and a penetrating puncture is performed from Jiache (ST6) to Dicang (ST4), from Dicang (ST4) to Quanliao (SI18) and from Quanliao (SI18) to Yingxiang (LI20). In the later stages (from the 8th to the 12th week), both acupuncture and moxibustion are applied on points of the affected side, and the points of the healthy side are punctured, too. The treatment is performed once daily and 12 sessions form one course. The patient should take two or three days rest during the courses of treatment.

[REMARKS]

1. Acupuncture and moxibustion can achieve a satisfactory result in treating this disease, but the key point of the treatment is to conduct it as early as possible. If timely and adequate treatment can be given, the recovery rate can be higher than 85%. Though the duration of the disease is different, the patient can recover in 10 days if the case is mild, but may not recover if the disease lasts longer than six months. For a few patients, there can be perverse facial paralysis which means the corner of the mouth deviates to the affected side, and some patients may suffer the sequelae of the facial spasm.

2. While both the acupuncture and moxibustion treatments are used, the patient should be told not to wash the face with cold water, and should wear a large gauze mask when he goes out to prevent a fresh attack of the facial meridians and collaterals by wind cold.

3. Massage can be combined to improve the therapeutic effect. Every morning and night, the patient should rub the hands to make them warm, then massage the face repeatedly so that the blood circulation can be improved.

FACIAL SPASM

[INTRODUCTION]

Tiredness, mental stress or autonomous movement aggravates a facial spasm. However, it stops after sleep. This disease mostly happens to the middle-aged people and more to female patients. It occurs mainly on one side of the face, and only a few patients get it on both sides. The reasons include obstruction of the facial meridians and collaterals due to invasion of the exogenous pathogenic wind and cold when the body constitution is weak; disturbance of the clear orifice by the stirred up endogenous wind, which is transformed from liver *yang* since *yin* is deficient and *yang* becomes hyperactive; and malnourishment of the facial muscles due to *yin* blood deficiency caused by overstrain and stress. The treatment principle is to eliminate wind and nourish the meridians and tendons. Points are mainly chosen from Yangming meridians, such as Sibai (ST2), Quanliao (SI18), Xiaguan (ST7), Dicang (ST4), Jiache (ST6), Ah-shi points, Hegu (LI4) and Taichong (LR3). Even needling technique is applied.

[CLINICAL EXPERIENCE]

1. CONVENTIONAL ACUPUNCTURE

(1) Penetrating Puncture

Points: Taiyang (Ex-HN5) to Jiache (ST6), Taiyang (Ex-HN5) to Quanliao (SI18), Taiyang (Ex-HN5) to Xiaguan (ST7), Dicang (ST4) to Yifeng (TE17), and Houxi to Laogong (PC8)

Technique: One to two pairs of points on the diseased side should be chosen each time. Every time, the penetration from Houxi (SI3) to Laogong (PC8) is conducted only on one side, while the left and right points are used alternately. Take 2- or 3-*cun* needles to perform the penetration at the subcutaneous or deeper level, giving strong stimulation, and retaining the needles for 20 to 30 minutes.

(2) Selection of Distal Point

Point: Yanglingquan (GB34), Zusanli (ST36), Baihui (GV20), Hegu (LI4) and Yamen (GV15)

Technique: Use points located on the four extremities bilaterally. Needle the points with the reinforcing technique, retaining the needles for 30 minutes after the arrival of *qi*. This method helps tonify *qi* and blood, dispel wind and stop the spasm. It is applied for a spasm caused by the blood deficiency.

(3) Shallow Needling

Point: Local affected region

Technique: Use 0.5 to 1-*cun* filiform needles (Size: Nos.30 to 32) to needle the local affected region shallowly at the skin level. The needle tip is placed just under the skin by stretching it, while the needle body is suspended but not falling off. Take 15 to 30 filiform needles according to the size of the diseased area, and insert them densely into the spasmodic region or puncture the skin of the affected area in a scattered pattern with needles 0.5 to 1 cm apart. Perform the treatment once a day, retaining the needles for 20 minutes. Ten sessions forming one course.

(4) Choosing Points on Healthy Side

Points: Fengchi (GB20), Yifeng (TE17), Dicang (ST4), Jiache (ST6), Taiyang (Ex-HN5), Xiaguan (ST7), Sibai (ST2), Yingxiang (LI20), Hegu (LI4) and Taichong (LR3)

Technique: Select the points of the face and head on the healthy side. Use points of the extremities bilaterally, and needle the points with the even method. Retain the needles for 30 minutes after obtaining the arrival of *qi*. The treatment is conducted once a day, 10 sessions making up one course.

2. MOXIBUSTION WITH MOXA STICK

Point: Local affected region

Technique: Take the region where the spasm occurs frequently, and apply suspended moxibustion with the moxa stick until the color of the skin has turned red. In general, each moxibustion treatment takes 15 minutes, and the treatment is carried out once a day. This method is applied for a facial spasm caused by the invasion of the pathogenic wind and cold or by blood deficiency.

3. AURICULAR THERAPY

Points: Eye, Cheek, Ear-shenmen, Mouth, Liver, Sub-cortex, Spleen and Ear Apex

Technique: Apply conventional acupuncture or the electro-auricular treatment first and then vaccaria seeds, selecting three to four points each time. Treat the ears alternately, giving the treatment once a day or once every other day, and retaining the needles for 40 minutes while applying gentle stimulation. Meanwhile, the bleeding of the ear apex should be conducted twice a week, or injection with the compound Radix Angelicae Sinesis performed alternately to points of the left and right ears should be combined if the therapeutic effect can be improved.

4. INTRA-DERMAL NEEDLING

Points: Reaction points on the local diseased region

Technique: Tap the diseased face once all over the affected region from up to down with the plum blossom needle along with gentle and flexible stimulation. Through the tapping is being carried out, the point that triggers the spasm is revealed. An intra-dermal needle is embedded in the point and the needle is fixed with tape. This intra-dermal needle is taken out three days later. The same method mentioned above is used to find other reaction points that may differ or be the same as the point found before. This method is good in the early stage of a spasm, and generally, the effect comes after seven embedding treatments have been applied.

5. NERVE-TRUNK NEEDLING

Point: Facial nerve trunk (the middle point of the line connecting the mastoidale and the mandibular condyloid process)

Technique: Insert a filiform needle (Size: No.28) to a depth of 1.5 to 2 cm. When the tip of the needle touches the facial nerve truck, pain in the deep part of the ear or pain on the face can be induced. Sometimes contraction of the facial muscles may occur. The needle is removed after the arrival of *qi*.

6. HYDRO-ACUPUNCTURE

(1) Injection with Vitamin B$_1$ and Vitamin B$_{12}$ Injection Fluid
Point: Ah-shi points, Quchi (LI11) and Hegu (LI4)

Technique: According to the size of the diseased region, choose one to two points locally for each treatment and use Quchi (LI11) and Hegu (LI4) alternately. Take 100 µg Vitamin B_{12} (1 contingent), mixing it with 2 ml Vitamin B_1, then inject the fluid into three to four points (0.2 to 0.5 ml into each facial point each time), and 0.5 to 1 ml into Hegu (LI4) and Quchi (LI11) each time. Inject the fluid between the skin and muscle layers on the facial points and in the muscle layer on Quchi (LI11) and Hegu (LI4) at a medium speed. The treatment is conducted once every other day.

(2) Injection with Ligustrazine

Points: Yifeng (TE17) and Xiaguan (ST7) (both on the diseased side)

Technique: Take 1 ml of ligustrazine and inject it into the points mentioned above separately, giving the injection once every other day. Stop the treatment if there is no improvement after five injections. There will be obvious pain in the local region when the injection is carried out.

7. ACUPUNCTURE AND MEDICINAL APPLICATION ON ACU-POINTS

Point: Sibai (ST2)

Technique: Take Sibai (ST2) of the diseased side, insert the needle from the lower part of Chengqi (ST1) at an angle of 45° to a depth of 0.8 to 1 *cun*, give a strong stimulation after gaining the arrival of *qi*, and manipulate the needles once every five minutes. The needles should be retained for 30 minutes, and the treatment is conducted once every other day. Seven sessions constitute one course. After needling, cut one Shangshizhitong Plaster into three to four pieces, and stick them on the skin from the nose bridge to the side of the face running over Chengqi (ST1), Sibai (ST2) and Juliao (ST3), respectively. Stretch the plasters slightly, and move them up or down on the following day to avoid skin allergy.

[REMARKS]

1. Facial spasm belongs to one of the intractable diseases. Acupuncture can relieve the symptoms.

2.   Conducting the treatment as early as possible is the key point. The longer the disease lasts, the poorer the therapeutic effect.

3.   The stimulation intensity of acupuncture technique is determined flexibly by the excess or deficiency condition of the disease. But in general, it is not common to apply the electro-acupuncture on the facial points of the affected side.

FACIAL PAIN

[INTRODUCTION]

Facial pain refers to the severe pain happening in a paroxysmal way, temporarily and repeatedly on the specific facial region. The pain mostly occurs in the forehead, cheek, upper and lower jaws. It mainly appears on one side of the face, and only a few patients get it on both sides. There are usually trigger points on the lateral side of such areas as the upper lip, nasal region, cheek, corner of the mouth and tongue. The pain will start when these regions are triggered slightly. In a severe case, the patient gets the pain when washing the face, brushing the teeth, talking, chewing and swallowing. The causative factors include the invasion of the exogenous pathogenic wind and cold, or the stagnation of liver *qi* transforming into liver fire, or the rising up of stomach fire transformed from heat since the food retention due to the improper food intake generates heat, or hyperactivity of fire due to the constitutional *yin* deficiency. These factors cause the obstruction of *qi* in the facial meridians or the burning of the facial meridians by heat. The treatment principle is to dredge the meridians and collaterals, promote the flow of *qi* and stop pain. The points are chosen from the local affected region, Yangming meridians and Jueyin meridians. For example, use Yangbai (GB14), Zanzhu (BL2) and Taiyang (Ex-HN5) to treat pain on the forehead; use Sibai (ST2), Quanliao (SI18), Yingxiang (LI20) and Juliao (ST3) to treat pain in the upper mandibular region; use Jiachengjiang, Xiaguan (ST7), Daying (ST5) and Yifeng (TE17) to treat pain in the lower mandibular region; use Fengchi (GB20), Waiguan (TE5) and Hegu (LI4) to treat pain due to the invasion of exogenous pathogenic wind and cold; use Yanglingquan (GB34) and Xingjian (LR2) to treat pain due to liver fire transformed from liver stagnation; use Quchi (LI11) and Neiting (ST44) to treat pain due to the rising up of stomach fire; use Zhaohai (KI6) and Sanyinjiao (SP6) and Taixi (KI3) to treat pain due to the hyperactive fire caused by *yin* deficiency. The needling technique applied is mainly the reducing technique, the even method should be applied for pain due to the hyperactivity of fire caused by *yin* deficiency, and moxibustion can be taken for the cold syndrome. This disease is equal to trigeminal neuralgia in modern medicine.

[CLINICAL EXPERIENCE]

1. CONVENTIONAL ACUPUNCTURE

(1) Needling with Heavy Stimulation

Points: Meichong (BL3) for the pain on the first branch, Sibai (ST2) for the pain on the second branch and Xiaguan (ST7) for the pain on the third branch.

Technique: Use a filiform needle (Size: No.28) with a length of 1-1.5 *cun*, insert it into Meichong (BL3) on the affected side at an angle of 30° to the medial and inferior direction to a depth of 0.3 *cun*. Lift and thrust the needle 20 to 50 times until there is a needling sensation like an electric shock radiating to the forehead. Insert the needle into Sibai (ST2) on the affected side at an angle of 45° to the oblique and upward direction to a depth of 0.5 *cun*, lifting and thrusting it 20 to 50 times until there is a needling sensation like an electric shock radiating to the upper lip. Insert the needle into Xiaguan (ST7) on the affected side toward the opposite sub-mandibular angle, lifting and thrusting it 20 to 50 times until there is a needling sensation like an electric shock radiating to the sub-mandibular region. The treatment is performed once every other day, 10 sessions forming one course. According to the statistics on 300 cases of trigeminal neuralgia, 138 cases were cured completely, making up 46%; 102 cases gained remarkable relief, 34%; (56 cases saw an improvement, 18.7%; and four cases saw no improvement, 1.3%. The effective rate was 98.7%.

(2) Needling the Ying (Spring) Point of Stomach Meridian

Point: Neiting (ST44)

Technique: Use a one-*cun* filiform needle and needling the point at an angle of 45° to a depth of 0.5 to 0.8 *cun*, applying rotating manipulation. During the needling manipulation, the patient feels a slightly cold sensation rising from the lateral side of the leg up to the abdomen, stomach and face. Finally the patient has a cool sensation in the mouth. Pain will be relieved quickly after the acupuncture treatment.

(3) Penetrating Puncture

Points: Neiguan (PC6) penetrating to Waiguan (TE5), Yangbai (GB14) penetrating to Yuyao (Ex-HN4), Shuaigu (GB8) penetrating to Taiyang (Ex-HN5), and Hegu (LI4) penetrating to Laogong (PC8).

Technique: After obtaining the arrival of *qi*, rotate needles a few minutes with strong stimulation. No needle retention is required.

(4) Deep Needling

Points: Foramen Supraorbitale, Foramen Infraorbitale and Foramen Mentale

Technique: Insert the needle into the foramen supraorbitale perpendicularly 1 to 1.2 *cun* deep. Insert the needle into the foramen infraorbitale at an angle of 45°, 1.2 to 1.4 *cun* deep, toward the unilateral mouth corner; and insert the needle into the foramen mentale at an angle of 20°, 1.2 to 1.4 *cun* deep, toward the unilateral Jiache (ST6). Deep needling applied on these points not only stops the pain, but also has a certain long-term effect.

(5) Tinggong (SI19) Needling

Point: Tinggong (SI19) (located on affected side).

Technique: Insert a one-*cun* needle (Size: No.30) perpendicularly, 0.6 to 0.7 *cun* deep, and retain it for 30 to 60 minutes, while manipulating once every 10 minutes by the even method. The needle can be retained up to several hours for a patient with prolonged or severe pain.

2. BLEEDING METHOD

Points: Taiyang (Ex-HN5), Jiache (ST6) and Dicang (ST4).

Technique: Prick the points with a three-edged needle, bleeding the points once every three days. After the bleeding treatment, the meridians and collaterals can be dredged, *qi* and blood circulation promoted, and the pain relieved.

3. ELECTRIC ACUPUNCTURE

Points: Yuyao (Ex-HN4), Sibai (ST2), Xiaguan (ST7), Jiachengjiang, Hegu (LI4) and Taichong (LR3).

Technique: Choose two points every treatment, and apply the dense-disperse wave with medium stimulation, retaining the needles for 15 to 30 minutes. Perform the treatment once a day.

4. AURICULAR THERAPY

Points: Liver, Gallbladder, Ear-Shenmen, Cheek, Brain and Kidney

Technique: Embed needles or Vaccaria seeds, treating the right and left ears alternately once every three to five days. The patient is told to press the points three to four times every day, two or three minutes each time.

5. HYDRO-ACUPUNCTURE

Points: Ah-shi points, Yuyao (Ex-HN4), Sibai (ST2), Xiaguan (ST7) and Jiachengjiang.

Technique: Choose two or three points every time and inject 0.5 ml VB_1 into each point. The treatment is conducted once every other day.

6. COMBINED TREATMENT

(1) Acupuncture Combined with Moxibustion

Points: Primary points: Sanjian (LI3), Hegu (LI4) and Toulinqi (GB15). Secondary points: Taiyang (Ex-HN5), Shangguan (GB3), Yangbai (GB14) and Zanzhu (BL2) for pain on the first branch of the trifacial nerve; Tongziliao (GB1), Sibai (ST2), Xiaguan (ST7) and Quanliao (SI18) for pain on the second branch; Jiache (ST6), Daying (ST5) and Xuanli (GB6), on the third.

Technique: Apply acupuncture first, then heavy moxibustion. After retaining the needles for 30 minutes, perform moxibustion on the facial painful points or acupoints for 40 minutes with the application of the moxa instrument once a day. If the treatment is given for seven to 10 consecutive days, a certain effect can be achieved.

(2) Acupuncture Combined with Pricking and Cupping

Points: Dazhui (GV14), Fengchi (GB20) (needled bilaterally), Hegu (LI4) (needled bilaterally), Xiaguan (ST7), Jiache (ST6), Sibai (ST2) and Heliao (LI19). All the points located on the affected side are applied in the treatment.

Technique: Puncture the points mentioned above with the filiform needles first, then apply the reducing needling method by rotation, retain the needles for 15 minutes, and manipulate them once every five minutes. Search for painful points on the affected side of the face after withdrawing the needles, choose two painful points and prick them with a three-edged needle. Then, cup the points pricked, letting out one to two ml of blood. It is better not to cause any bruising when the cupping is performed. The treatment is conducted once a day or once every other day, 10 sessions forming one course.

[REMARKS]

1.   Acupuncture treatment is certainly effective to relieve primary trigeminal neuralgia. A further examination should be taken to diagnose if it is secondary trigeminal neuralgia when there is sensory dysfunction, deviation of the mouth and a mass on the neck.

2.   The block therapy performed with procaine or the therapy with integrated Chinese and Western medicine can be conducted if the effect of the acupuncture treatment is not satisfactory.

HEADACHE

[INTRODUCTION]

Headache, a commonly seen subjective symptom, is found in

many acute and chronic diseases. Clinically, it is divided into ones due to invasion of the exogenous pathogens and ones due to internal injury. The headache due to invasion of the exogenous pathogens refers to the one occurring when such exogenous pathogens as wind, cold, damp and heat disturb the clear orifice, the attack of this headache is sudden and is characterized by severe and constant pain accompanied by chills and fever. The treatment principle should be to relieve the exterior syndrome and stop pain. The points of the three *yang* meridians are taken as the main points, including Fengchi (GB20), Fengmen (BL12), Taiyang (EX-HN5), Hegu (LI4), Waiguan (TE5) and Lieque (LU7). If it is caused by wind cold, moxibustion is combined; if it is caused by wind heat, Dazhui (GV14) and Quchi (LI11) are added; and if it is caused by wind damp, Yinlingquan (SP9), Fenglong (ST40) and Touwei (ST8) are adopted. The headache due to internal injury usually occurs because of dysfunction of the zangfu organs. When the liver is damaged by emotional disturbance, liver stagnation gives rise to fire that will disturb the clear orifice; or when liver and kidney *yin* is deficiency, liver *yang* becomes hyperactive; or when the spleen fails to carry out transportation and transformation, phlegm and damp are produced from the interior and they obstruct *yang*; or when there is improper food intake and overstrain and stress damaging the spleen *qi*, so that it fails to transform *qi* and blood, *qi* and blood are deficient and cannot nourish the brain; or when there is the congenital deficiency, kidney essence deficiency, or insufficient brain marrow, headache occurs. The treatment principle is to regulate *qi* to stop pain, such points as Baihui (GV20), Fengchi (GB20) and Taiyang (EX-HN5) being used. In case of the flaring up of liver fire, Xingjian (LR2) and Yanglingquan (GB34) are combined; in case of hyperactivity of liver *yang*, Taichong (LR3) and Sanyinjiao (SP6) are united; in case of *qi* and blood deficiency, Zusanli (ST36) and Pishu (BL20) are added; in case of the retention of phlegm damp in the interior, Fenglong (ST40) and Yinlingquan (SP9) are used; and in case of the kidney deficiency, Shenshu (BL23) and Taixi (KI3) are adopted. Apart from what has been mentioned above, depending on the location of the headache, other points can be added. This disease is commonly found in vascular headache, catatonic headache, hypertension, and some intra-cranial diseases.

[CLINICAL EXPERIENCE]

1. CONVENTIONAL ACUPUNCTURE

(1) Penetrating Puncture

Points: Fengchi (GB20) to Fengfu (GV16), Sizhukong (TE23) to Shuaigu (GB8), Touwei (ST8) to Qubin (GB7), Hegu (LI4) and Yanglingquan (GB34).

Technique: Needle the points with the reducing technique, performing the treatment once every other day. It is mainly indicated for migraine.

(2) Combination of Distal and Adjacent Points

Points: Fengchi (GB20) and Jinmen (BL63).

Technique: Use Fengchi (GB20) of the diseased side and distal Jingmen (BL63) bilaterally. The points are needled with the reducing technique. This method is very effective to treat vascular headache.

(3) Selecting One Point Only

Point: Baihui (GV20)

Technique: Needle the point horizontally 1 to 1.5 *cun* deep, puncturing the point along the running course of the meridian from the front to the back for excessive syndrome and from the back to the front for deficient syndrome.

(4) Puncturing Positive Reaction Points

Points: Vertex and forehead.

Technique: Flat nodes can be found on the areas mentioned above, and hurt when finger pressure and thumbnail pressure are exerted on them. The headache will be relieved afterwards. Filiform needles are taken to puncture the nodes. The rotating technique is used and the needles are manipulated intermittently for 10 to 20 minutes. The treatment is performed once a day, and the headache will be relieved or will disappear after the flat nodes disappear.

(5) Penetrating Puncture on Points of Different Meridians

Points: Tianshu (ST25) and Huangshu (KI16).

Technique: Press Tianshu (ST25) with the thumb of the left hand and Huangshu (KI16) with the middle finger of the left hand. Hold the needle with the right hand and insert it into Tianshu (ST25) to a depth of 0.8 *cun*. After the arrival of *qi*, lift the needle up to the region of 0.5 *cun* in depth, turning it horizontally toward Huangshu (KI16). After penetrating to Huangshu (KI16) and rotating the needle slightly, retain the needles for 20 minutes after the arrival of *qi*. This method is used to treat headache caused by retention of phlegm.

(6) Needling Four Wind Points

Points: Fengchi (GB20), Fengfu (GV16), Yifeng (TE17) and Fengmen (BL12)

Technique: When Fengchi (GB20) is needled, the direction of the tip of the needle should be pointed toward the opposite eyeball or zygoma. The point is needled 1.2 to 1.5 *cun* deep with reinforcing and reducing methods achieved by lifting, thrusting and rotating. The needling sensation will reach the forehead or the orbital region from Fengchi (GB20) along the occiput and vertex of the head. When Yifeng (TE17) is needled, the direction of the needle should be pointed toward the contralateral processus mastoideus. The point is needled 2 to 2.5 *cun* deep. The needling sensation will radiate to the throat and root of the tongue. This method is used to treat all kinds of headache.

(7) Needling Geshu (BL17) – Influential Point of Blood

Technique: Puncture Geshu (BL17) bilaterally, needle the point at an angle of 75° to 1 *cun* in depth, and turn the needle obliquely toward the vertebrae, and perform the lifting, thrusting and rotating manipulation until there is numbness. Retain the needles for 30 minutes. Conduct the treatment once every day, 10 sessions being one course. This method is indicated for vascular headache.

(8) Using Mainly Huatuojiaji (EX-B2) Points

Points: Huatuojiaji (EX-B2) lateral to the 5th, 7th, 9th, and 11th thoracic vertebrae.

Technique: The patient should take a sitting posture first and then extend his head slightly. Fengchi (GB20) is punctured horizontally with a 1.5-*cun* filiform needle toward the opposite eye corner to a depth of 1 *cun*. The reducing technique achieved by rotation is performed after the arrival of *qi*. The needling sensation should reach the opposite eye corner or Taiyang (EX-HN5) along the running course of the Shaoyang meridian, then the needle is withdrawn. The patient should lie prone for the needling of Huatuojiaji (EX-B2). Huatuojiaji (EX-B2) is punctured with 1.5-*cun* filiform needles from the place lateral to the lower border of the spinous process, the tips of the needles are pointing obliquely toward the vertebrae, and the needle bodies are at an angle of 75° with the skin. The point is needled to 1 *cun* in depth. The needling sensation should transmit along the vertebrae up and down, or along the ribs. Reducing manipulation is performed after the arrival of *qi*. Retain the needle for 30 minutes. The treatment is conducted once every other day for vascular lateral headache.

2. MOXIBUSTION

Points: Yangbai (GB14), Zanzhu (BL2), Taiyang (EX-HN5), Sizhukong (TE23) and Ah-shi points

Technique: One to three points are selected each time. Burning rush moxibustion is performed, and the treatment is conducted once every other day. Usually improvement is obtained after one to two sessions. In order not to burn the patient's hair, the doctor can make a hole in a piece of cardboard and place the hole right over the point, after which he can perform the moxibustion treatment.

3. BLEEDING METHOD

(1) Bleeding Sishencong (EX-HN1)

Technique: After regular sterilization, prick Sishencong (EX-HN1) with a three-edged needle. Sometimes blood will flow out immediately; otherwise, the point should be squeezed to cause bleeding. It is not necessary to let out a big amount of blood. Headache caused by excessive heat is treated with this method.

(2) Bleeding Taiyang (EX-HN5)

Technique: Prick the congested veins found around Taiyang (EX-HN5) with a three-edged needle to cause bleeding. Before the treatment is conducted, a towel can be put on the neck of the patient. The two ends of the towel may be held with the hands and twisted hard so that the congested veins become more distinctive. With some patients, the blood spurts out after the bleeding is completed; with others, there is scant blood or even no blood flowing at all. In the latter case, we can draw blood with a small cup. In general, pain stops after the blood flows out. This method is used for the lateral headache located on both sides of the head.

(3) Bleeding Weizhong (BL40)

Technique: After performing local regular sterilization, find the veins around Weizhong (BL40) that have the blood stasis inside and bleed with a three-edged needle.

4.　ELECTRIC ACUPUNCTURE

Points: Main points: Taiyang (EX-HN5), and Anmian[2]. Supplementary points: Combining Yintang (EX-HN3), Shangxing (GV23) or Yangbai (GB14) for frontal headache; using the penetrating puncture from Touwei (ST8) to Hanyan (GB4) for migraine; adopting Baihui (GV20) or Sishencong (EX-HN1) for vertex headache; and adding Naohu (GV17) and Fengchi (GB20) for occipital headache.

Technique: Tell the patient to lie supine. Perform lifting, thrusting and rotating manipulation on the points, and retain the needles for 20 minutes after arrival of *qi*. Use G6805 electric stimulator, applying continuous wave of a high frequency. The treatment is performed once every day and is used to treat severe headache.

5.　NEEDLING NERVE TRUNK

(1) Needling Point on Auriculotemporal Nerve

Point: The point is in the groove anterior to the tragus and posterior to the arteria temporalis superficials.

Technique: At first, touch the arteria temporalis superficialis anterior to the tragus to feel the pulsation, and needle the point slightly posterior to the artery perpendicularly, 0.2 to 0.3 *cun* deep. Turn the needle body up and down. There will be a sensation like an electric shock radiating to the temporal region when the auriculotemperal nerve is stimulated. This method is used for migraine.

(2) *Needling Point on Greater Occipital Nerve*

Point: The point is 1.5 *cun* lateral posterior to the crossing point of the line joining the two processus mastuideus and the posterior mid-line.

Technique: After locating the point accurately, needle it perpendicularly 0.5 to 0.8 *cun* deep, and turn the needle body left and right. When the greater occipital nerve is stimulated, there will be a sensation like an electric shock radiating to the back of the occiput. This method is indicated for occipital headache.

6. AURICULAR THERAPY

(1) *Puncturing Auricular Points*

Points: Forehead, Occiput, Sub-cortex, Brain and Ear Apex.

Technique: Choose one to two pairs of points each time, and perform filiform needle acupuncture with a medium amount of stimulation after applying local sterilization. Retain the needles 30 to 60 minutes. Conduct the treatment once every day and 10 sessions make up one course.

(2) *Bleeding Back of the Ear*

Point: Blood vessels of the artery on the back of the ear.

Technique: Perform the massage on the auricle of the patient to cause congestion in the blood vessels. After applying regular sterilization on the place to be incised, fix the blood vessel with the left hand, hold the knife in the right hand and cut the blood vessel on the back of the auricle, letting out one to two ml of blood. Then press the incised blood vessel with antiseptic gauze to stop bleeding. Conduct the treatment once every day, treating one ear each time. Four to six sessions make up one course. It is forbidden to use this method to treat a patient with hemorrhagic diseases or women patients experiencing pregnancy or menstrual periods.

7. HYDRO-ACUPUNCTURE

Points: Taiyang (EX-HN5), Yintang (EX-HN3) and Fengchi (GB20)

Technique: Use either 0.25 to 1% of procaine solution, or the mixture of 3.5 ml of 0.25% procaine and 0.5 ml of caffeine, and inject 0.5 to 1 ml injection fluid into each point. Conduct the treatment once every day or once every other day.

8. MEDICINAL APPLICATION ON ACU-POINTS

Points: Yintang (EX-HN3) and Taiyang (EX-HN5)

Technique: Take three slices of fresh ginger, and wrap them separately with mulberry paper. Use water to make the mulberry paper wet and heat them up in hot ashes. Apply one wrapped slice on Yintang (EX-HN3) and one on each Taiyang (EX-HN5) until they are cool. At the end, take a belt to bind the head and fix the wrapped ginger slices in place. This method is used for headache caused by wind and cold.

[REMARKS]

1. Acupuncture treatment is certainly effective to relieve headaches caused both by the invasion of the exogenous pathogenic factors and internal injuries.

2. When treating headaches, some doctors prefer to use more points of *yang* meridians, especially the points on the head and distal points on the four limbs.

3. Electric acupuncture should be used cautiously when the patient who has a headache and hypertension is treated.

4. The effect of this treatment can be improved if combined with massage.

HYPOCHONDRIAL PAIN

[INTRODUCTION]

Hypochondrial pain generally refers to the pain appearing unilaterally or bilaterally on the hypochondrial and costal regions, and is a common clinical subjective symptom. It is pointed out in *Miraculous Pivat, Five Evils* that: "Once there are pathogens in the liver, there is hypochondrial pain." The liver is closely related to the gallbladder.

The liver meridian is distributed in the hypochondrial and costal regions, while the gallbladder meridian runs inside the hypochondrial region and passes through the floating rib. All of this confirms that hypochondrial pain is closely related to the liver and gallbladder. The causative factors of hypochondrial pain include mainly the stagnation of liver *qi*, stagnation of *qi* and blood, accumulation of damp and heat, or deficiency of liver blood. The treatment principle is to regulate the liver and gallbladder. Such points as Qimen (LR14), Riyue (GB24), Zhigou (TE6), Yanglingquan (GB34) and Taichong (LR3) are taken as the primary points. Other points like Neiguan (PC6), Xiaxi (GB43) and Ganshu (BL18) are used to promote the free flow of liver *qi* and remove liver stagnation in the case of the liver *qi* stagnation; Dabao (SP21), Geshu (BL17), Jingmen (GB25) and Sanyinjiao (SP6) to regulate *qi* and activate blood in the case of the *qi* and blood stagnation; Yinlingquan (SP9) and Xingjian (LR2) to clear heat and eliminate dampness in the case of the accumulation of damp heat; Ganshu (BL18), Pishu (BL20), Gushu (BL17) and Zusanli (ST36) to tonify *qi* and blood in the case of the blood deficiency. This disease is commonly seen in the diseases of liver, gallbladder, pleurae and intercostal neuralgia diagnosed in terms of modern medicine.

[CLINICAL EXPERIENCE]

1. CONVENTIONAL ACUPUNCTURE

(1) Penetrating Puncture

Point: Penetrating from Qiuxu (GB40) to Zhaohai (KI6)

Technique: Use the point on the right side to treat the pain on the left side, and the point on the left side to treat the pain on the right side. Insert a 2 *cun* filiform needle into Qiuxu (GB40), penetrating toward Zhaohai (KI6), which is located 1 *cun* below the tip of the medial melleous. The needling treatment works when the patient has had the needling sensation or radiating sensation in the points. Other points are combined according to different clinical manifestations.

(2) Needling Xinshu (Bl15), Zhigou (TE6) and Shenmen (HT7)

Technique: Needle points bilaterally and perform the treatment once every day. Ten sessions constitute one course. This method has certain effects to treat post-operative intercostal neuralgia.

2. ELECTRIC ACUPUNCTURE

Point: Jiaji (EX-B2)

Technique: Choose appropriate Jiaji (EX-B2) relevant to the painful region, and use one-*cun* filiform needles to puncture the points bilaterally. Connect the electric stimulator to the needles, applying medium stimulation for 20 to 30 minutes.

3. SCALP ACUPUNCTURE

Points: Contralateral thoracic area and sensory area for body trunk

Technique: Insert needles along the scalp, applying strong stimulation or electric stimulation.

4. AURICULAR THERAPY

Point: Liver, Gallbladder, Ear-Shenmen and Chest

Technique: Choose the points on the affected side, and apply strong stimulation to treat excessive syndrome and mild stimulation to treat deficient syndrome, retaining the needles for 30 minutes. Alternatively, apply intra-dermal needling or auricular seed embedding therapy.

5. CUTANEOUS PUNCTURE

Points: Ah-shi points, Back-shu points and Jiaji (EX-B2) relevant to the Ah-shi points

Technique: Tap the points with a subcutaneous needle; then perform cupping on the local region.

6. MEDICINAL APPLICATION ON ACU-POINT

Points: Zhongmen (LR13) and Jingmen (GB25)

Technique: Grind equal amounts of Baijiezi and Wuzhuyu into powder and then sieve powder and water into a paste. During the treatment, apply the paste on the points, changing it when it becomes dry. Perform the treatment several times a day. This method is used to treat hypochondrial pain accompanied by belching.

7.   COMBINED TREATMENT

(1) Acupuncture Combined with Bleeding Method

Points: Zhigou (TE6) and Weizhong (BL40)

Technique: Needle bilateral Zhigou (TE6), bleeding bilateral Weizhong (BL40). This method is used to treat migrating pain in the chest, difficult speech due to cough and inability to turn the body.

(2) Acupuncture Combined with Plum-Blossom Treatment and Cupping

Points: Neiguan (PC6) and Yanglingquan (GB34)

Technique: Insert the needle with rotation into Neiguan (PC6) of the affected side, performing the lifting and thrusting manipulation to make the needling sensation radiate to the upper extremities. Tell the patient to breathe deeply. While penetrating the needle transversely from Yanglingquan (GB34) to Yinlingquan (SP9), apply the rotating manipulation to make the sensation travel upward and downward. Retain the needles for 30 to 60 minutes, manipulating them once every five minutes. After taking the needles out, tap the most painful region with a plum-blosson needle lightly at first, but gradually more strongly until the local skin turns red and bleeds slightly. After that, apply cupping for 10 to 15 minutes. Take off the cups when the skin color turns purplish red. The needling treatment is performed once a day, and the cupping treatment is done once every other day. Six days of the treatment form a course, and the interval between two courses is two days.

[REMARKS]

1.   Acupuncture treatment can achieve a better effect in relieving hypochondrial pain. However, a clear diagnosis should be made and treatment determined on the basis of the etiology so as to obtain long-term effects.

2.   The emotional changes of the patient relate closely to this disease. Therefore, the patient should keep a good mood and seek to remain in good psychological condition.

LOWER BACK PAIN

[INTRODUCTION]

Lower back pain is also known as spinal pain of the lower back. The pain is located in the spinal area in the unilateral or bilateral lower back. It is held in traditional Chinese medicine that lower back pain is usually caused by the invasion of pathogenic cold and damp, kidney deficiency and overstrain and stress or stagnation of blood due to sprain and contusion. The symptoms of lower back pain caused by cold and damp are heaviness and cold pain in the lower back; the pain becomes aggravated on cloudy and rainy days or during the change of the seasons. The symptoms of lower back pain caused by kidney deficiency are soreness, weakness and dull pain. Lower back pain caused by blood stagnation due to sprain and contusion is manifested by pricking and fixed pain, and an inability to turn the body. The treatment principle is to dredge the meridians and collaterals, and tonify kidney *qi*. The points are mainly selected from Foot Taiyang Meridian and Governor Vessel, such as Shenshu (BL23), Yaoyangguan (GV3), Weizhong (BL40), Mingmen (GV4), Zhishi (BL52), Taixi (KI3), Ahshi points and so on. Acupuncture and moxibustion are used together, or cupping therapy can be combined. Reducing manipulation is applied to treat the excessive syndrome while reinforcing manipulation is used to treat the deficient syndrome. Lower back pain is the main symptom seen in the protrusion of lumbar inter-vertebral discs, lumbar posterior-articular disturbance, acute lumbar sprain, chronic lumbar muscle over strain and other diseases diagnosed in modern medicine.

[CLINICAL EXPERIENCE]

1. CONVENTIONAL ACUPUNCTURE

(1) Needling Renzhong (GV26)

Technique: With the patient in a sitting posture, the needle is inserted with rotation slowly to a depth of 0.2 *cun*. When the patient feels local numbness and distension, the needle is rotated two or three minutes continuously with large amplitude. The patient is then asked to turn the lumbar region forward, backward, left and right, and the needle is then retained for 15 minutes. The needle is manipulated once or twice during retention, while the patient is told to move the lumbar region at the same time. The needle is removed when the pain disappears. This method is effective to treat spinal pain in the lower back.

(2) Needling Fengfu (GV16)

Technique: The patient is asked to take a sitting posture first and then lower his head slightly. A 1.5-*cun* (Size: No.30) needle is inserted to a depth of 0.3 *cun*, and then 0.5 *cun* deep at a 45° angle downward. Afterwards, the needle is rotated to increase the stimulation until the needling sensation radiates to the lower back. It is then retained for a further 10 minutes. After the needle is taken out, if other points like Shenshu (BL23) and Weizhong (BL40) are needled as well, the effect of the treatment is better. This method is used to treat lower back pain caused by sprain and contusion wind-damp.

(3) Needling Houxi (SI3)

Technique: Puncture the unilateral Houxi (SI3) perpendicularly with a two-*cun* filiform needle, needling the points to a depth of 1-2 *cun*. Perform reducing manipulation while rotating the needle. Tell the patient to turn the lumbar region. Take the needle out after patient has freedom of movement. Most patients will recover from lower back pain after receiving 1-2 sessions. This method is indicated for acute lumbar sprain.

(4) Needling Tianzhu (BL10)

Technique: The patient is asked to sit straight and extend his head. The one-*cun* filiform needles are inserted into bilateral Tianzhu (BL10) to a depth of 0.5-1 *cun*. Retain the needles for 15 minutes after arrival of *qi*. This method is used to treat acute bilateral lumbar sprain.

(5) Needling Yanglao (SI6)

Technique: The patient is told to stand, lift up the upper arm slightly, flex the elbow and turn the palm to face the chest. A 1.5-*cun* filiform needle is inserted into unilateral Yanglao (SI6). The needling sensation may radiate to the elbow. After the arrival of *qi*, the patient is asked to move the lumbar region. In general, lower back pain can be relieved immediately. The needle is manipulated a few times during the 30-minute retention. This method is used to relieve acute lumbar sprain.

(6) Needling Jiaji (EX-B2)

Technique: The patient is told to lie prone. Jiaji (EX-B2) relevant to the painful points are selected, and a filiform needle (Size: No.26 or 28) is inserted quickly. The Jiaji (EX-B2) lateral to the lumbar vertebrae 1-3 are punctured 1.5 to 2 *cun* deep; the Jiaji (EX-B2) lateral to the lumbar vertebrae 4-5 are punctured 2 to 2.5 *cun* deep. The needles are thrust up and down, left and right to make the needling sensation radiate down to the heel, and are retained for 30 minutes after arrival of *qi*. This method is used to treat all kinds of lower back pain.

2. MOXIBUSTION

(1) Moxibustion Performed with Moxa Box

Point: Local region of low back pain

Technique: The patient is told to lie prone. A two-*cun* moxa stick is taken, and both ends are lit at the same time before it is placed in the moxa-box. Afterward, the moxa-box is put over the local region of the lower back. This method is mostly combined with acupuncture treatment to treat both acute and chronic lower back pain.

(2) Moxibustion on Warming Needle

Points: Shenshu (BL23), Dachangshu (BL25), Zhishi (BL52), Yaoyangguan (GV3) and Ah-shi points

Technique: The patient is asked to lie recumbent after the arrival of *qi*. A one-*cun* moxa stick is put on the handle of the needle, and the end closer to the skin is ignited. Two moxa sticks are applied in every session. This method is suitable to treat both acute and chronic lower back pain.

2. ELECTRIC ACUPUNCTURE

(1) Puncturing Zhishi (BL52)

Technique: The patient is asked to extend his fingers slightly. The points to be located are 1.5 *cun* anterior to the dorsal transverse crease of the wrist and are the middle points of the space between the second and third metacarpal bones and between the fourth and fifth metacarpal bones. One-*cun* needles (Size: No.30) are inserted into the bilateral points. The direction of the needle is perpendicular or slightly oblique toward the carpal bone. Then the electric stimulator is connected to the needles after arrival of *qi*, the electric intensity being determined by the patient's tolerance. This method is suitable to treat acute lumbar sprain.

(2) *Puncturing Yaotongxue (EX-UE7)*

Technique: The patient is asked to extend his fingers slightly. The relevant points are located 1.5 *cun* anterior to the dorsal transverse crease of the wrist, and they are the middle points of the spaces between the second and third metacarpal bones and the fourth and fifth metacarpal bones. One-*cun* needles (Size No.30) are inserted into the bilateral points. The direction of the needle is perpendicular or slightly oblique toward the carpal bone. Then, the electric stimulator is connected to the needles after the arrival of *qi*, the electric intensity determined by the patient's tolerance. This method is suitable to treat acute lumbar sprain.

3. BLEEDING METHOD

Points: Weizhong (BL40) and Renzhong (GV26)

Technique: A three-edged needle is used to prick Weizhong (BL40) to cause slight bleeding. A one-*cun* filiform needle (Size No.26) is taken to puncture Renzhong (GV26) quickly to let out blood. The method treats local pain in the lower back caused by wind cold obstruction in the meridians and collaterals.

4. AURICULAR THERAPY

Points: Lumbar Vertebra, Abdomen, Ear-Shenmen and External Genitalia

Technique: Needle points with 0.5-*cun* filiform needles, applying heavy manipulation. Rotate the needles while asking the patient to move the lower back. Manipulate the needle with the amplitude from small to big until the pain is relieved or has disappeared, retaining the needles for 30 to 60 minutes, or applying the needle-embedding method. This treatment is suitable for acute lumbar strain.

5. ORBITAL ACUPUNCTURE

Points: Bilateral middle and lower Jiao areas

Technique: Insert one-*cun* filiform needles into the areas mentioned above to a depth of 0.2 *cun*. This method is suitable for the treatment of the protrusion of lumbar discs, and it has good effect for motor recovery.

6. HYDRO-ACUPUNCTURE

Point: Chengshan (BL57)

Technique: Inject Chinese Angelica Root Extract fluid into Chengshan (BL57) bilaterally with 2 ml fluid into each point, performing the treatment once a day or once every other day.

7. CATGUT-EMBEDDING ON ACU-POINT

Points: Jiaji (EX-B2), and points of the relevant parts of the bladder meridian

Technique: Choose Jiaji (EX-B2) and bladder meridian points in correspondence to the affected region, performing regular sterilization and local anesthesia. Thread a puncture needle with two or three *cun* long surgical catgut, puncturing the needle perpendicular to a certain depth, and embedding the surgical catgut in the points. After taking the needle out, bandage the point with antiseptic gauze. Select two or three points every time and perform the treatment once a week. This method is used to treat the lumbar hyper-osteogenesis.

8. MEDICINAL APPLICATION ON ACU-POINT

Point: Yaoyan (EX-B7)

Technique: Prepare Danggui (Chinese angelica) 50 g, Honghua (safflower) 30 g, Ruxiang (frank incense) 20 g, Moyao (myrrh) 20 g and Chuanniuxi (Radix jurineae) 15 g, soak them in 300 ml of vinegar for four hours, then pour the mixture into a pot and heat it until it boils. Soak gauze in the vinegar, place it on the points while hot, and change the gauze when it turns cold. The treatment should last three to four hours every time and should be given once a day. This method is suitable to treat lower back pain caused by the stagnation of blood that has the symptoms of pricking and fixed pain.

9. COMBINED TREATMENT

(1) Acupuncture Combined with Cupping

Points: Tenderness points lateral to spinal column

Technique: Insert a 1.5-*cun* filiform needle into the tender points lateral to the spine, and perform lifting, thrusting and rotating manipulations. Manipulate the needles for five to 10 minutes continuously, and then perform cupping 15 minutes after taking the needles out. This method is applied in the treatment of lumbar muscular fibrositis.

(2) Acupuncture Combined with Infra-red Light

Points: Tenderness points and other ones lateral to the lumbar sacral vertebrae

Technique: Use 1.5-*cun* filiform needles to puncture three to four points, and apply lifting, thrusting and scraping needling manipulation. Retain the needles for 20 to 30 minutes, further manipulating the needles once every five to 10 minutes, combined with infra-red radiation for 30 minutes. The treatment should be performed once a day, 10 sessions forming one course, with a two or three day break between courses. This method is suitable for the treatment of spinal joints disorders.

(3) Acupuncture Combined with Moxibustion

Points: Shenshu (BL23), Weizhong (BL40), Fuliu (KI7) and Dadu (SP2)

Technique: Insert filiform needles, 1 to 1.5 *cun* in length, into the points mentioned above, retain them for 30 minutes after the arrival of *qi*, and apply moxibustion on Shenshu (BL23) and Dadu (SP2) after the needles are taken out. Use three moxa cones on each point. This treatment is good for lower back pain causing an inability to stand.

(4) Acupuncture Combined with Intradermal Needle

Points: Mingmen (GV4) and Zulinqi (GB41)

Technique: Puncture bilateral Zulinqi (GB41) at first, and retain the needles for 15 minutes after the arrival of *qi*. Rotate both needles for one minute simultaneously once every five minutes. After the needling treatment, the pain should be gone and the patient should have freedom of motion. Then, insert the intra-dermal needle into Mingmen (GV4) and retain it for two or three days. This method is suitable for lower back pain caused by baby delivery.

[REMARKS]

1. Acupuncture has a certain effect in treating lower back pain and can be relieved by it alone. If the patient suffers from a secondary lower back pain, an accurate diagnosis should be made, and other combined therapies applied.

2. Applying massage and hot compression treatments on the local painful region will help stop the pain.

3. The effect comes quicker in a patient with acute lower back pain. For a patient with chronic lower back pain, since the relapse of the disease occurs repeatedly, the treatment course lasts longer.

SCAPULOHUMERAL PERIARTHRITIS

[INTRODUCTION]

Clinically, scapulohumeral periarthritis is chiefly manifested as unilateral or bilateral shoulder joint pain and movement limitation. It is usually encountered among the patients around 50 years of age, hence is also known as "50-year-old shoulder disorder." Chinese medicine ascribes this condition to the invasion of pathogenic wind, cold and damp at the meridians of the shoulder region when an individual's *qi* and blood are deficient, and the nutrient and defensive *qi* are not strong enough to control the body surface; or because of over-exertion, sprain and contusion which lead to stagnation of *qi* and blood in the shoulder region. Treatment is to eliminate wind, disperse cold, resolve damp and remove obstruction from the collateral, as well as regulate the flow of *qi* and blood. Points are mainly selected from three *yang* meridians, i.e., Jianyu (LI 15), Jianliao (TE 14), Jianzhen (SI 9), Binao (LI 14), Quchi (LI 11) and Hegu (LI 4).

[CLINICAL EXPERIENCE]

1. CONVENTIONAL ACUPUNCTURE

(1) Penetrating Tiaokou (ST 38) and Chengshan (BL 57)

Technique: Puncture Tiaokou (ST 38) with a two-*cun* filiform needle toward Chengshan (BL 57), 1.5-1.8 *cun* deep so as to penetrate the two points. Apply twisting, reducing manipulation to the points. Meanwhile, tell the patient to exercise the affected arm. After five minutes, remove the needle if any pain is felt. Jianyu (LI 15), Jianliao (TE 14), Jianneiling (Extra), Hegu (LI 4), and other acupoints may also be needled.

(2) Penetrating Jianzhen (SI 9) and Jiquan (HT 1)

Technique: Use a two-*cun* filiform needle and puncture Jianzhen (SI 9) toward Jiquan (HT 1) to penetrate the two points. Make the needling sensation radiate to the fingers. Retain and rotate the needle for three to five minutes.

(3) Puncturing Yinlingquan (SP 9) and Xinshexue [directly below Fengchi (GB 20), 1.5 cun inferior to the posterior hairline, at the same level with the transverse spinous process of the 4th cervical vertebra].

Technique: First, puncture Yinlingquan (SP 9) of the healthy side perpendicularly 1.5-2.5 *cun* deep, and conduct lift-thrust-rotating-reducing manipulation to cause strong stimulation. Concurrently, instruct the patient to exercise the upper limb. Remove the needle when the pain is alleviated, then needle Xinshexue (extra) of the affected side 1.5-2 *cun* deep toward the transverse spinous process of the 4th cervical vertebra. After the needling sensation is obtained, ask the patient to slowly exercise the affected arm. Remove the needle immediately when functional improvement of the arm appears.

(4) Puncturing Shangshandian [location: 3 cun lateral to the Adam's apple (LI 18) and 1 cun inferolateral to it, at the posteri-

or border of m. sternocladomastoidus, at the intersecting point directly below the ear lobe and the posterior border of sternocladomastoidus]. Locate the point while the patient is sitting with the head facing straight forward.

Technique: After routine disinfection of the point, take a 1.5-*cun*, needle (Size No.32), and slowly insert it in the precisely located point. In general, the insertion is not more than 0.5 *cun* deep. Then, apply sparrow-pecking manipulation with the needle tip directed at the affected region. The needling is considered effective if the electric shock sensation radiates to the fingertips, and the needle is not retained in the point after the needling sensation is obtained.

(5) Puncturing Yanglingquan (GB 34) and Taichong (LR 3)

Technique: Treat the points on the affected side, first puncturing Yanglingquan (GB 34), and then Taichong (LR 3). While the point is being needled, instruct the patient to exercise the affected limb. This treatment is aimed at regulating the flow of *qi* in the liver meridian so as to relax the muscles and tendons, activate the flow of *qi* and blood in the meridians and collaterals, and relieve pain.

2. MOXIBUSTION

(1) Warm Needle Moxibustion

Points: Jianyu (LI 15), Jianzhen (SI 9), Jianliao (TE 14), Binao (LI 14), Jianjing (GB 21) and Quchi (LI 11).

Technique: Needle the points of the affected side. Place a 1.5-*cun* moxa stick respectively on the handle of needles at the shoulder region points, then ignite the moxa. Apply the treatment once a day, 10 sessions constituting one course, with a break of three to five days between two courses.

(2) Moxibustion with Moxibustioner

Points: Jianzhen (SI 9), Jianyu (LI 15), Binao (LI 14), Naoshu (SI 10) and Jianjing (GB 21).

Technique: Load the moxibustioner with moxa wool and powder of Chinese drug, and then ignite the moxa wool. Fix the moxibustioner to the obvious tender spot of the shoulder. In order to avoid overheating the point, place a few layers of gauze between the skin and the moxibustioner. Apply for 30 minutes, once every other day. Ten sessions constitute one course.

3. BLEEDING METHOD

Points: Local: Jianzhen (SI 9), Jianyu (LI 15), Jianqian (Extra) and local region of the posterior aspect; distal: Chize (LU 5), Quchi (LI11) and Quze (PC 3).

Technique: Prick the selected points and the stagnant vein around the point with a three-edged needle to cause bleeding. After the bleeding of the pricked points ceases, apply cupping for five minutes. Treat once every 10-15 days, in each session bleeding all the local points and one of the distal points.

4. ELECTRIC ACUPUNCTURE

(1) Jiaji Point

Technique: Select Jiaji points of the upper thoracic region. After routine disinfection of the points, pinch the point with the thumb and index finger of the left hand and insert rapidly and subcutaneously a three-*cun* filiform needle (Size: No.28) held in the right hand to the point. The needle inserted is parallel with the spine. After the needling sensation is obtained, continuously manipulate the needle to make the sensation radiate to the shoulder or the back. Then insert the needle to the point on the other side in the same way. After the needling sensation appears at the points of both sides, connect the electro-stimulator to the needle handle, and set the stimulator to the continuous wave mode, with frequency of 100-150 times/sec. Adjust the volume of the stimulation to the tolerance of the patient. Retain the needles for 15 to 30 minutes, applying the treatment once a day. Advise the patient to do functional exercises in addition to the acupuncture treatment.

(2) Shousanli (LI10) and Local Region

Technique: Needle Shousanli (LI 10) on the affected side and the tender spot of the shoulder region. After the needling sensation is obtained, retain the needles in the points for 20 minutes. Concurrently, connect the needle to the semi-conductor electro-stimulator. Set the instrument in the continuous mode of stimulation. Give the treatment once daily, 10 sessions constituting one course.

5. HOT-RED NEEDLING

Points: Peripheral points of the shoulder region

Technique: Conduct routine disinfection of the point. Heat a thick needle made of a special material over a fire until it turns red, then immediately puncture the point, with the needle staying in the point merely 0.5 sec. After puncturing the point, use a piece of dry cotton to press the needling hole so as to minimize the after-effects of the puncture. In general, for acute condition the puncture should be shallow, and for the chronic cases, the puncture deeper. In each session, puncture five points on the shoulder region. Treat once every three to five days.

6. AURICULAR THERAPY

Points: Shoulder, Shoulder Joint, Clavicle, Adrenal Gland, Liver, Spleen and Sub-cortex.

Technique: In each session, select three to four points, puncturing them with the filiform needle. Apply the treatment once every other day. It is also possible to alternate the treatment by applying seeds to the points, which is performed once a week. During the treatment, when the auricle becomes congestive and feverish, ask the patient to exercise the affected limb moderately. The exercise should not be strenuous, otherwise the shoulder pain may get worse.

7. ORBITAL ACUPUNCTURE

Points: Upper triple energizer area, large intestine area and small intestine area

Technique: Puncture the point shallowly with one-*cun* needles without manipulation. Retain the needles in place for five minutes. Apply the treatment once every three days.

8. SCALP ACUPUNCTURE

Points: Anterior oblique line of vertex-temporal [middle 1/3 of the line from Qianding (GV 21) to Xuanli (GB 6)].

Technique: Select the contralateral line of the affected side, needle the point with a 1.5-*cun* filiform needle (Size: Nos.28 to 32), the insertion being 1 *cun* deep. Retain the needle for over an hour after the needling sensation is obtained. Manipulate the needle once every 10-20 minutes. Meanwhile, ask the patient to exercise the shoulder. Treat once every other day, 10 sessions constituting one course.

9. LASER THERAPY

Points: ① Jianzhen (SI 9), Jianneiling (Extra), Tianzong (SI 11), Tiaokou (ST 38) and Ah-shi. ② Jianneiling (Extra) and Ah-shi. ③ Jianyu (LI 15), Binao (LI 14), Ah-shi and Tiaokou (ST 38)

Technique: In each session, select one group of points according to the pathological condition, irradiate the points with He-Ne laser irradiator, and make the laser beam directly irradiate the skin of the points via the fiber in the tube. Generally, irradiate each point within five minutes. Conduct the treatment once a day, 10 sessions constituting one course.

10. HYDRO-ACUPUNCTURE

(1) Compound Chinese Angelica Root Extract Injection

Points: Jianyu (LI 15), Jianliao (TE 14), Binao (LI 14) and Ah-shi.

Technique: Inject 4 ml of compound Chinese Angelica Root Extract fluid into the above respective points. Inject once daily, 10 sessions constituting one course.

(2) Injection of Dexamethasone Phosphate and Vitamin

Points: Tender points of the shoulder region

Technique: Inject 2 ml of dexamethasone phosphate injection and 2 ml vitamin B12 into the tender points of the shoulder region. It is appropriate to inject the liquid into the point between the periosteum and bursa submuscularis. Inject 1-2 ml into each point, and perform treatment once a week. Four sessions constitute one course, with a seven-day break between courses.

11. COMBINATION OF ACUPUNCTURE AND MOXIBUS-TION WITH CUPPILNG

Points: Jianyu (LI 15), Jianliao (TE 14), Jianneiling (extra), Jianzhen (SI 9), Jianzhongshu (SI 15), Quchi (LI 11) and Hegu (LI 4)

Technique: In each session, select four or five points. Conduct acupuncture with mild stimulation, manipulate the needle in the twisting technique and add a 1.5-*cun* long moxa stick to the needle to apply warm needle moxibustion twice on each point. After needle removal, apply 10 minutes of cupping at the local region. Give the treatment once a day.

[REMARKS]

1. Acupuncture exerts immediate satisfactory therapeutic effect on this disease.

2. The patient should be encouraged to do some functional exercises, which, however, should not be overdone, five to 10 minutes being the maximum. It is beneficial to associate the treatment with massage.

CERVICAL SPONDYLOPATHY

[INTRODUCTION]

Clinically, cervical spondylopathy, which is classified into cervical, radical, spinal cord, vertebroarthrial, sympathetic and mixed patterns, is manifested as headache, numbness, and pain of neck, arm and hand, associated with dizziness, lassitude, nausea, visual disturbance, etc. Some patients may also be troubled with obvious muscular atrophy. Chinese medicine regards it as being induced by weakness of the liver and kidneys with deficiency of essence and blood, which deprive the meridians and collaterals of nourishment; or by invasion at the meridians and collaterals by exopathogens of wind, cold and damp, resulting in the obstruction of *qi* and blood circulation that blockades the meridians and collaterals. Treatment of the disease is directed toward removing exopathogens, warming the meridians and collaterals, moving *qi* and blood so as to resolve blood stasis, and tonifying *qi* and blood. Points of local region Governor vessel, Shaoyang and Yangming meridians are commonly selected, such as neck Jiaji, Fengchi (GB 20), Dazhui (GV 14), Jianyu (LI 15), Jianjing (GB 21), Tianzhong (SI 11), Quchi (LI 11), Waiguan (TE 5), Zusanli (ST 36) and Juegu (GB 39).

[CLINICAL EXPERIENCE]

1. CONVENTIONAL ACUPUNCTURE

(1) Selection of Governor Vessel Points

Points: Shenting (GV 24), Shangxing (GV23), Xinhui (GV 22), Qianding (GV 21) and Baihui (GV 20)

Technique: Conduct horizontal insertion toward the back with a filiform needle, which is inserted subcutaneously 1 *cun* inside the point. Retain the needles in place for 20 minutes. Apply the treatment once a day, five sessions constituting one course.

(2) Selection of Points from Three Yang Meridians of Hand and Foot.

Points: Fengchi (GB 20), Shousanli (LI 10), Waiguan (TE 5), Jianjing (GB 21), Yanglingquan (GB 34) and Juegu (GB 39).

Technique: Needle the points with even movement, and retain the needle for 30 minutes. In the procedure, puncture Fengchi (GB 20) first, then the distal points.

(3) Mainly Selecting Four "Tian" Points

Points: Tianzhu (BL 10), Tianliao (TE 15), Tianzong (SI 11), Tianjing (TE 10) and Jiafeng (tender point along the medial border of the scapula).

Technique: Needle Jiafeng perpendicularly 0.3 *cun* deep and other points in conventional technique. Apply moderate stimulation to the points. Retain the needle for 15 minutes. Conduct the treatment once a day or once every other day, 10 treatments being one course. For neck pain, the effective treatment rate is 97.6%.

(4) Combining the Principal Point with Supplementary Points

Points: Main point: Dazhui (GV 14). Supplementary points: Jianyu (LI 15) and Quchi (LI 11) for shoulder, arm pain and numbness; Waiguan (TE 5) and Hegu (LI 4) for finger numbness.

Technique: Rapidly puncture Dazhui (GV 14), and then slowly push the needle down to 1.5-*cun* depth (depending on the body composition of the patient) to cause needling sensation. At the time of insertion, the needle is inserted slightly upward. After the sensation is obtained, guide the needle tip downward. Then, with the thumb and index finger, apply rapid lift-thrust stimulation in small amplitude so as to induce soreness and numbness moving down along the Governor Vessel. Thereafter conduct rhythmic rotating manipulation, through which the patient feels the needling sensation radiating to the abdomen and thigh. Manipulate the needle for about 30 seconds. The needle is then retreated subcutaneously, its tip being guided toward the affected side. Conduct lift-thrust and rotating manipulation as above for one minute to induce soreness and numbness to the shoulder and arm, then remove the needle. Needle the supplementary points in a conventional way. Apply the treatment twice a week, 10 sessions constituting one course. It is considered ineffective if three courses of treatment have been applied without pronounced improvement of the condition.

2. MOXIBUSTION

(1) Warm Needle Moxibustion

Point: Neck Jiaji

Technique: Select Neck Jiaji points level with cervical vertebrae 3, 4 for neck pain and occipital pain; select those level with CV 4, 5 for pain radiating along lateral aspect of the upper arm and radial side of the forearm; for pain and numbness radiating along the above mentioned line and to the thumb and index finger, select Jiaji points level with CV 5, 6; and select those level with CV 6, 7 for the numbness radiating along the arm to the index finger and middle finger. Choose Jiaji in line with CV7 and T1 for numbness and pain extending to the small finger. In the treatment, insert a 1.5-*cun* filiform needle into each point by twisting technique. After the needling sensation is obtained, apply even movement manipulation, and then retain the needle. Place a moxa stick to the handle of the needle, and ignite from the bottom (the end near the skin). Treat each point with two pieces of moxa stick to cause skin redness in the local area. Apply the treatment once a day, 10 treatments constituting one course.

(2) Moxibustion with Moxa Box

Points: Neck Jiaji and tender spot

Technique: Instruct the patient to assume prone posture with the neck exposed. Put two ignited pieces of 2-*cun* moxa stick into the box. Place the box over the neck for moxibustion.

(3) Indirect Moxa Cone Moxibustion Insulated with Ginger

Points: Main point: Neck Jiaji. Supplementary points: Dazhui (GV 14), Jianjing (GB21) and Jianyu (LI 15).

Technique: Select three to five points in each session and conduct indirect moxibustion. Treat each point with five cones in total. Apply the treatment once a day, 10 sessions constituting one course.

3. BLEEDING METHOD

Point: Taiyang (Extra) and Chize (LU 5)

Technique: Prick the points bilaterally with a three-edged needle to cause bleeding. This method may alleviate neck pain, numbness, etc.

4. Puncturing the Nerve Trunk

Point: Jingcongdian (the middle point of the posterior border of m. sternocladomustoidus)

Technique: The patient should be in a sitting position, with the head turned to the opposite site of the point to be punctured. After the needle is punctured into the point, turn it to the posterosuperior direction to induce electric sensation to the occipital region; then, change the direction of the needle posteroinferiorly to cause the electro-shock sensation to radiate to the clavicle and shoulder region. Soon after the needling sensation is obtained, remove the needle. Apply the treatment once a day, 10 treatments constituting one course.

5. ELECTRIC ACUPUNCTURE

Points: Neck Jiaji, Tianzhu (BL 10), Fengchi (GB20), Dazhui (GV 14), Dazhu (BL 11), Jugu (LI 16), Quchi (LI 11), Waiguan (TE 5) and Hegu (LI 4).

Technique: In each treatment, select five or six points, which should be rotated. Take Jiaji point as the principal one and the distant point as the supplementary one. After the needling sensation is detected, connect the electro-stimulator to the needles with the negative pole to the principal point and the positive pole to the supplementary point. Set the frequency at 200-250 times/min and the volume to a comfortable level for the patient. Treat once daily, each session lasting for 30 minutes. A total of 15 sessions constitute one course, and there should be a break of four to five days between courses. The effective treatment rate for cervical spondylosis is 93 %.

6. HYDRO-ACUPUNCTURE

Point: Neck Jiaji (CV 3-7)

Technique: Select compound red sage injection or Guning injection for hydro-acupuncture. In each treatment choose 1 or 2 points and inject 1-2 ml to each point. Generally, after two to four courses of treatment, the pain should be basically under control and functional activity steadily improved.

7. ELECTRO-STIMULATION THERAPY

Points: Neck and scapular region

Technique: Place one electrode at the side of the 4th and 5th cervical vertebrae, but later on move the electrode along the supraspinous muscle; lay another electrode at Jianzhen (SI 9) and move it later on to the deltoid muscle, the lateral border of greater pectoral muscle and the medial aspect of the scapula. Apply electro-stimulation with the electrode for about one minute at each location.

[REMARKS]

1. For this condition, acupuncture therapy is obviously effective for alleviating headache, neck, shoulder and back pain as well as pain

of the upper limb.

2. According to the pathological condition of the patient, massage, traction, iontophoresis and functional exercises may be combined with acupuncture treatment, so that the clinic therapeutic effect will be improved.

TORTICOLLIS

[INTRODUCTION]

Torticollis is clinically manifested as an awry neck with stiffness, soreness and pain, and inability to turn the neck freely; in severe cases, the pain may involve the shoulder, back and upper limb of the affected side. It is usually induced by an awkward sleeping position, by neck sprain or attack of wind and cold, which disturbs the normal movement of *qi* and blood in the meridians and collaterals, leading to *qi* and blood stagnation and resulting in muscular spasm. Treatment is directed toward relaxing the muscles and facilitating blood circulation, dispersing wind and opening the collaterals. The points of the Governor Vessel, of Taiyang and Shaoyang meridians are chiefly selected in the treatment, such as Fengchi (GB 20), Tianzhu (BL 10), Dazhui (GV 14), Juegu (GB 39), Houxi (SI 3), Waiguan (TE 5) and Luozhen (extra). Acupuncture of the reducing technique, moxibustion and/or cupping may be applied together.

[CLINICAL EXPERIENCE]

1. CONVENTIONAL ACUPUNCTURE

(1) Puncturing Luozhen (extra)

Points: Luozhen (located some 0.5 *cun* proximal to the metacarpophalangeal joint of the 2nd and 3rd metacarpal bones)

Technique: Puncture the point 0.5-0.8 *cun* deep and manipulate the needle continuously in a twirling technique until the symptoms are alleviated or disappear, then remove the needle. Treat the left point for an inability to turn the neck to the right and vice versa.

(2) Selection of Distal Point

Points: Xuangzhong (GB 39) and Lieque (LU 7)

Technique: If the awry neck is toward the left, puncture the point on the right side, and vice versa. Puncture Xuangzhong (GB 39) perpendicularly 0.8 *cun* deep in the reducing method, and Lieque (LU7) obliquely 0,5 *cun* deep. Retain the needles for 10 to 20 minutes.

(3) Needling Associated with Movement of the Affected Region

Point: Xiadu (located between the heads of the 4th and 5th metacarpal bones)

Technique: Needle the point on the affected side with oblique insertion 1-1.2 *cun* deep toward the palm. After the needling sensation is obtained, conduct lift-thrust and twirling manipulation with big amplitude for one or two minutes, while telling the patient to move the neck. Retain the needle in place for 10 to 15 minutes. Generally, one or two treatments should be sufficient to cure the disorder.

(4) Puncturing Yanglao (SI 6)

Technique: Needle the point on the left side for pain on the right side of the neck, and vice versa. Apply strong stimulation to the point with lift-thrust and twirling manipulation. Instruct the patient to turn the neck while stimulating the point. This treatment has satisfactory effect.

(5) Puncturing Houxi (SI 3) Bilaterally

Technique: Needle the point perpendicular 0.3-0.5 *cun* deep with strong stimulation. After the needle sensation of soreness, numbness and distension appears, retain the needle in the point for 20 minutes. Meanwhile, ask the patient to move the neck, or connect the electro-stimulator to the needle. One or two treatments may cure the disorder.

(6) Combination of the Anterior and Posterior Points

Points: Chengjiang (CV 24) and Fengfu (GV 16)

Technique: Puncture Chengjiang (CV 24) first, and then Fengfu (GV 16). Needle the two points in the reducing method. After the needling sensation is obtained, retain the needle in the point for five minutes.

2. MOXIBUSTION

(1) Mild Warmth Moxibustion with Moxa Stick

Points: Local tender spot, Fengchi (GB 20), Tianzhu (BL10), Jianzhongshu (SI 15), Dazhui (GV 14) and Houxi (SI 3).

Technique: Treat mainly the local points. In each session, select three or four points and conduct moxibustion over each point for 15 to 30 minutes. Treat once or twice a day, three treatments constituting one course.

(2) Warm Needle Moxibustion

Points: Ah-shi in the local area, Fengchi (GB 20), Dazhui (GV 14) and Dazhu (BL 11).

Technique: After needling sensation is obtained, put a 1.5-*cun* moxa stick on the handle of the needle, and light. Treat each point with two moxa sticks in one treatment and conduct the treatment once a day. For severe case, perform the treatment twice a day.

3. ELECTRIC ACUPUNCTURE

Points: Luozhen (extra) and Houxi (SI 3)

Technique: Puncture the bilateral points perpendicularly with filiform needles and connect the electric stimulator to the bilateral points after the needling sensation of soreness and numbness and pain are obtained. Apply the electro-stimulation for 15 to 20 minutes with a frequency of 40-50 times /min. Set the intensity of the stimulation to the tolerance of the patient. Instruct the patient to move the neck during needle retention.

4. AURICULAR THERAPY

Points: Neck, cervical vertebra and tender spot. Add liver and gallbladder points for problems with the Shaoyang meridian, and the small intestine and bladder for problems with the Taiyang meridian.

Technique: Apply strong stimulation to the point with filiform needles, which should be retained for 60 minutes. During the period of retention, instruct the patient to move the neck. Generally, the symptom will be obviously alleviated after needling. However, the symptoms may relapse when the needles are being removed. It is, therefore, advisable to retain the needles for a longer period of time rather than remove them shortly after needling.

5. CUTANEOUS PUNCTURE

Points: Fengfu (GV 16), Yamen (GV 15) Fengchi (GB 20), Tianzhu (BL 10), Jianjing (GB 21) and Jianwaishu (SI 14).

Technique: Apply the treatment in the order of puncturing from the upper point to the lower point, and from the medial to the lateral. It is appropriate to tap the points until the skin becomes red, but without bleeding. Combination of cutaneous tapping with cupping may enhance the therapeutic effect.

6. MAGNETIC THERAPY

Points: Tender point of the neck and Wailaogong (extra)

Technique: Conduct the treatment with a magnetic vibrator that exerts dual effect, magnetism and massage, achieving rapid pain relief and anti-inflammation effect. Treat each point for 15 minutes and once a day.

7. HYDRO-ACUPUNCTURE

Points: Ah-shi, neck Jiaji and Fengchi (GB 20).

Technique: Select two to three points each time. Inject compound red sage root extract, 0.5 ml, into each point. Apply the treatment once every other day.

8. ELECTRO-STIMULATION THERAPY

Points: ① Yanglao (SI 6), Xinshe (located directly below Fengchi (GB 20), 1.5 *cun* posterior to the posterior hairline), Waiguan (TE 5) and Jianzhongshu (SI 15). ② Fengchi (GB 20), Jianjing (GB 21) and Jianwaishu (SI 14).

Technique: Use induced current stimulator to stimulate the points rhythmically with the positive pole connected to the points of Group 1, and negative pole to Group 2, each time stimulating gently for three to five seconds. Treatment is conducted once a day and five to 10 minutes in total. Three to five sessions constitute one course.

9. FINGER ACUPOINT PRESSURE

Points: Tianzhu (BL 10), Fengfu (GV 16) and Tianzong (SI 11).

Technique: Treat the points of the affected side. Press Tianzhu (BL 10) with the thumb and Fengfu (GV 16) with the index finger of one hand, and press Tianzong (SI 11) with the thumb of the other hand. While pressing, knead the point as well. The acupoint pressure will induce obvious soreness and a numbness sensation. Apply acu-pressure of the three points simultaneously for five minutes, by which time the symptoms will be alleviated.

Point: Shousanli (LI 10)

Technique: Apply acu-pressure with thumb at Shousanli (LI 10) of the affected side for five to10 minutes so as to produce soreness, numbness, distension and pain in the local region. Instruct the patient to move the neck left and right.

10. BLEEDING METHOD ASSOCIATED WITH CUPPING AND MOXIBUSTION

Points: Tender spot, Fengchi (GB 20) and Jianjing (GB 21) (selecting all the points on the affected side)

Technique: Find out the obvious tender spot on the affected side of the neck, and conduct conventional disinfection of the point to be bled. Make three to five pricks rapidly with a three-edged needle at the tender spot to let out 2-5 ml of blood. Wipe away the blood and add cup with the flash fire cupping method to the pricked point. Retain the cup at the point for 10 to 20 minutes, during which prick Fengchi (GB 20) and Jianjing (GB21) to let out blood. After the cup has been removed, apply mild warmth moxibustion with a moxa stick at the cupped area. Conduct the treatment once a day. In general, one to three sessions can cure the illness.

[REMARKS]

1. Acupuncture and moxibustion are quite effective therapies for

torticollis. Generally speaking, only one to three sessions of therapy may heal the acute condition, but chronic case needing a few more treatments can also be managed with better therapeutic effect.

2. In the treatment of an acute condition, the distal point is needled first in the reducing method, while the patient is instructed to move the neck. After manipulation, the needle is retained for 10 to 15 minutes. Then, the local point is punctured as well. This method may increase the therapeutic effect.

BACK PAIN

[INTRODUCTION]

This condition is induced either by exogenous or endogenous factors. The exogenous factor mainly refers to the pathogenic wind-cold invading the Taiyang Meridian, causing blockage in the meridians and collaterals, so that circulation of *qi* and blood becomes retarded, and stiffness and pain of the back with involvement of neck and scapula appear. The endogenous factor refers to *qi* and blood stagnation, which is frequently the cause with an old or weak patient who usually suffers from some chronic disease. As *qi* of the old or weak patient is generally deficient, the blood lacks the energy so the circulation is sluggish, resulting in *qi* and blood stagnation; and backache ensues, which is characterized by aggravation of pain after sleep and alleviation after motor activities. Treatment of this condition is aimed at removing the obstruction from the meridians and collaterals with the points Dazhui (GV 14), Shenzhu (GV 12), Zhiyang (GV 9), Jiaji of the back region, Ah-shi, Weizhong (BL 40) and Kunlun (BL60). In the treatment, the reducing method is applied for excess syndrome and reinforcing technique for deficiency syndrome. Moreover, moxibustion or cupping may be added in addition to acupuncture. In modern medicine back pain is often seen in the spondylitis, displacement of spine, occult cleft spine, etc.

[CLINICAL EXPERIENCE]

1. CONVENTIONAL ACUPUNCTURE

(1) Puncturing Two Points
Points: Dazhui (GV 14) and Zhongzhu (TE 3)
Technique: Tell the patient to sit erect. Puncture Dazhui (GV 14) 0.5-1 *cun* deep with needle tip slightly upward. After needling sensation is obtained, remove the needle. Puncture Zhongzhu (TE 3) perpendicularly with the needle retained in the point for 20 minutes. This method is indicated for heaviness of the back.

(2) Puncturing Single Point
Point: Jingqu (LU 8)
Technique: Puncture the point bilaterally 0.3 *cun* deep, and manipulate the needle with the twirling method for two minutes. This is used for back spasms.

(3) Combination of Anterior Point and Posterior Point
Points: Yamen (GV 15) and Renzhong (GV 26)
Technique: Puncture Yamen (GV 15) 0.5 *cun* deep; manipulate the needle in the rotating method for one minute. Puncture Renzhong (GV 26) 0.2 *cun* deep and conduct twirling manipulation for one minute. This method is applicable for stiff back.

(4) Contralateral Puncture
Point: Location in the thoracic region corresponding to the tender spot in the back
Technique: Find out the tenderest spot in the back, and then puncture the point in the thoracic region corresponding to the tender spot. The more accurate the location, the more effective the treatment is. Needle the point obliquely or superficially. Deep insertion of the needle is not allowed.

2. MOBILE CUPPING

Point: Pain spots at the back
Technique: Tell the patient to take a prone position. Put some Vaseline or massage lotion on the back. Apply cupping with a cup on the back with weak suction to the skin. With the help of Vaseline lubrication move the cup up and down to cause redness of the skin.

This method is applicable for the back pain over a large area.

3. HOT-RED NEEDLE PUNCTURING

Points: Jiaji points of the affected region

Technique: Select a needle 0.5 mm in diameter for hot-red needling therapy. Heat the needle over an alcoholic burner, and puncture the bilateral Jiaji points of the affected region deeply and rapidly. Treatment is conducted once every other day, with seven treatments making up one course. This is used for hyper plastic rachitis and tuberculosis of the spine. In the treatment, apply strict disinfection of the point and tell the patient to protect the punctured hole from infection. The needle must be fired until it is bright red, otherwise it will be difficult to insert it into the point and remove it out without cause severe pain. Needle removal should be done rapidly and forcefully so as to avoid it sticking to the muscle.

4. HYDRO-ACUPUNCTURE

Points: Shenshu (BL 23) and Dachangshu (BL 25)

Technique: Mix 2 ml of compound Chinese Angelicae Synesis injection, 2 ml of Guning injection, 100 ml of vitamin B_1, and 0.1 ml of vitamin B_{12} and inject the mixture into the bilateral points of Shenshu (BL 23) and Dachangshu (BL 25). Inject once a day or once every other day. It is suitable for regressive rachitis.

5. COMBINATION OF ACUPUNCTURE AND MEDICINAL APPLICATION ON ACU-POINT

Points: For medicinal application (moxibustion): the affected region of the spine; for acupuncture: Dazhu (BL 11), Yanglingquan (GB 34), Xuanzhong (GB 39), Fengchi (GB 20), Fengfu (GV 16), Shengzhu (GV 12), Waiguan (TE 5), Fengshi (GB 31), Zusanli (ST 36) and Sanyinjiao (SP 6).

[REMARKS]

1. It takes a relatively a long period of treatment to obtain therapeutic effect for back pain encountered in hyperplasic rachitis and spinal hypertrophy, etc.

2. The patient should avoid getting cold or living in a moist place.

SCIATICA

[INTRODUCTION]

Sciatica may be classified into two patterns, namely, the primary and the secondary. However, according to the affected location, it may be classified into nervous root and nervous trunk patterns. This condition is mainly manifested as pain of the lower back and leg that radiates from the unilateral side of the lower back and buttock to the posterior aspect of the thigh, popliteal space, the lateral aspect of the low leg to the lateral side of foot. The pain may differ in nature and intensity, being aggravated by a cough or forceful exertion in bending the lower back. Chinese medicine attributes the disease to exposure of wind-cold-damp that blockades the meridians and collaterals causing impairment of *qi* and blood circulation. It may be induced by falling down or by sprain and contusion, so that the meridians and collaterals are injured and the circulation of *qi* and blood obstructed. Treatment is directed toward eliminating wind and cold, removing damp and opening the collateral, moving *qi* and blood with the points chiefly selected from Taiyang and Shaoyang meridians of foot, such as Shenshu (BL 23), Dachangshu (BL25), Baliao (BL 31-34), Huantiao (GB 30), Zhibian (BL 54), Chengfu (BL 36), Yinmen (BL 37), Weizhong (BL 40), Yanglingquan (GB 34), Chengshan (BL 57), Juegu (GB 39) and Kunlun (BL 60). Treatment is conducted in a combination of moxibustion with acupuncture, the latter applied in the reducing technique.

[CLINICAL EXPERIENCE]

1. CONVENTIONAL ACUPUNCTURE

(1) Puncturing Weizhong (BL 40) While Raising the Leg
   Points: Dachangshu (BL 25), Zhibian (BL 54), Weizhong (BL 40)

and Yanglingquan (GB 34)

Technique: Ask the patient to assume a prone position, and puncture Dachangshu (BL 25) perpendicularly with a filiform needle, 2-2.5 *cun* deep, in the reducing technique. Guide the needle sensation to radiate downward to the heel or the toes. Puncture Zhibian (BL 54) perpendicularly 3-3.5 *cun* deep to cause the needle sensation down to the toes with contraction of the leg three times. Instruct the patient to change position from prone to supine and puncture Weizhong (BL 40) while the leg is up. Manipulate the needle in the lift-thrust reducing technique to cause a sensation extending to the toes and induce contraction of the lower limb three times. Needle Yanglingquan (GB 34) in a supine position obliquely downward to a depth of 2 *cun* with the lift-thrust reducing technique to make the sensation move to the toes. For a stubborn case, add Renzhong (GV26), which is needled with sparrow pecking manipulation technique until the eyes are full of tears.

(2) Puncturing Huanzhongshang (extra)

Point: Huanzhongshang [located 2.5 *cun* superior to Huantiao (GB 30)].

Technique: Tell the patient to lie down in a recumbent position. Puncture deeply to a depth of 4-6 *cun* to cause the needle sensation down to the toes. Apply the needling once daily.

(3) Puncturing Xiashandian (extra) and Other Points

Points: Main points: Xiashandian [located 6 *cun* lateral to the 4th caudal vertebra, 3 *cun* lateral to Zhibian (BL 54) at the border of middle gluteal muscle, least gluteal muscle, greater sciatic notch, forming a triangle with Zhibian (BL 54) and Huantiao (GB 30)]. Supplementary points: Wangu (SI 4), Yanglingquan (GB 34) and Kunlun (BL 60).

Technique: While puncturing Xiashandian point, the patient is standing in front of an object which is as high as the hip, with the head bending down and the feet 30 cm apart. The lower legs extend with backward force, the hands are on the front object, and the buttock muscles are relaxed. When the patient is standing steadily, start the needling. Use a 4-6 *cun* needle (Size: Nos.28-30) to puncture the point, making the needle sensation radiate to the heel and toes without retaining the needle in the point. Puncture other points in conventional way and retain the needles in the points for 20 to 30 minutes.

(4) Puncturing the Tender Spot

Point: Tender spot in lumbosacral and buttock regions.

Technique: Instruct the patient to assume a prone position, and press both sides of the lumbosacral vertebrae to find the tender spots. Puncture the tender spots of the lumbosacral region 0.8-1.2 *cun* deep in lift-thrust and needle hand scraping manipulation. Retain the needle for 15 to 30 minutes, re-manipulating the needle once every five to 10 minutes. Conduct the treatment once a day. When the symptoms are alleviated, give treatment once every other day, 10 sessions constituting one course. This method is mainly applied for sciatica resulting from lumbar vertebral hyperplasia and prolapse of the lumbar intervertebral disk.

(5) Selecting Shu-Stream Point

Points: Zhongzhu (TE 3) and Houxi (SI 3)

Technique: Puncture Zhongzhu (TE 3), the Shu-Stream point of Triple-Energizer meridian of Hand Shaoyang, and Houxi (SI 3) respectively with a one-*cun* filiform needle. Stimulate the points strongly and retain the needle in place for 20 minutes.

(6) Puncturing Shuangyang (extra)

Point: Shuangyang [2 points located respectively one *cun* above and one *cun* below the mid-point between Huantiao (GB 30) and Fengshi (GB 31)]

Technique: Conduct conventional disinfection of Shuangyang, then needle the points respectively to a depth of 2.5-3 *cun* with moderate stimulation. Guide the needling sensation of the upper point to the lumbar and hip region and the lower point down to the toes. Retain the needle for 10 to 20 minutes. Give treatment once a day, 10 sessions constituting one course. After the removal of the needles, apply flash-fire cupping for 10 minutes.

(7) Heat Producing Needling

Points: Zhibian (BL 54) and Ah-shi

Technique: Ask the patient to adopt a prone position. Locate the point precisely. Puncture Zhibian (BL 54) and the tender point at the buttock region perpendicularly with a filiform needle so that the needling sensation radiates to the lower limb, and conduct "setting the mountain on fire" (heat producing) manipulation so as to activate blood circulation and resolve blood stasis. This is applied for sciatica induced by hernia of the intervertebral disk.

2. MOXIBUSTION

Points: Shenshu (BL 23), Dachangshu (BL 25), Baliao (BL 31-34), Huantiao (GB30), Chengfu (BL 36), Yanglingquan (GB 34), Yangjiao (GB 35) and Xuanzhong (GB39).

Technique: After the needling sensation is obtained in the acupuncture treatment, apply warm needle moxibustion on three to five points selected from the above prescription in each session. Usually the moxibustion lasts 20 minutes. Give treatment once a day, 10 treatments making up one course.

3. CUPPING

Point: Painful region of the affected side

Technique: First apply flash cupping at the painful region of the lumbus and the painful region of the lower limb so as to cause warmth and slight redness of the skin, then leave a few cups at the tender spots for 10 to 15 minutes.

4. BLEEDING

Points: Yaoshu (GV2), Weizhong (BL 40), Yangjiao (GB 35) and Qiuxu (GB 40).

Technique: Prick the points of the affected side with a three-edged needle to let out blood. In the first session, pain remission is achieved by letting off much blood. Conduct the treatment once a day. After the pain eases, apply bleeding once every other day.

5. STIMULATING NERVE TRUNK WITH ELECTRIC ACU-PUNCTURE

Point: Projecting point of sciatic nerve (Located slightly inferior to 1/3 of the line between posterosuperior iliac spine and greater trochanter), Weizhong (BL 40) or Chengshan (BL 57).

Technique: In puncturing the projecting point of the sciatic nerve, use a 4-*cun* needle to puncture the point at an angle of 70°, the needle tip slightly toward the medial of the buttock, and the electric-like needle sensation radiating down to the toes. Then, use the electric stimulating apparatus to perform electro-stimulation with the negative pole connected to the projecting point and the positive pole to Weizhong (GL 40) or Chengshang (BL 57). Apply the treatment once a day, each session lasting 10 or 15 minutes.

6. AURICULAR THERAPY

Point: Sciatic nerve

Technique: Needle the ear point of the affected side first. If there is no effect, or the effect is not satisfactory, needle the point in the other ear. Apply strong stimulation to the point and retain the needle for one or two hours. During the needle retention period, instruct the patient to move the affected limb so as to increase the therapeutic effect. Conduct the treatment once daily or once every other day. In general, the initial treatment is very effective, but after some sessions, the effect of the therapy is not so obvious as that of the early day treatment.

7. HYDRO-ACUPUNCTURE

Points: Huantiao (GB 30) and Yinmen (BL 37)

Technique: Puncture Huantiao (GB30) or Yinmen (GL 37) with the injection composed of 2 ml of Chinese Angelicae Synesis, 100 mg of vitamin B_1 and 10% glucose liquid to make 20 ml volume in total. The needle used in the treatment is same as that used for lumbar puncture.

8. COMBINED TREATMENT

(1) Contralateral Puncture and Cupping

Point: The contralateral point on the healthy side corresponding to the tender spot of the affected limb.

Technique: The patient is in a prone posture with the lower limbs extending straight. The practitioner uses his/her thumb or index finger to press-push from Chengfu (BL 36) down to Kunlun (BL 60) to find the tender spot. In searching for the tender spot on the lower limb, lay stress on the posterior lateral aspect of the thigh, lateral side of the popliteal space, posterior lateral aspect of the lower leg as well as the buttocks and lumbosacral region. The contralateral point on the healthy side corresponding to the tender spot on the affected side is the location to be treated. The proper depth of puncture is that at which the needling sensation is obtained. Retain the needle for 30 to 60 minutes, manipulating the needle every 10 to 20 minutes. Concurrently, apply cupping over the tender region of the affected side along the lateral posterior aspect of the buttock, the thigh and the lower leg for 10 to 15 minutes. Apply the treatment once a day, 10 sessions constituting one course, with a break of three to five days between courses,

(2) Electric Acupuncture Combined with Moxibustion

Points: Group 1: Shenshu (BL23), Baliao (BL 31-34), Zhibian (BL 54), Weizhong (BL 40), and Chengshan (BL 57). Group 2: Huantiao (GB30), Fengshi (GB 31), Yanglingquan (GB 34), Juegu (GB 39) and Kunlun (BL 60). Group 3: Biguan (ST 31), Zusanli (ST 36), Shangjuexue (ST 37) and Chongyang (ST 42).

Technique: In the first session, puncture two or three points of Group 1; in the 2nd session, treat two or three points of Group 2; and, in the 3rd session, needle two or three points of Group 3. After conventional electro-acupuncture treatment, add a moxa box containing two pieces of 1.5-*cun* ignited moxa stick over the treated points. The treatment is completed when the moxa sticks burn off.

(3) Acupuncture Combined with Infrared Radiation

Points: Shenshu (BL 23), Huantiao (GB30), Chengshan (BL 57) and Kunlun (BL 60), all the points treated bilaterally.

Technique: Instruct the patient to take a prone position. Apply strong manipulation to the respective points three times after the needling sensation is obtained. Retain the needles for 30 minutes, and concurrently add infrared radiation to the painful region of the affected limb. Conduct the treatment once every other day.

[REMARKS]

1. Acupuncture exerts anesthetic effect in varying degrees on sciatica induced by various causes. Of the cases treated, sciatic neuritis is treated with best therapeutic effect. However, the therapeutic effect is not so good for nerve root pressed type sciatica, especially those patients suffering from prolapse of the lumbar intervertebral disc. If naprapathy is added, the effect will be improved.

2. If electro-stimulation is applied to the nerve trunk, the stimulation should not too strong, so as to avoid impairing the nerve.

3. In the acute stage of the condition, the patient is advised to take bed rest. When the condition is better, the patient is encouraged to combine some proper motor activities in addition to acupuncture treatment.

4. The lower limbs and the lumbar region should be kept warm. It is better for the patient to lie on a hard bed (wood bed) and have a small cushion under the lumbus while lying on the back.

SEMINAL EMISSION

[INTRODUCTION]

Seminal emission refers to the outflow of seminal fluid in the absence of sexual activities. In Chinese medicine it is called *yijing* when it happens during dreaming and *huajing* (spermatorrhea) in conscious state. Clinically, it is associated with headache, insomnia, lassitude, soreness of the lower back, etc. In Chinese medicine the mechanism of the diseases is attributable to the incomplete closure of the seminal chamber, the condition being either of deficiency or excess. The deficient condition may be induced by indulgence in sexual activity that impairs the kidneys, and the seminal chamber is not well closed; or consumption of heart *yin* leads to the *yin* deficiency and hyperactivity of fire, so that there is disharmony between the heart and the kidneys and the seminal chamber is disturbed by the fire. The excess variety is provoked by downward flow of damp-heat to the lower energizer to disturb the seminal chamber. As a result, the seminal chamber fails to be controlled and seminal emission arises. Treatment of the illness is directed toward tonifying the kidneys and tranquilizing the mind, consolidating the seminal chamber and clearing damp-heat. Back-Shu points and the points from the bladder meridian, the Conception Vessel and the three *yin* meridians may be selected, such as Shenshu (BL 23), Guanyuan (CV 4), Sanyinjiao (SP 6) and Taixi (KI 3). For the syndrome of kidney deficiency with weak restriction of the seminal chamber, Zhishi (BL 52), Mingmen (GV 4), and Qihai (CV 6) are added and treated both by acupuncture and moxibustion. For the pattern of disharmony between the heart and the kidneys, Shenmen (HT 7), Xinshu (BL 15), and Zhongfeng (LR 4) are supplemented and treated with needling alone. For the downward flow of damp-heat syndrome, which is essentially handled by needling, Baliao (BL 31-34), Yinlingquan (SP 9) and Neiting (ST 44) are added in the treatment. For excess syndrome, reducing technique is applied, and the deficiency variety is managed with reinforcing technique. In modern medicine, neurosis, spermatocystitis, orchitis and prostatitis may be encountered with seminal emission.

[CLINICAL EXPERIENCE]

1. CONVENTIONAL ACUPUNCTURE

(1) Reducing Method of Filiform Needle Puncture
  Points: Guanyuan (CV 4) and Xingjian (LR 2)
  Technique: Puncture Guanyuan (CV 4) with a 1.5-*cun* needle and guide the needling sensation to the external genitalia region. Needle Xingjian (LR 2) with a one-*cun* needle. Puncture the two points with the reducing method. Apply the treatment once daily for five days in succession. This method is conducted for long-term seminal emission in dreaming.

(2) Reinforcing Method of Filiform Needle Puncture
  Points: Yingu (KI 10) and Zhishi (BL 52)
  Technique: While locating Yingu (KI 10), ask the patient to assume a supine posture with knees flexed and soles facing each other.

Puncture the point between two tendons, and apply reinforcing manipulation after the needling sensation is obtained. Retain the needle for 15 minutes, and then puncture Zhishi (BL 52) in the reinforcing method after the patient changes from a supine to a prone position. Retain the needle for 15 minutes.

(3) Puncturing the Point in Twisting Method
   Point: Huiyin (CV1)
   Technique: Tell the patient to assume a supine posture with the lower limbs slightly bent. Puncture the point perpendicularly 1.5-2 *cun* deep, manipulating the needle in the twisting method without lift-thrust manipulation. Needling stimulation tolerable to patient is regarded as appropriate. Apply the treatment once a day or once every other day. In each session, keep the needle in the point for 20-30 minutes, and manipulate it once every five to seven minutes.

(4) Puncturing Before Sleep
   Points: Sanyinjiao (SP 6), left side
   Technique: Conduct the treatment for 30 minutes prior to sleep. Needle the point of the left side, retaining the needle for 15-20 minutes, during which apply the rotating method of reinforcement. Giving the treatment every evening for three to five days in succession is beneficial for spermatorrhea during dreaming.

(5) Puncturing Baliao (BL 31-34) as the Main Points
   Points: Main point: Baliao (BL31-34). Supplementary points: Guanyuan (CV 4), Zhongji (CV 3), Mingmen (GV 4) and Shenshu (BL 23) for kidney deficiency; Qimen (LR 14) and Sanyinjiao (SP 6) for liver *qi* stagnation syndrome; Zusanli (ST 36), Zhongwan (CV 12) and Sanyinjiao (SP 6) for spleen deficiency syndrome; Shenmen (HT 7) and Neiguan (PC 6) for heart deficiency; Zusanli (ST 36) and Yinlingquan (SP 9) for damp-heat pattern.
   Technique: Locate Baliao (BL 31-34) with the help of the middle finger lying at the spinous process of the 2nd sacral vertebra, the small finger being at the hiatus sacralis. Moreover, keep the index finger, middle finger, ring finger and the small finger equally spaced apart. The points are located where the fingertips point. Insert the needle into Baliao (BL 31-34) swiftly, conducting lift-thrust and rotating ma-

nipulation for three to five seconds. Treat the other points either in reducing manipulation for the excess syndrome or reinforcing technique for the deficiency syndrome based on the pathological condition.

2. MOXIBUSTION

(1) Moxibustion at Ququan (LR 8)
Point: Ququan (LR 8)

Technique: Conduct moxibustion at Ququan (LR 8) with five to 10 cones in one session. Apply the treatment once every other day.

(2) Indirect moxibustion insulated with salt
Point: Shenque (CV 8)

Technique: Take proper amount of table salt, grinding it into powder, and lay the salt on the navel. The salt surface should be level with the abdominal skin. Place five to 30 moxa cones in the size of a soybean or half core of a date onto the salt. Apply the treatment once a day or once every other day. Ten treatments constitute one course, with a break of five days between courses.

3. AURICULAR THERAPY

Points: Seminal Chamber (Jinggong), Endocrine, Kidney, Heart, Mid-tragus

Technique: In each session, puncture two to three points with filiform needles, applying strong stimulation for spermatorrhea in dreaming and mild stimulation for spermatorrhea happening in a conscious state. Retain the needles for 20-30 minutes. Conduct the treatment once a day, 10 treatments making up one course. It is also applicable to embed the intradermal needle into the points for three to five days.

4. CUTANEOUS NEEDLE THERAPY

Point: The back and the lumbar portion of the Governor Vessel and the bladder meridian

Technique: Apply mild tapping with a cutaneous needle along the selected portion of the meridians until the skin becomes slightly red. Conduct the treatment once a day or once every other day for 20 minutes.

5. HYDRO-ACUPUNCTURE

Points: Qihai (CV 6), Zhongji (CV 3) and Guila (ST 29).

Technique: Inject the mixture containing 100 ml of vitamin B_1, 0.1 ml of vitamin B_{12}, 2 ml of compound Chinese Angelica Synesis injection, and 1 ml of 1% procaine into 2 of the points listed above in each session. Treat the points in turn and conduct the treatment once a day.

6. MEDICINAL APPLICATION ON ACU-POINT

Point: Siman (KI 14)

Technique: Grind Chinese gall (Galla Chinensis) into fine powder and turn the powder into paste with normal saline solution. Put the paste onto a 3-4 cm-long plaster, and stuck it to Siman (KI 14). Change the medicinal plaster once every three days, three treatments constituting one course. A total of 35 cases were treated with this therapy over two or three courses, and the therapy was remarkably effective for nine cases, effective for 19 cases and not effective for seven cases.

[REMARKS]

1. Acupuncture exerts better therapeutic effect for this disorder.

2. It is preferable for the patients to adopt a recumbent posture during sleep and avoid pressing the penis by clothes or bedding. For severe case, it is advisable for the patient to sleep with the knees bent and use a wide band to hold the neck, putting the other end of the band downward around the legs so as to prevent them from extending while the patient is sleeping soundly.

IMPOTENCE

[INTRODUCTION]

Impotence refers to the inability of the young or the middle-aged man whose penis fails to become erect, or the erection is so weak that normal sexual activity is disturbed. Concomitantly, it may be associated with dizziness, tinnitus, seminal emission during dreaming, pre-ejaculation, etc. Clinically, more deficiency syndromes of the condition are encountered than excess ones. In Chinese medicine it is attributable to a decline of vital gate fire, deficiency of *qi* and blood, downward flow of damp-heat leading to sluggish tendons so that the penis fails to become erect. Treatment is directed toward tonifying *qi* and reinforcing kidneys. Points may be selected from the meridian of foot Shaoyin, the Conception Vessel, such as Shenshu (BL 23), Guanyuan (CV 4) and Sanyinjiao (SP 6). For the syndrome of decline of vital gate fire, Mingmen (GV 4) and Yaoyangguan (GV 3) are added; for deficiency of *qi* and blood syndrome, Pishu (BL 20), Weishu (BL 21) and Zusanli (ST 36) are added; and for the pattern of damp-heat in the lower energizer, Zhongji (CV 3), Yinlingquan (SP 9), Baliao (BL 31-34) and Neiting (ST 44) are supplemented. In the treatment of deficiency syndrome, the reinforcing method is adopted with heavy moxibustion; and for excess syndrome, the reducing technique is employed. Modern medicine regards this disease as sexual neurosis. It is often associated with some chronic deficient disorders.

[CLINICAL EXPERIENCE]

1. CONVENTIONAL ACUPUNCTURE

(1) Selection of Point from the Lower Abdomen
Point: Qugu (CV 2)
Technique: Puncture the point with a 1.5-2 *cun* needle. Conduct lift-thrust and twisting technique to cause the needling sensation radiate to the penis. Sometimes the glans penis may feel numb, and the penis may become erect. In the treatment, other points may be added based on the variety of syndrome.

(2) Selection of Point from the Sacral Region
Point: Ciliao (BL 32) bilateral
Technique: Instruct the patient to take a prone posture. Puncture the point 4 *cun* deep. An electric feeling may radiate down to the perineum, the external genitalia or the penis. Retain the needle for 20

minutes, and manipulate the needle once or twice.

(3) Selection of Point from the Buttocks

Point: Huanzhongshang [2.5 *cun* superior to Huantiao (GB 30)]

Technique: Puncture the point obliquely with a 5-*cun* filiform needle toward the external genitalia to a depth of 4 *cun*. Apply sparrow-pecking manipulation once or twice without twisting the needle. Remove the needle when the needling sensation reaches the external genitalia.

(4) Selection of Yangwei Point, etc.

Points: Yangwei [2.5 *cun* superior to Shenshu (BL 23), 1 *cun* lateral to the Governor Vessel], Zhongji (CV 3), Sanyinjiao (SP 6) and Zusanli (ST 36).

Technique: Needle the points with moderate stimulation. For a strong person, strong stimulation may be applied. Conduct the treatment once a day.

2.   MOXIBUSTION

(1) Moxa Cone Moxibustion

Point: Guanyuan (CV 4)

Technique: Instruct the patient to adopt a supine posture. Use some cold moxa wool to make medium-sized cones. Put a moxa cone on Guanyuan (CV 4) to perform the treatment, which is completed with 150-180 cones in one session. Apply the treatment once a week, three sessions constituting one course, and a break of one week between courses. Two courses of this therapy have been conducted in 12 cases, of which seven were cured, three showed remarkable effect, and two improved.

(2) Warming Needle Moxibustion

Point: Guanyuan (CV), Zhongji (CV 3), Taixi (KI 3) and Huiyin (CV1)

Technique: Puncture the points in an even movement except Huiyin (CV1). After the needling sensation is obtained, retain the needle and add three to five moxa cones in succession onto the handle of the needle for warming. Treat Huiyin (CV1) with a moxa stick that is held over the point. Apply the treatment once every other day.

3. SCALP ACUPUNCTURE

Points: Bilateral foot sensory area and reproductive area
Technique: Conduct the treatment once a day, seven sessions forming one course.

4. CUTANEOUS PUNCTURE

Point: Huiyin (perineum region), lumbosacral region, medial aspect of thigh
Technique: Use a plum-blossom needle to tap the above regions respectively until the skin becomes red. Apply the treatment once every other day, 10 sessions constituting one course.

5. NEEDLE EMBEDDING METHOD

Point: Sanyinjiao (SP 6)
Technique: Ask the patient to adopt a supine posture. After conventional disinfection of the point, press the perineum region with the left thumb, and instruct the patient to breathe in as much as possible and concentrate his attention on the balanus. Hold hemostatic forceps with the right hand to clap the intradermal needle, which is then embedded into Sanyinjiao (SP 6) and then somewhat rotated and kneaded so as to induce slight needling sensation. Treat both sides of the point with the intradermal needle, which is fixed with adhesive tape. Press the perineum for five minutes. The embedded needle is retained in the point for three days. After the removal of the needles, the following three days should be free of treatment.

6. HYDRO-ACUPUNCTURE

(1) Placental Injection

Points: Guanyuan (CV4) and Zhongji (CV 3)
Technique: Inject 2 ml of placental injection into one of the two points. In each session, inject one point, alternate the points and apply the treatment once every other day. Twenty sessions constitute one course.

(2) Strychnine Injection

Point: Baliao (BL 31-34)

Technique: Inject Baliao (BL 31-34) respectively with the mixture of 2 ml of strychnine, and 30 ml of 5% glucose injection. Insert the syringe needle into the foraminea sacralia posterior, and slowly push the injection into the point. The patient may experience soreness and distending sensation, and sometimes the sensation radiates to the pudendum. Apply the injection once every other day, three treatments constituting one course, with a seven-day break between courses.

7. PRICKING METHOD

Points: Shenshu (BL 23), Mingmen (GV 4), Baliao (BL 31-34), Sanjiaoshu (BL 22), Guanyuan (CV4), Dazhui (GV 14), Dazhu (BL 11) and Changqiang (GV 1).

Technique: In each session select two or three of the above points, although additional points may be added in accordance with the syndrome. Apply the treatment mainly with the Tiaoti or Tiaobai method. Treat each spot with the Tiaobai method for 5 minutes. For the deficiency patient, use a thin needle to apply the Tiaojin method, and moxibustion may be added. Prick once every three to five days, three to five treatments forming one course. This method exerts better effect for patients of hypo-sexual function and infertility due to oligospermia.

8. AURICULAR THERAPY

Points: Seminal Chamber, External Genitalia, Testis and Endocrine

Technique: Select two to four points in each session. Puncture the points in mild stimulation, retaining the needles for 20 minutes. It is also possible to treat the points with embedding needle or with semen vaccaria that is stuck to the point with adhesive tape.

[REMARKS]

1.   As this disease is mainly attributable to functional disturbance, and the patients tend to suffer fear and anxiety, it will be beneficial if the doctor provides some psychological care to the patient so as to relieve this mental stress, and offers suggestions on proper sexual activity that will favor recovery.

2. During the period of treatment, sexual activity should be restricted in order not to influence the therapeutic effect.

3. If the impotence is secondary, resulted from paraplegia or prostatitis, the primary disease should be actively treated.

MALE INFERTILITY

[INTRODUCTION]

Male infertility is often induced by oligospermia, deformity of sperms, asthnospermia, ejaculation spermatism, etc. Chinese medicine ascribes this condition to congenital deficiency, non-recovery of chronic or severe illness, or frequent masturbation, all of which lead to deficiency of kidney essence and declining of vital gate fire. Reinforcing the kidney and tonifying kidney essence may treat the condition. The Front-mu and Back-shu points as well as some points from the Conception Vessel and the Shaoyin meridian may be selected, such as Shenshu (BL 23), Zhishi (BL 52), Mingmen (GV 4), Baliao (BL 31-34), Guanyuan (CV 4), Zusanli (ST 36), Sanyinjiao (SP 6) and Taixi (KI3). Needling in reinforcing technique is applied, and heavy moxibustion is added on the points of the trunk. Clinically, male infertility may be sometimes attributable to kidney and liver *yin* deficiency with hyperactivity of "minister fire," for which nourishing *yin* and reducing the fire should be the therapeutic principle, and Ganshu (BL 18), Shenshu (BL 23), Yanglingquan (GB 34), Sanyinjiao (SP 6), Taichong (LR 3) and Taixi (KI 3) are punctured with even movement manipulation.

[CLINICAL EXPERIENCE]

1. CONVENTIONAL ACUPUNCTURE

(1) Reinforcing Method with Lift-Thrust and Twisting Manipulation
   Points: ① Mingmen (GV4), Shenshu (BL 23), Zhishi (BL 52) and Taixi (KI 3). ② Guanyuan (CV 4), Qihai (CV6), Zusanli (ST 36) and

Sanyinjiao (SP 6).

Technique: Rotate the two groups of points, and apply the treatment once a day. Puncture the points superficially with thin needles, and conduct lift-thrust, twisting reinforcing manipulation. The treatment has certain effect for oligospermia, asthnospermia attributable to kidney *yang* deficiency and vital gate fire declining patterns.

(2) Reducing Method with Lift-Thrust and Twisting Manipulation
   Points: Zhongji (CV3), Xingjian (LR 2) and Sanyinjiao (SP 6)

Technique: Treat the points on both sides with the reducing method of lift-thrust twisting manipulation. Retain the needles for 20 minutes. Give the treatment once daily, five treatments constituting one course, with a break of two to three days between courses. This method is applicable for ejaculation spermatism attributable to liver *qi* stagnation transforming into fire.

2. MOXIBUSTION

(1) Moxibustion with Moxa Stick
   Points: Zhongji (CV 3) and Sanyinjiao (SP 6)

Technique: Apply indirect moxibustion with a moxa stick that is held about 1 *cun* over the skin and moved up and down. Treat Zhongji (CV3) and bilateral Sanyinjiao (SP 6) respectively for five to seven minutes. Apply the treatment once every other day, 14 treatments forming one course, with a seven-day break between courses.

(2) Indirect Moxibustion Insulated with Ginger
   Points: Guanyuan (CV 4), Shenque (CV 8), Shenshu (BL 23), Mingmen (GV 4) and Zhishi (BL 52).

Technique: In each session, select two to three points, each of which is treated with five cones. In accordance with the pathological condition, large or medium-sized or small moxa cones may be used. Treat once a day, 10 sessions forming one course, with a five-day break between courses.

(3) Indirect Moxibustion Insulated with Salt, Ginger and Pericardium Zanthoxyli
   Point: Shenque (CV 8)

Technique: First fill the umbilicus with clean dry salt and treat the point with seven cones. Afterward, remove the salt from the point and put 21 pieces of Pericardium zanthoxyli into it and cover it with a ginger slice, then continue the moxibustion with another 14 cones. After the treatment, use plaster to cover the point. The moxa cone used in the treatment should be the size of a finger, 0.5-0.6 *cun* high.

3. COMBINED TREATMENT

(1) Electro-Acupucture with Moxibustion

Points: ① Guanyuan (CV 4), Zhongji (CV 3), Qugu (CV 2) and Sanyinjiao (SP 6). ② Huiyin (CV1), Huiyang (BL 35), Ciliao (BL 32) and Shenshu (BL 23).

Technique: The two groups of point may be used in rotation. Apply the treatment once a day, five treatments making up one course. Needle the points with a filiform needle first, then connect bilateral Sanyinjiao (SP 6) and Ciliao (BL 32) to the electro-stimulator for 20 minutes. Shenshu (BL 23), Guanyuan (CV 4) and Zhongji (CV3) may be treated with moxa in the box. This method is applicable for ejaculation spermatism.

(2) Acupuncture and Massage

Points: Zhongji (CV 3), Taixi (KI3), Zhaohai (KI 6) and Huiyin (CV 1).

Technique: Needle Zhongji (CV 3), Taixi (KI 3) and Zhaohai (KI 6) with even movement manipulation, retaining the needles after the needling sensation is obtained. After needling, apply moxibustion with moxa stick and massage alternately on Huiyin (CV1) for some 30 minutes. Apply the treatment once every other day, 10 treatments constituting one course, with a six-day break between courses.

[REMARKS]

1. This illness needs a relatively long period of treatment. The patient should be encouraged to have over six courses of treatment before deciding it is not effective.

2. During the treatment period, sexual activity is forbidden, and the patient is advised to take an optimistic attitude toward his problem and believe it can be cured.

UROSCHESIS

[INTRODUCTION]

In Chinese medicine, uroschesis is classified into deficiency pattern and excess pattern. The deficiency pattern usually arises when kidney *qi* of the elderly becomes deficient, the vital gate fire declines and the micturing function of the bladder is impeded; or it is due to weakness of *qi* in the middle energizer so that the transmitting function of the bladder is feeble, resulting in urinary retention. The deficiency condition is chiefly manifested as dribbling micturation, urinary discharge lacking force, soreness and weakness of the lumbus and knees and pale complexion. The excess pattern is principally induced by downward flow of damp-heat in the middle-energizer to the bladder impeding its micturing function; or it is elicited by traumatic injury and lower abdominal surgery leading to stagnation or obstruction of the meridians and collaterals, influencing the bladder's micturing function and causing urinary retention. Clinically, this pattern is marked by obstruction of urination and failure of exerted efforts to induce it, associated with low abdominal distension, spasms and pain. Treatment is aimed at warming the spleen and kidneys, clearing damp-heat and regulating the passage of fluids. The front-Mu and back-Shu points as well as points from the Conception Vessel may be selected as the principal points, e.g., Pangguangshu (BL 28), Zhongji (CV 3), Weiyang (BL 39) and Sanyinjiao (SP 6). For deficiency pattern, Pishu (BL 20), Shenshu (BL 23), Shenque (CV 8), Guanyuan (CV 4), Zusanli (ST 36) and Taixi (KI 3) may be added and needled with the reinforcing method; moxibustion is also adopted in the treatment. For excess syndrome, Yinlingquan (SP 9), Yingu (KI 10), Baliao (BL 31-34), Xingjian (LR 2) and Duiduan (GV 27) may be added and punctured with reducing technique. Urinary retention caused by various factors may be treated with reference to this introduction.

[CLINICAL EXPERIENCE]

1. CONVENTIONAL ACUPUNCTURE

(1) Penetrating Puncture
Points: Zhongji (CV 3) to Qugu (CV2)
Technique: Instruct the patient to adopt a prone position. Puncture Zhongji (CV 3) perpendicularly 1.5 *cun* deep with a two-*cun* needle. If there is an empty feeling under the needle, lift-thrust it slowly a few times. The sore and distending sensation may extend to the genital or perineum region. Then, lift the needle to the subcutaneous level and puncture deeply toward Qugu (CV 2). After that, slowly lift-thrust the needle. Repeat the above lift-thrust manipulation three to five times and the patient may have the desire to urinate; if there is no such desire, retain the needle for five to 10 minutes and then repeat the above manipulation.

(2) Reinforcing and Reducing Method with Slow and Rapid Manipulation
Points: Pianli (LI 6, bilateral), Lieque (LU7, bilateral), Ququan (LR 8, right), Yinlingquan (SP 9, right) and Taixi (KI 3, right).
Technique: Needle Taixi (KI 3) with the reinforcing method of slow-rapid manipulation, and other points with reducing slow-rapid manipulation.

(3) Method of Strong Stimulation
Points: Hegu (LI 4) and Sanyinjiao (SP 6).
Technique: After needling bilateral Hegu (LI 4) and Sanyinjiao (SP 6), apply strong manipulation of the needle to the points for two minutes. Retain the needles for five minutes. This method was applied in 86 cases, and an immediate effect was obtained in the treatment of all.

(4) Puncturing Lumbosacral Region
Points: Zhibian (BL 54), Mingmen (GV 4), Baliao (BL 31-34) and Yaoqi (below the spinous process of the 2nd sacral vertebra).
Technique: Puncture Bilateral Zhibian (BL 54) with a three-*cun* needle and guide the sensation to the testes and urethra. Retain the needles for 20 minutes. Treat the other points with a sharp hook nee-

dle. It is applicable for urinary retention caused by simple hyperplasia of prostate.

2. MOXIBUSTION

(1) With Moxa Stick

Points: Mingmen (GV 4) and Guanyuan (CV4).

Technique: Apply sparrow-pecking moxibustion with moxa stick for five to 10 minutes at each point. Apply the treatment twice a day.

(2) With Moxa Cone Insulated with Salt

Point: Shenque (CV 8)

Technique: Use salt to fill the umbilicus and apply 21 large cone moxibustion continuously until urination appears. When micturation occurs, stop the treatment.

3. ELECTRIC ACUPUNCTURE

Point: Shuidao (ST 28)

Technique: Use a long needle to puncture the point bilaterally. Needle the point two or three *cun* deep to join Qugu (CV 2), and then apply electro-stimulation to the point for 15 to 30 minutes.

4. PRICKING METHOD

Points: Dachangshu (BL 25) and Pangguangshu (BL 28)

Technique: Find the pigmentation spots around Dachangshu (BL 25) and Pangguangshu (BL 28). Prick the spots with a three-edged needle. The pigmentation spot is usually gray-brown or gray-white, slightly protruding from the skin. It is as big as the head of pin, and the color does not change when it is pressed. This method is applied for urinary retention induced by senile hypertrophy of the prostate.

5. CUTANEOUS PUNCTURE

Points: The courses of Conception Vessel, the kidney meridian and the stomach meridian at the abdominal region.

Technique: Tap the meridians with a cutaneous needle using moderate force. Apply the treatment two or three times a day.

6. SCALP ACUPUNCTURE

Point: Urinary and genital area (bilateral).

Technique: Puncture the area obliquely with a 1.5-*cun* filiform needle (the needle is inserted 1 *cun* in the cutaneous region) toward the posterior and parallel with the middle line of the head. Apply reducing manipulation to the needle and connect it to the electrostimulator for 20 minutes. This is set in dense-disperse pattern of stimulation, with the intensity adjusted to the patient's endurance. The treatment is given once a day.

7. HYDRO-ACUPUNCTURE

Point: Ciliao (BL 32), bilateral

Technique: Inject 0.5 mg of meostigmine respectively to the bilateral point once a day. Sometimes, one treatment cures the problem.

8. LASER THERAPY

Points: Zhongji (CV 3) and Longmen (middle point of the lower border of syphysis pubica).

Technique: Use the He-Ne laser needle, which is kept 5-10 cm away from the point, to radiate each point respectively for 10 minutes. Apply the treatment once a day. Meanwhile, apply a hot compress at the lower abdomen. This method was applied for 15 cases of postpartum urinary retention, and all were cured.

9. MEDICINAL APPLICATION ON ACU-POINT

(1) Application of Scallion

Point: Shenque (CV 8)

Technique: Take a proper amount of scallion, remove its peel and pound it into a mash, which is placed on the point. Usually 24-48 hours later urination may appear. At the beginning, there is a dribble, then smooth urination as a stream gradually occurs.

10. COMBINATION OF ACUPUNCTURE WITH MOXIBUSTION

Point: Sanyinjiao (SP 6) bilateral

Technique: Puncture bilateral Sanyinjiao (SP 6) deeply with a two-*cun* filiform needle. After the needling sensation is obtained, retain the needle for 15 minutes. After the removal of the needles, apply indirect moxibustion with moxa stick held over the point for three minutes. This method is applied for postpartum urinary retention.

[REMARKS]

1.   Acupuncture is an effective therapy for urinary retention. It is particularly good for patients of nervous and functional disturbance. For obstructive urinary retention, comprehensive treatment in accordance to the causative factors should be applied.

2.   If the bladder is overfilled with urine and acupuncture fails to induce micturation, immediate urethral catheterization should be made. However, in the next session treatment by acupuncture may be used first.

3.   When the bladder is overfilled with urine, acupuncture should be made shallowly and obliquely. Deep and perpendicular insertion of needle is forbidden.

EDEMA

[INTRODUCTION]

Edema in Chinese medicine is mainly ascribed to wind-damp of external origin that attacks the lungs leading to obstruction of the fluid passage, or to deficiency of the spleen in transportation and transformation, or to dysfunction of the kidneys in governing the opening and closing, meaning the fluid fails to be well distributed and discharged out of the body, but is, instead, retained in the muscles and skin. Clinically, this disorder is classified into *yang* edema and *yin* edema. *Yang* edema, with relatively abrupt onset, usually first affects the face and head, and then evolves to the region above the lower back, affecting the lung. Treatment of *yang* edema is directed toward activating the lung's dispersal function, so as to remove the exopathogens from the body surface, eliminate wind and promoting diuresis. Points are mainly selected from Taiyin meridians and Yangming meridians of hand and foot combining with Back-Shu points, such as Feishu (BL 13), Sanjiaoshu (BL22), Fengchi (GB 20), Pianli (LI 6), Yinlingquan (SP 9) and Hegu (LI 4), which are needled with reducing technique. *Yin* edema with slow onset appears initially on the dorsum of the foot, extending obviously to the region below the lower back. The affected organs are principally the spleen and kidneys. Principle of treatment for *yin* edema is warming the spleen and kidney *yang* to assist the removal of water. Points of the Conception Vessel, the Yangming meridian and the Shaoyin meridian of the foot are chosen with relevant Back-Shu points, e.g., Pishu (BL 20), Shenshu (BL 23), Shuifen (CV 9), Qihai (CV 6), Yinlingquan (SP 9), Zusanli (ST 36) and Taixi (KI 3), which are punctured with the reinforcing method and treated also by moxibustion. This condition is encountered in acute and chronic nephritis and some cardiac diseases, as well as dystrophic edema of modern medicine.

[CLINICAL EXPERIENCE]

1. CONVENTIONAL ACUPUNCTURE

(1) Combination of Reinforcing and Reducing Method

Points: Shuifen (CV 9), Neiguan (PC 6), Sanyinjiao (SP 6), Shenshu (BL 23) and Pishu (BL20).

Technique: Puncture Sanyinjiao (SP 6), Shenshu (BL 23) and Pishu (BL 20) with lift-thrust and twirling reinforcing manipulation. Needle Shuifen (CV 9) and Neiguan (PC 6) with the reducing method of the same manipulation. This method was once applied for chronic nephritis patient attributable to wind edema with phlegm heat disturbing the heart for one month; the amount of urine was greatly increased and general edema disappeared.

(2) Puncturing Ah-shi Point

Point: Tender spot in the renal region

Technique: Ask the patient to adopt a prone position and find the tender spot in the renal region besides the spine. Select two or three spots for needling according to the size of the tender region. Puncture the tender spot 0.8-1.2 *cun* obliquely at an angle of 30° toward the spine. Retain the needle for 30-60 minutes, during which period manipulate the needles once every 10-15 minutes. The treatment is indicated for pyelonephritis. Apply the treatment once a day for acute cases and once every other day for chronic cases.

2. MOXIBUSTION

(1) *Warming Needle Moxibustion*

Points: Pishu (BL 20), Zusanli (ST 36), Yinlingquan (SP 9) and Taibai (SP 3).

Technique: Remove the needle from Pishu (BL 20) after the point is punctured with needling sensation. Retain needles in the other points after the needling sensation is obtained for 20 minutes. Meanwhile, put a piece of moxa stick onto the handle of each needle. This method is used for edema due to deficiency of the spleen with excessive dampness.

(2) *Moxibustion with Cones*

Point: The point inferior to the medial malleolus

Technique: For general edema with facial puffiness, apply moxibustion with three cones at the junction of the red and white skin below the medial malleolus.

3. CUTANEOUS PUNCTURE

Points: Points of the bladder meridian on the back

Technique: Tap gently with a cutaneous needle up and down the first lateral line and the second lateral line of the bladder meridian on the back until the skin becomes reddish.

4. AURICULAR THERAPY

Point: Kidney

Technique: Find out the point of lower electrical resistance or tenderness at the kidney point of the two auricles. Puncture the points with a filiform needle and retain the needle for four to six hours. Apply the treatment once a day, seven sessions constituting one course. During the treatment, administration of diuretics may be stopped. This therapy is indicated for chronic nephritis.

5. MEDICINAL APPLICATION ON ACU-POINTS

(1) Application of Castor Seed
Point: Yongquan (KI 1)

Technique: Pound 50 kernels of castor beans and three to five macrostem onions (Bulbus Allii Macrostemi) into paste and lay on bilateral Yongquan (KI 1). Treat the patient once a day and apply the treatment continuously for a few days.

6. COMBINED TREATMENT

(1) Combination of Acupuncture with Moxibustion
Points: Feishu (BL 13), Pishu (BL 20), Shenshu (BL 23), Qihai (CV 6), Yinlinquan (SP 9) and Shuifen (CV9).

Technique: Apply strong moxibustion with a piece of moxa stick at Shuifen (CV9) for five to 10 minutes. Needle Qihai (CV 6) with lift-thrust manipulation with no retention of the needle at the point. Puncture other points with the reinforcing method of lift-thrust and twirling manipulation, and apply warm needle moxibustion. This is indicated for edema due to spleen and kidney *yang* deficiency.

(2) Combination of Acupuncture with Infra-Red Radiation
Point: Renal area

Technique: Select two or three points in the tender region of the renal area. Needle the points with lift-thrust twirling manipulation and retain the needles for 30-60 minutes; concomitantly, add infrared radiation. A total of 78 chronic pyelonephritis cases were treated with this method, of which 69 were cured, making up 88.5%.

[REMARKS]

1. Deep puncture is forbidden in the renal region so as to avoid injuring the kidneys.

2. The patient is advised to take rest during the period of treatment and stick to a low salt diet.

STRANGURIA

[INTRODUCTION]

In Chinese medicine, frequent, urgent and dribbling urination with lower abdominal spasms and urethral stabbing pain is regarded as stranguria. This condition is ascribed to damp-heat collecting in the lower energizer, which impedes the micturing function of the bladder; or it stems from deficiency of the spleen and kidneys, the latter's function of separating the clear from the turbid being disturbed. Clinically, there are five patterns classified, namely Relin (stranguria due to heat), Shilin (induced by the passage of urinary stones), Xuelin (complicated by hematuria), Qilin (caused by disorder of *qi*), and Gaolin (marked by chyluria). Clinically Relin is manifested as burning and stabbing pain in the urethra, with scanty yellow turbid urine; Shilin is marked sometimes by a stone in the urine and lower abdominal and penis distension and spastic, stabbing pain; Xuelin is revealed by urgent, frequent urination and bloodstained urine; Qilin is manifested by weak urination with intermittent urine; and Gaolin produces cloudy urine like rice-washing water, and irritating urethral pain. Treatment of stranguria is directed toward normalizing the function of the bladder, promoting diuresis and relieving pain. In the treatment, Back-Shu and Front-Mu points and points of the three *yin* meridians may be mainly selected, such as Pangguangshu (BL 28), Zhongji (CV 3), Sanyinjiao (SP 6) and Taichong (LR 3). For Relin, Quchi (LI 11), Waiguan (TE 5) and Hegu (LI 4) may be added; for Shilin, Weiyang (BL 39) and Rangu (KI 2) may be selected as well; for Xuelin, Xuehai (SP 10) and Geshu (BL 17) may be supplemented; for Qilin, Shenshu (BL 23), Taixi (KI 3) and Qihai (CV6 with moxa) are added; and for Gaolin, Pishu (BL 20), Shenshu (BL 23), Zusanli (ST 36) and Guanyuan (CV4 with moxa) are added. The excess syndrome is managed with reducing technique, and the deficiency syndrome with the reinforcing method. Urinary tract infection, acute and chronic prostatitis and chyluria of modern medicine may be treated with reference to this introduction. Urinary system stones will be discussed separately in the book.

[CLINICAL EXPERIENCE]

1. CONVENTIONAL ACUPUNCTURE

(1) Selecting Points in the Sacral Region

Point: Baliao (BL 31-34)

Technique: In each session, select two pairs of the points and puncture them deeply. Retain the needle for 30 minutes after a relatively strong sensation is obtained; and electro-stimulation may be added.

(2) Selecting Extra Point

Point: Xiazhibian (Extra)

Technique: The patient is placed in a recumbent posture with the lower leg extended on the bed, and the upper leg flexed, the popliteal region of the upper leg is at an angle of 130°, and the trunk of the patient is slightly bent toward the chest. The posture should be correctly assumed. A side of an equilateral triangle is measured between the anterosuperior iliac spine and the middle point of the greater trochanter, and the junction of the other two sides of the triangle is the location of the point.

Puncture the point with a filiform needle (Size: No.28), 3.5 to 5 *cun* long, insert it obliquely, 10 degrees anterior toward the ventral. Apply lift-thrust and twirling manipulation, and the sensation will immediately radiate to the lower abdomen, the genitalia and the perineum region. Retain the needle for two or three minutes, then remove it.

(3) Application of Strong Stimulation

Points: Shenshu (BL 23), Zhubin (KI 9), Fuliu (KI 7), Guilai (ST 29), Feiyang (BL 58) and Zhongji (CV 3).

Technique: Apply the treatment once a day with strong stimulation, 10 sessions constituting one course. This method is used for urinary tract infection.

(4) Selecting Group of Points

Points: ① Guanyuan (CV 4), Zhongji (CV3), Yinlingquan (SP 9) and Sanyinjiao (SP 6). ② Huiyin (CV1) and Shenshu (BL 23)

Technique: The two groups of points may be used in rotation.

Apply the treatment once a day. Needle the points in reducing technique without retention of the needles. Puncture Huiyin (CV 1) perpendicularly two or three *cun* deep with a 3-4 *cun* needle (Size: Nos.26-28). When the patient feels soreness and a distending sensation, apply lift-thrust manipulation three to five times before removing the needle. Puncture other points in a conventional way. This method is applicable for chronic prostatitis.

2.   MOXIBUSTION

(1) Moxibustion with a Moxa Stick

Point: Zhongji (CV 3)

Technique: Ask the patient to adopt a supine posture. Use a moxa stick to apply circular movement over the point for 40 minutes. Apply the treatment twice a day for urethral syndrome. After the treatment, the patient's symptoms may see obviously remission or disappear.

(2) Warming Needle Moxibustion

Points: Shenshu (BL 23), Pangguangshu (BL 28), Ciliao (BL 32) Zhongji (CV3) and Guanyuan (CV4).

Technique: After the needling sensation is obtained, apply moxibustion with three to five pieces of moxa sticks on each point. Give the treatment once daily, 10 sessions constituting one course. This is applicable for chronic urocystitis and chronic pyelonephrosis.

(3) Moxibustion with Moxa Cone

Point: Zhongfeng (LR 4)

Technique: For the five patterns of stranguria, apply moxibustion with 14 cones on the point located on a small vessel, one-*cun* antero-inferior to the medial malleolus.

(4) Salt Insulated Moxibustion

Point: Shenque (CV 8)

Technique: Parch table salt warm and fill the umbilicus with it. Apply moxibustion with seven large cones on the point. Treat the patient once a day for hesitant, dribbling and painful urination. If the treatment combines Sanyinjiao (SP 6) treated with moxa cone, the effect will be better.

3. CUTANEOUS PUNCTURE

Point: Guanyuan (CV 4), Qugu (CV2), Guilai (ST 29), Shuidao (ST 28), Groin, Ququan (LR 8), Sanyinjiao (SP 6) and Jiaji (14th-21st vertebrae).

Technique: Use a cutaneous needle to tap the points along the course of the meridian from any direction, upper or lower, until the skin becomes red. This is used for chronic prostatitis.

4. AURICULAR THERAPY

Points: Kidney, Bladder, Sanjiao (triple energizer), Urethra, Subcortex, Endocrine and Shenmen.

Technique: In each session treat three to five points with filiform needles and retain the needles for 20 minutes, or treat all the points with Semen Vaccaria. Treat the patient once daily, 10-15 sessions constituting one course, with three to five days between courses. This is applicable for a patient suffering from chyluria.

5. LASER THERAPY

Point: Huiyin (CV 1)

Technique: Insert a hollow needle that contains optical fiber with a diameter of 80 micron inside into the prostate cavity via Huiyin (CV1) and radiate it with He-Ne laser.

6. HYDRO-ACUPUNCTURE

Points: Auricular, Kidney, Bladder, Sub-cortex, Shenmen.

Technique: Apply the treatment once a day, in each session injecting 0.1 ml of mixture of vitamin B1 and B12 into each point. Eight treatments form one course, with a break of three days between courses. This has definite effect for chyluria .

7. MEDICINAL APPLICATION ON ACU-POINT

Point: Shenque (CV 8)

Technique: Grind some alum (Alumen) into a fine powder, to which is added wheat flour or scallion, and put it onto the point. This is quite effective for urethritis.

[REMARKS]

1.   Acupuncture has certain effect for urinary infection, chronic prostatitis and chyuria. Medicinal herbal therapy may be combined.

2.   As far as diet is concerned, it is better to have red-bean porridge, lotus root starch, lotus seeds, apples and pears, and avoid spicy and irritating food.

DIABETES MELLITUS

[INTRODUCTION]

This condition is manifested mainly in excessive drinking of fluid, polyphagia, polyuria and emaciation. Clinically as the symptoms vary in degree, it may be classified into three patterns: upper Xiao, middle Xiao and lower Xiao. The disease may be induced by prolonged or drastic emotional changes leading to liver *qi* stagnation that transforms into fire, counteracting on the lungs and consuming lung *yin*; or it may be caused by improper diet such as eating much greasy and sweet food which produces heat in the spleen and stomach, transforming into dryness and impairing the body fluids; or it may be provoked by indulgence in sexual activity that consumes kidney *yin* leading to deficiency. Upper Xiao is marked by polydipsia, drinking excessive fluids, dry mouth and tongue. Middle Xiao is characterized by an immense increase in appetite, accelerated digestion and frequent hunger. Lower Xiao is chiefly manifested as frequent and urgent urination with milky urine. Treatment is directed toward nourishing *yin* and moistening the dryness. Back-Shu points may be selected as the main points, such as Feishu (BL 13), Yishu (Extra), Shenshu (BL 23), Sanyinjiao (SP 6), etc. For upper Xiao, Xinshu (BL15), Taiyuan (LU 9), Shaofu (HT 8) and Yuji (LU 10) are added; for middle Xiao, Weishu (BL 21) and Neiting (ST 44) are supplemented; and for Lower Xiao, Ganshu (BL 18), Zhaohai (KI 6), Taixi (KI 3) and Rangu (KI 2) are added.

[CLINICAL EXPERIENCE]

1. CONVENTIONAL ACUPUNCTURE

(1) Mainly Selecting Back-Shu Points

Points: Weiguanxiashu (1.5 *cun* lateral to the lower border of the spinous process of the 8th thoracic vertebra), Feishu (BL 13), Pishu (BL 20), Shenshu (BL 23) and Sanyinjiao (SP 6)

Technique: Puncture the Back-Shu points with a one-*cun* filiform needle to a depth of 0.5-0.8 *cun* to obtain a needling sensation. When it appears, retain the needles in the points for 20 minutes. Apply the treatment once a day. For severe thirst, add Lianquan (CV 23); for hunger pangs soon after eating, add Zhongwan (CV 12); for ulceration in the mouth, add Tongli (HT5), Hegu (LI 4) and Zhaohai (KI 6); for blurred vision, add (Yanglao (SI 6) and Guangming (GB 37).

(2) Selecting Points from the Liver and Kidney Meridians

Points: Xingjian (LR 2) and Yongquan (KI 1).

Technique: It is recorded in *Bai Zheng Fu (Rhyme Prose for 100 Disorders)* that "Xingjian (LR 2) and Yongquan (KI1) are indicated for Xiaoke due to depletion of kidney." Xingjian (LR2), the Ying-Spring point, has the action of clearing heat and reducing fire, Yongquan (KI 1), the Jing-Well point, the son point of the kidney meridian, has the action of heat clearing, *yin* nourishing and kidney reinforcing. Puncturing the point in a conventional way will treat lower Xiao attributable to the syndrome of *yin* deficiency and *yang* hyperactivity.

2. MOXIBUSTION

(1) Moxibustion with Moxa Cones

Points: Xiaochangshu (BL 27), Dazhui (GV 14), two small fingers and two small toes

Technique: Apply moxibustion with a few score cones on Xiaochangshu (BL 27) for thirst and 10 cones respectively on two small fingers and two small toes and Dazhui (GV 14) for urgent urination.

(2) Indirect Moxibustion Insulated with Ginger

Points: ① Zusanli (ST 36) and Zhongwan (CV 12). ② Mingmen (GV 4), Shenzhu (BL 10) and Pishu (BL 20). ③ Qihai (CV6) and

Guanmen (ST 22). ④ Jizhong (GV 6) and Shenshu (BL 23). ⑤ Huagai (CV 20) and Liangmen (ST 21). ⑥ Dazhui (GV 14) and Ganshu (BL18). ⑦ Xingjian (LR 2), Zhongji (CV3) and Fuai (SP 16). ⑧ Feishu (BL 13), Geshu (BL 17) and Shenshu (BL 23)

Technique: Conduct moxibustion once daily, treating one group of points in each session, with the eight groups selected in turns. The fresh ginger slice used in the treatment is 3-4 mm thick, 2 cm in diameter; the moxa cone is of 1.5×2 cm^2, 0.5 g. Treat each point with 10-30 cones. Needling is also added on other points in accordance with the pattern of the disease.

3. CUTANEOUS PUNCTURE

Points: The first and second lateral lines of the bladder meridian on the back

Technique: Tap the meridian gently with a cutaneous needle. Apply the treatment once a day or once every other day, and each session lasts five to 10 minutes. Ten sessions constitute one course of treatment.

4. AURICULAR THERAPY

Points: Pancreas, Endocrine, Kidney, Sanjiao, Ear Vagus Root, Shenmen, Heart and Liver.

Technique: Puncture the points with a filiform needle once every other day, or treat the point with Semen Vaccaria once every three to five days. In each treatment, select three to five points.

5. HYDRO-ACUPUNCTURE

Points: Feishu (BL 13), Pishu (BL 20), Shenshu (BL 23), Weiguanxiashu (1.5 *cun* lateral to the lower border of the spinous process of the 8th thoracic vertebra).

Technique: Select two points in each session, injecting each point with 2-3 ml of astragalus root injection. Apply the treatment once a day.

6. COMBINED TREATMENT

Acupuncture and Moxibustion Combined with Tuina

Points: Jianjing (GB 21), Taodao (GV 13), Ganshu (BL 18),

Shenshu (BL 23), Sanjiaoshu (BL 22), Zhongwan (CV 12) and Yin-jiao (GV 28).

Technique: Instruct the patient to take a sitting posture, and apply massage on the spine first. Then, puncture the points on the back with needles retained for 15 minutes. After the removal of the needles, let the patient lie face up and puncture the points of the abdomen. For a chronic case, apply moxibustion on the abdominal points.

[REMARKS]

1. Acupuncture exerts better therapeutic effect for early stage and mild diabetes mellitus.

2. With lower body resistance, the diabetic is liable to infection, so caution must be taken to conduct strict disinfection in acupuncture treatment.

3. The diabetic tends to have numbness of the limbs, pain and cataracts, thus relevant points for these problems may be treated as well if these symptoms are present.

MALARIA

[INTRODUCTION]

Malaria is characterized by alternation of chills and fever, headache, sweating and regular attacks and remission. Clinically, it may be quotidian, tertian or quartan. This condition, often occurring in summer and autumn, is considered to be induced by a malarial pathogenic factor associated with wind, cold, summer heat, damp or pestilential pathogen that reside in the Shaoyang meridian, the intermediate region of interior and exterior of the body, entry and exit between Ying (nutrient or *yin*) and Wei (defensive or *yang*) system. When the pathogen is in *yin*, chills appear, and in *yang*, fever occurs, and the attack arises when the body resistance combats with the pathogens. Treatment is directed toward harmonizing Shaoyang and eliminating the malarial pathogenic factor. Points are mainly selected from the Governor Vessel, Hand Taiyang and Shaoyang meridians, e.g., Dazhui (GV 14), Houxi (SI 3), Jianshi (PC 5) and Hegu (LI 4). Acupuncture is made in reducing technique; and the therapeutic effect improved if the treatment is applied one or two hours before full onset of an attack.

[CLINICAL EXPERIENCE]

1.   CONVENTIONAL ACUPUNCTURE

(1) Puncturing Mainly the Tender Spots of the Spine

Points: The tender spots of thoracic vertebra No.1 to lumbar vertebra No.5 (T1- L5), Dazhui (GV 14), Taodao (GV 13), Neiguan (PC 6), Jianshi (PC 5), Quchi (LI 11) and Fuliu (KI 7).

Technique: The patient first adopts a prone position. Search for the tender spots from T1 to L5 with the palm side of the thumb in even force. Puncture the tender spots, Dazhui (GV 14) and Taodao (GV13) with strong stimulation, but not retaining the needles in the points. Treat other points with lift-thrust and twisting method, and retain the needles for 20 to 30 minutes. Apply the treatment two or three hours before the attack, conducting continuously   for three to six days.

(2) Selecting Points from the Unilateral Side

Points: Houxi (SI 3), Jianshi (PC5) and Zusanli (ST 36).

Technique: Apply the treatment two hours prior to the attack. First puncture Houxi (SI 3) to a depth of 0.5 *cun*, then puncture Jianshi (PC 5) 0.8 *cun* deep, finally needle Zusanli (ST 36) 0.8 *cun* deep. In one session, puncture the points on one side, and rotate to the points on the other side in the next session. The needles are retained for 15 to 30 minutes. If necessary, apply heat producing needling before the attack and cool-producing needling during it.

(3) Selecting Nüemen Point

Point: Nüemen (located in the depression of the bone juncture between the middle finger and ring finger, i.e., the depression distal to the 4th and 5th metacarpophalangeal joint) while locating the point, ask the patient to keep the four fingers close together, and make a loose fist.

Technique: After conventional disinfection of the point, puncture it with a 1-1.5 *cun* needle at an angle of 15° and 0.8-1.0 *cun* deep. Conduct reducing manipulation of twisting. When relatively strong stimulation is obtained, retain the needle for 20 to 30 minutes. During this period, twirl the needles once every five to 15 minutes to maintain the soreness and distending sensation.

2. BLEEDING METHOD

(1) Bleeding Shenzhu (GV 12)

Technique: It exerts better effect if the treatment is made one-hour-and-a-half before the attack. The patient is in sitting posture with the back facing the practitioner. Select the point below the third thoracic vertebra. After routine disinfection, pinch the skin of the point with the left hand, and prick the point 0.1 *cun* deep with a three-edged needle held in the right hand. Then use the thenar minor of one hand to press the Fengfu (GV 16), and the thenar minor of the other hand to press the caudal region, with both hands pushing toward the needling hole. Repeat the pushing about 10 times until three to five drops of blood are squeezed out of the needling hole. Wipe away the blood.

(2) Bleeding Shixuan (extra) and Weizhong (BL 40)

Technique: When the patient has chills that suggests an attack, prick Shixuan (extra) and Weizhong (BL 40) bilaterally with a three-edged needle to let out blood. This method may stop the attack and be applicable for the patient with a relatively good constitution.

3. AURICULAR THERAPY

Points: Adrenal Gland, Subcortex and Endocrine
Technique: Puncture the points bilateral two to six hours prior to the attack with strong stimulation, retaining the needles in the points until one to two hours after the attack. During retention, apply twisting manipulation a few times.

4. MEDICINAL APPLICATION ON ACU-POINTS

Point: Dazhui (GV 14)

Technique: Pound one or two hot peppers into a mash, and place this on Dazhui (GV 14) two hours prior to the attack. The mixture should be fixed on the point for three to four hours.

5. COMBINED TREATMENT

Points: Dazhui (GV 14), Jianshi (PC 5), Fuliu (KI 7) and Shendao (GV 11).

Technique: Apply five-cone moxibustion on Dazhui (GV 14), and needle Jianshi (PC 5) 0.5 *cun* deep with twisting manipulation for one minute. Then, apply moxibustion with three moxa cones respectively on Jianshi (PC 5) and Fuliu (KI 7) and two or three cones on Shendao (GV 11).

[REMARKS]

1. Acupuncture has good therapeutic effect for malaria, but the time of treatment must be well selected.

2. After the patient is cured, he or she should avoid taking cold, uncooked and greasy food for two weeks, otherwise their intake may cause a relapse.

JAUNDICE

[INTRODUCTION]

Clinically, jaundice of *yin* and *yang* types is classified. Jaundice of the *yang* type is mostly caused by the attack of exogenous pathogenic damp and heat, which are retained in the liver and gallbladder, and lead to abnormal circulation of bile, resulting in exudation. The clinical manifestations of this type include bright yellow skin like the color of an orange, fever, thirst, yellow sticky coating on the tongue and soft rapid pulse, referring to heat and excess syndromes. The treatment principle is to smooth the liver *qi*, benefit the gallbladder, clear away heat and resolve damp. The points are mainly selected from Governor Vessel, Foot-Jueyin, Hand and Food Shaoyang meridians, such as Dazhui (GV14), Zhiyang (GV7), Waiguan (TE5), Wangu (SI4), Zhongchong (PC9), Yanglingquan (GB34), Yinlingquan (SP9) and Xingjian (LR2), which are punctured by reducing needling technique. Jaundice of the *yin* type is mainly caused by improper food intake, hunger and overeating or excessive mental activity and fatigue, which damage the spleen and stomach, leading to dysfunction of transportation and transformation, production of internal damp transforming into cold, retention of cold and damp in the Middle Energizer blocking the secretion of bile, resulting in exudation and yellow skin. The clinical manifestations include dark yellow skin, aversion to cold, anorexia, no taste and thirst, pale tongue with a sticky coating, soft and moderate pulse, referring to cold and deficiency syndromes. The treatment principle is to strengthen the spleen, benefit the gallbladder, and eliminate cold and damp by the warming method. The points are mainly selected from Foot-Yangming and Taiyin meridians and Back-Shu points, such as Pishu (BL20), Danshu (BL19), Qihai (CV6), Zusanli (ST36), Yinlingquan (SP9) and Sanyinjiao (SP6), which are punctured by reinforcing needling technique with both acupuncture and moxibustion. The treatment of jaundice is taken as the reference for acute and chronic hepatitis, cirrhosis and cholecystitis in modern medicine.

[CLINICAL EXPERIENCE]

1. CONVENTIONAL ACUPUNCTURE

(1) Penetrating Method

Points: Yanglingquan (GB34) to Yinlingquan (SP9), Taichong (LR3) to Yongquan (KI3) and Zusanli (ST36).

Technique: Even and reducing needling techniques by lifting, thrusting and rotating methods are applied for mild and severe cases respectively. Needles are manipulated once every five minutes and retained for 30 minutes. Quchi (LI11), Hegu (LI4) or Dazhui (GV14) are supplemented for fever; Zhongwen (CV12) and Neiguan (PC6) for vomiting; and Tianshu (ST 25) and Dachangshu (BL 25) for abdominal distention and constipation.

(2) Puncturing Back-Shu Points

Points: Ganshu (BL18), Danshu (BL19), Pishu (BL20) and Weishu (BL21) combining with Zusanli (ST36) and Taichong (LR3).

Technique: To take a one-*cun* filiform needle to puncture Back-Shu points and Taichong (LR3) and a 1.5-*cun* needle to puncture Zusanli (ST36). Apply reducing technique for jaundice of the *yang* type and acupuncture and moxibustion for the *yin* type. The treatment is given once every other day.

(3) Puncturing Five-Shu Points

Points: Zhongfeng (LR4), Houxi (SI3), Hegu (LI4) and Zusanli (ST36)

Technique: Zhongfeng (LR4) is the Jing-River point of the liver meridian; Houxi (SI3), the Shu-Stream point of the small intestine meridian; Hegu (LI4), the Yuan-Primary point of the large intestine meridian; and Zusanli (ST36), the He-Sea point. The points on one side are selected every day and bilateral points are applied alternately and punctured by reducing technique. The penetrating method is applied from Houxi (SI3) to Laogong (PC6) or from Hegu (LI4) to Laogong (PC6). The treatment is given once a day, retaining needles for 20 minutes, with a two-week treatment making up one course.

(4) Combination of Chief and Supplementary Points

Points: Main points: Quchi (LI11), Xuehai (SP10), Taichong (LR3), Ququan (LR8), Zhongwan (CV12), Zusanli (ST36), Gongsun (SP4), Taixi (KI3) and Sanyinjiao (SP6). Supplementary points: Zhigou (TE6) and the point located 2 *cun* above the medial malleolus added for pain in the liver region, Zhongwan (CV12), Tianshu (ST25), Yinlingquan (SP9) and Pishu (BL20) for abdominal distention; Jianli (CV11), Gongsun (SP4) and Chengshan (BL 57) for anorexia; Tianshu (ST25), Zhongwan (CV12), Zusanli (ST36), Zhangmen (LR13) and Pigen (3.5 *cun* lateral to the spinal process of the 1st lumbar vertebra) for swelling of the liver and spleen.

Technique: To apply moxibustion on Pigen point and puncture the other points. The treatment is given once a day for the syndromes in the later stage of hepatitis.

2. MOXIBUSTION

(1) Moxa on a Single Point
Point: Zhiyang (GV9)

Technique: Apply seven moxa cones on Zhiyang (GV9) to remove jaundice by causing sweating.

(2) Moxa on Double Points
Points: Ganshu (BL18) and Zusanli (ST36)

Technique: Apply direct moxibustion with small cones once a day, five to seven cones on each point, and once every other day after 10 treatments.

(3) Cupping
Points: ① Dazhui (GV14), Ganshu (BL18), Qimen (LR14) and Weishu (BL21). ② Shenzhu (GV12), Danshu (BL19) and Pishu (BL20).

Technique: Apply the two groups of points alternately in each treatment once a day and retain the cups for 20 minutes.

(4) Auricular Therapy
Points: Main points: Liver, Gallbladder, Spleen and Stomach. Supplementary points: Pancreas and Spleen added for anorexia, Ear-Shimen and Subcortex for pain in the liver region, Sub-cortex, Pancreas and Large Intestine for abdominal distention, Ear-Shimen, Heart and Subcortex for insomnia and liver *yang* and Ear Apex for the high transaminase.

Technique: Needle the auricular points on the bilateral sides, four to six points selected in each treatment with moderate stimulation. Apply the therapy once every day or once every other day, the needles retained for one hour. Ten days of treatment make up one course. Alternatively, apply seed-pressing technique with Semen Vaccaria, or inject 100 mg of Vitamin B_{12} on the liver, gallbladder and spleen once a day for 10 days. This therapy is suitable for chronic hepatitis and the early stages of cirrhosis.

(5) Hydro-acupuncture
i) Injection of Radix Isatidis
Points: Ganshu (BL18), Danshu (BL19), Qimen (LR14), Riyue (GB24) and Zhongzhu (TE3)

Technique: Inject two or three points in each treatment, 0.5 to 1 ml for each. Apply the treatment once every day for 10 days.

ii) Injection of Vitamin B$_{12}$

Point: Ganshu (BL18)

Technique: In each treatment, 1 ml of Vitamin B$_{12}$ is injected on Ganshu (BL18) of either side. The syringe needle is inserted on the point precisely and injects the medicine slowly after the patient feels sourness, numbness and distention by gently rotating the needle. Twenty treatments make a course and there should be a rest period of one to two weeks before treatment resumes. This therapy is suitable for protracted and chronic hepatitis.

iii) Injection of Radix Salviae Miltiorrhizae

Point: Zusanli (ST36)

Technique: Inject 1 ml of Radix Salviae Miltiorrhizae on Zusanli (ST36), alternately being sides. The treatment is applied once a day and 30 days make up a course. This therapy is suitable for protracted and chronic hepatitis.

(6) Catgut-embedding Method

Points: Sanyinjiao (SP6) and Qimen (LR14) only on the right side.

Technique: Inject 1 ml of 2% procaine in the points, about 1 *cun* deep, then insert the triangular suture needle (Size: No.0) with surgical catgut from the lower part of the point and out of it from the upper part, about 1 cm deep and 1 to 1.5 cm long. The two ends of the catgut are slightly beneath the skin. Dress and sterilize the area. Avoid water for three days to prevent infection. This therapy is suitable for chronic hepatitis. Generally, in two weeks of catgut embedding, the distending pain in the liver region is reduced or disappears, and one month later the positive index of liver functions are reduced by differing degrees.

(7) Laser Therapy

Points: Ganshu (BL18), Zusanli (ST36) and inguinal lymph nodes (corresponding to BL13).

Technique: Radiate the point by He-Ne laser with 2 mw output power and 15 to 30 cm far from the point. Each point is radiated for 10 minutes each time, alternately. Ten treatments make up one course.

[REMARKS]

1. The therapeutic result is effective in the treatment of jaundice by acupuncture, but strict sterilization of the medical instrument is required to prevent cross-infection.

2. The patient suffering from jaundice should rest in a lying position, keep a good mood with rich nutrient and also undertake some physical exercise under the guidance of a physician.

INTOXICATION

[INTRODUCTION]

Clinically, carbon monoxide poisoning and food poisoning are commonly seen. Chinese medicine believes that poison in the body may cause disturbance of *qi* and blood circulation, abnormal ascending and descending of *qi* of Zangfu organs, failure by the clear *yang* to ascend, and upward perversion of the turbid *qi*, disturbing the mind and resulting in a series of symptoms. A mild case is treated mainly by regulating *qi* activity of Zangfu organs by Baihui (GV20), Taiyang (Ex-HN5), Neiguan (PC6), Zhongwan (CV12), Quchi (LI11), Hegu (LI4), Zusanli (ST36) and Taichong (LR3). A severe case is treated by opening the orifice, detoxification and regaining consciousness by Suliao (GV25), Renzhong (GV26), Neiguan (PC6), Shenque (CV8) and 12 Jing-well points.

[CLINICAL EXPERIENCE]

1. CONVENTIONAL ACUPUNCTURE

(1) Puncturing Suliao (GV25)

Points: Suliao (GV25), Ex-HN3 (Yintang), penetrating puncture from GV 23 (Shangxing) to Baihui (GV20) and Neiguan (PC6)

Technique: Adopt the sparrow-pecking needling on Suliao (GV25) to induce tearing, needle obliquely on Yintang (Ex-HN3) by lifting and thrusting technique to cause reducing, horizontally puncture from

Shangxing (GV23) to Baihui (GV20), 2.5 to 3 *cun* deep, with rotating technique to cause reducing; perpendicularly puncture on Neiguan (PC6) by rotating, lifting and thrusting technique to cause reducing. Lifting, thrusting and rotating needling technique is applied repeatedly during needle retention. The therapy is given for mild cases of carbon monoxide poisoning.

(2) Puncturing Dazhui (GV14) and Dazhu (BL11)

Points: Dazhui (GV14), Dazhu (BL11), Geshu (BL17), Pishu (BL20), Shenshu (BL23), Zhongwan (CV12), Qihai (CV6), Zusanli (ST36), Sanyinjiao (SP6), Xuanzhong (GB39) and Taixi (KI3).

Technique: Five to seven points are selected alternately in each treatment and punctured by reducing needling technique. The needles are retained for 30 minutes to regulate and tonify *qi* and blood, nourish *yin* and benefit marrow. The therapy is given for chronic benzene poisoning. The treatment is given once a day and 20 treatments make up one course.

(3) Puncturing Zanzhu (BL2), Renzhong (GV26) and Daling (PC7)

Points: Zanzhu (BL2), Renzhong (GV26) and Daling (PC7).

Technique: Strong stimulation is applied on the points by rotating needles for five minutes until consciousness is slightly regained. Then let the patient take some fresh radish juice with warm water to calm the mind, open the orifice and relax the chest. The therapy is given for gas poisoning manifested as loss of consciousness, unclear mind and generally red skin.

2. BLEEDING METHOD

(1) Bleeding on Shixuan (Ex-UE11) and Quze (PC3)

Technique: Take a three-edged needle or a syringe needle to prick Shixuan (Ex-UE11) and Quze (PC3) to get three to five ml of blood. Generally, the points on one side are pricked, and the bilateral points are only applied to relatively severe case. The therapy is given for gas poisoning.

(2) Bleeding on Zhongchong (PC9) and Shaoshang (LU11)

Points: Main points: Zhongchong (PC9) and Shaoshang (LU11). Supplementary points: Shenque (CV8), Shuifen (CV9), Yinjiao (CV7) and Huangshu (KI16). All the points are selected bilaterally.

Technique: Take a three-edged needle to prick Zhongchong (PC9) and Shaoshang (LU11) bilaterally to cause bleeding until blood turns from purplish toe light red. For severe case, the supplementary points are pricked, 0.1 to 0.4 cm deep and cupping is applied on the points around the umbilicus to get few blood. The therapy is given for acute food poisoning.

3. ELECTRIC ACUPUNCTURE

Points: Quchi (LI11), Hegu (LI4), Neiguan (PC6), Zusanli (ST36) and Xiajuxu (ST37).

Technique: Electric stimulation is applied by the electric pulse apparatus on Quchi (LI11), Hegu (LI4), Zusanli (ST36) and Xiajuxu (ST37) after the arrival of *qi* for 20 minutes. The therapy is given for the mild case of food poisoning.

4. AURICULAR THERAPY

Points: Main points: Kidney, Sub-cortex and Liver. Supplementary points: External Ear and Shenmen for tinnitus and deafness; Forehead, Occiput, Shenmen and Heart for insomnia and dream-disturbed sleep; Forehead, Occiput and Taiyang for headache; and Stomach and Sympathetic for vomiting.

Technique: Strong stimulation technique by rotating the needle is applied on the points of both ears after perpendicular insertion, which must not penetrate the ear cartilage. The therapy is given once a day, retaining the needle for two to four hours and rotating the needle three or four times at regular intervals. Twelve treatments make one course, with a two- or three-day interval between courses. The therapy is given for dizziness, nausea and vomiting caused by streptomycin poisoning.

5. SCALP ACUPUNCTURE

Points: Metal-emotional area (corresponding to Lateral Line 1 of Neck).

Technique: A filiform needle (Size: No.28) is inserted swiftly

216

along the muscular layer of the scalp with the tip of needle to the back, about 1 *cun* deep. The electric acupuncture apparatus is attached on the needle handle after rotating for one minute, 20 times/second. Frequency, continuous wave at a level determined by the patient's tolerance is applied for 20 minutes each time. The therapy is given for the mild poisoning and sequelae.

6.   COMBINED TREATMENT

(1) Puncturing, Cupping and Bleeding

Points: Dazhui (GV14), Yongquan (KI1) and Fengfu (GV16)

Technique: Prick Dazhui (GV14) for three to five seconds with a three-edged needle after routine sterilization, then cup the point by a large size glass jar to get 5 to 10 ml of blood. The reducing needling technique by rotating, lifting and thrusting method is applied on Yongquan (KI1) and the sparrow-pecking technique applied to Fengfu (GV16), which is located with the patient in a sitting position with the head lowered. The needle is inserted for 2 *cun* deep and withdrawn until numbness and electric sensation are present. The therapy is given for food poisoning.

(2) Combination of Acupuncture and Moxibustion

Points: Zhongwan (CV12), Neiguan (PC6), Zusanli (ST36), Weizhong (BL40), BL 57 (Chengshan) and Shenque (CV8).

Technique: Apply indirect moxibustion with salt on Shenque (CV8) for 15 to 30 minutes, and at the same time, puncture Zhongwan (CV12), Neiguan (PC6) and Zusanli (ST36) with the patient in a lying position. When the condition is relieved, Weizhong (BL40) and Chengshan (BL57) are punctured. The therapy is for food poisoning.

[REMARKS]

1.   Relatively good therapeutic results are achieved for opening the orifice, detoxification and sequelae of poisoning diseases by acupuncture and moxibustion, but the combination of Chinese and Western medicine is adopted for severe poisoning.

2.   The patient with poisoning sequelae should build up confidence

of conquering the disease, keep a good mood and undertake functional exercise in combination with the treatment to promote recovery.

COLLAPSE SYNDROME

[INTRODUCTION]

Collapse syndrome is mainly manifested as sudden fainting, loss of consciousness and extreme cold in the four limbs. Generally, the duration of fainting is short and there are no hemiplegia, aphasia and deviation of mouth and eye, but death may result. There are four types of collapse syndrome, commonly named as *qi*, blood, phlegm and food-related types, differentiating into excess and deficiency syndromes in the clinic. Excess syndrome is treated by Shuigou (GV26) and Neiguan (PC6) mainly to regain consciousness and open the orifice in an emergency; Taichong (LR3) is supplemented for collapse syndrome of the *qi* type; Xingjian (LR2) and Yongquan (KI1) for blood type; Juque (CV14) and Fenglong (ST40) for phlegm type; and Zhongwan (CV12) and Zusanli (ST36) for the food-related type. Deficiency syndrome is treated by Baihui (GV20) and Qihai (CV6) mainly to rescue *yang* from collapse and Shenque (CV8) and Zusanli (ST36) are supplemented for the *qi* type and Guanyuan (CV4) for blood type. The treatment therapy in the chapter is taken as a reference for shock, collapse syncope, summer collapse, hypoglycemic coma and hysterical coma in modern medicine.

[CLINICAL EXPERIENCE]

1. CONVENTIONAL ACUPUNCTURE

(1) Puncturing Suliao (GV25)

Points: Main points: Suliao (GV25) and Neiguan (PC6). Supplementary points: Shaochong (HT9), Shaoze (SI1), Zhongchong (PC9), Yongquan (KI1) and the auricular point for increasing blood pressure.

Technique: The chief points are punctured at first with filiform needles, but if there is no result within half an hour, one to two supplementary points are added to give moderate stimulation. The needles are retained and rotated intermittently for one to two hours, then removed until the condition of the case is relieved. The therapy is given for shock due to various reasons.

(2) Puncturing Renzhong (GV26) and Neiguan (PC6)

Technique: The patient adopts a lying position with the head lowered. Lifting, thrusting and rotating technique is applied on Renzhong (GV26) and rotating technique on Neiguan (PC6). Constant stimulation is given until the blood pressure increases. The needles are removed until the four limbs become warm. The therapy is given for shock.

(3) Penetrating Puncturing from Houxi (SI3) to Laogong (PC8)

Points: Penetration puncturing from Houxi (SI3) to Laogong (PC8) and Zusanli (ST36).

Technique: Strong stimulation is applied on the bilateral points, the needles being retained for a severe case. The therapy is given for convulsion.

(4) Penetrating Puncturing from Kunlun (BL60) to Taixi (KI3)

Technique: Penetrating puncturing from Kunlun (BL60) to Taixi (KI3) with strong stimulation is applied for high fever and hysterical syncope and syncope without definite reason. Generally, the needles are retained for three to five minutes until consciousness returns.

(5) Puncturing Weizhong (BL40)

Points: Weizhong (BL40), Zhiyang (GV9), Zuqiaoyin (GB44), Dadun (LR1) and Changqiang (GV1).

Technique: Either strong stimulation with a filiform needle or the bleeding method with three-edged needle is applied. The treatment is given for fainting due to blood stasis in the brain and intracranial hypertension.

(6) Puncturing Jing-Well Points

Points: Shaoshang (LU11), Shangyang (LI1), Guanchong (TE1), Shaoze (SI1)) and Yongquan (KI1).

Technique: A one-*cun* filiform needle is applied to strongly stimulate bilateral Jing-Well points. Blood pressure can be effectively increased. The treatment is given for all kinds of shock.

2. MOXIBUSTION

(1) Indirect Moxibustion with Salt by Moxa Cones

Point: Shenque (CV8)

Technique: With the patient in a lying position, the umbilicus is filled with salt, and then a moxa cone the size of a soybean or half of a date kernel is placed on it. In each treatment, five to 30 cones are prepared until the pulse is restored and the patient sweats. The therapy is given for collapse of *yang* and *yin*.

(2) Direct Moxibustion with Moxa Cones

Point: Guanyuan (CV4)

Technique: Five to 20 big cones are applied on the point with the patient lying down. This method is for all kinds of shock.

3. BLEEDING METHOD

Points: Shangyang (LI1) and Shixuan (Ex-UE11)

Technique: Prick the above-mentioned points with a three-edged needle or a syringe needle to cause a little bleeding. The therapy is given for collapse due to over-indulgence of food and drink.

4. HYDRO-ACUPUNCTURE

Points: Dazhui (GV14), Quchi (LI11) and Hegu (LI4)

Technique: Inject the above-mentioned points successively with Injection for Regaining Consciousness with Calculus Bovis, 4 ml, one to two times a day. The dosage is reduced to half for children. The therapy is given for fainting due to high fever.

5. AURICULAR THERAPY

Points: Main points: Adrenal, the point for increasing blood pressure, Subcortex and Heart. Supplementary points: Shenmen, Sympathetic and Liver.

Technique: Two to four commonly used points are selected on both ears alternately and needled with strong stimulation, retaining them for one to two hours. The therapy is applied one to two times a day.

6. FINGER ACU-PRESSURE

Point: Tiantu (CV22)

Technique: Press Tiantu (CV22) with the thumb for several minutes. The therapy is given for collapse of the phlegm type.

7. COMBINATION OF ACUPUNCTURE AND MOXIBUSTION

(1) Indicating Hemorrhagic Shock

Points: Yinbai (SP1) and Sanyinjiao (SP6)

Technique: Puncture bilateral Sanyinjiao (SP6) at first, then simultaneously apply moxibustion on Yinbai (SP1) with a moxa stick for 30 to 60 minutes until the limbs turn warm. The pulse is restored and consciousness gradually returns.

(2) Indicating Colic Caused by Ascaris

Points: Baihui (GV20), Shenque (CV8), Guanyuan (CV4), penetrating puncturing from Neiguan (PC6) to Waiguan (TE5), Zusanli (ST36) and Liangmen (ST21).

Technique: Moxibustion with the moxa stick is given above Baihui (GV20), Shenque (CV8) and Guanyuan (CV4) for 30 minutes in total. Then acupuncture is applied on the rest points bilaterally until the limbs turn warm and consciousness returns, retaining the needles for 30 minutes.

[REMARKS]

1. Since collapse syndromes refer to critical emergencies, if the treatment result by acupuncture and moxibustion for such an emergency is not remarkable, comprehensive therapy should be adopted.

2. For the most urgent conditions, finger acu-pressure is applied on Renzhong (GV26) and Neiguan (PC6) instead of needling.

SUNSTROKE

[INTRODUNTION]

The disease is commonly caused by disturbance of *qi*, blood, *yin* and *yang* due to invasion of pathogenic summer heat because of staying in a high-temperature condition or exposure to the burning sun for a long time in summer. Clinically, the disease is divided into mild and severe cases. The mild case is due to summer heat combining with damp stagnation in the muscles and skin, manifested as dizziness, headache, fever, slight sweating, vomiting, irritability and thirst, and is treated by eliminating the exterior syndromes, clearing away summer heat, harmonizing the Middle Energizer by the points on Governor Vessel, Hand and Foot-Yangming and the pericardium meridians, i.e., Dazhui (GV14), Hegu (LI4), Xiangu (ST43), Neiguan (PC6), Zusanli (ST36) and Yinlingquan (SP9). A severe case is due to the extreme burning of summer heat blocking the pericardium, manifested as a extreme high fever, anhydrosis, burning heat of the muscles and skin, red face and eyes, irritability, restlessness and loss of consciousness, and is treated by clearing away summer heat, calming down the mind and opening the orifice by the points on Governor Vessel, Foot-Taiyang and the pericardium meridians, i.e., Baihui (GV20), Renzhong (GV26), Shixuan (Ex-UE11), Quchi (LI11), Quze (PC3) and Weizhong (BL40) punctured with reducing and bleeding techniques.

[CLINICAL EXPERIENCE]

1. CONVENTIONAL ACUPUNCTURE

(1) Regaining Consciousness and Opening the Orifice
   Points: Renzhong (GV26) and Neiguan (PC6)
   Technique: Puncture bilateral Neiguan (PC6) perpendicularly, 1 to 1.5 *cun* deep with reducing technique by the combination of rotating, thrusting and lifting needle for one minute; then puncture Renzhong (GV26) with sparrow-pecking technique until tears appear in the eyes.

(2) Puncturing Five Heart Points
   Points: Baihui (GV20) (the heart of the vertex), bilateral Laogong (PC8) (the heart of the hand) and bilateral Yongquan (KI1) (the heart of the sole).
   Technique: Take one-*cun* filiform needles to puncture the above-

mentioned points with reducing technique on Laogong (PC8) and Yongquan (KI1). The treatment is given for severe sunstroke.

2. BLEEDING METHOD

(1) Bleeding Renzhong (GV26), Quze (PC3) and Weizhong (BL40)

Technique: Prick the points with a three-edged needle to cause bleeding for loss of consciousness due to sunstroke.

(2) Bleeding Shixuan (Ex-UE11)

Technique: Prick Shixuan (Ex-UE11) with a three-edged needle or thick needle to cause bleeding for a high fever due to sunstroke.

3. PLUM-BLOSSOM NEEDLING METHOD

Points: Points on Governor Vessel

Technique: Tap with strong stimulation from Fengfu (GV16) to Shenzhu (GV12) along the Governor Vessel for mild sunstroke.

4. AURICULAR THERAPY

Points: Ear-apex, Shenmen, Adrenal, Heart and Occiput

Technique: The filiform needles are applied to strongly stimulate the points bilaterally, retaining them for 20 minutes. The bleeding method is applied on the Ear-apex.

5. SCRAPING THERAPY

Technique: A smooth and even-edged pottery or porcelain spoon dipped in vegetable oil or water is applied to scrape the bilateral sides of the spine, neck region, inter-thoracic costal spaces, shoulders, arms, cubital fossa and popliteal fossa until the skin turns purplish. The treatment is given for mild sunstroke.

6. COMBINED TREATMENT

(1) Combination of Acupuncture and Moxibustion

Points: Baihui (GV20), Neiguan (PC6) and Qihai (CV6)

Technique: Even needling technique is applied by filiform needles on Baihui (GV20) and Neiguan (PC6) and moxibustion with the moxa stick applied on Qihai (CV6) to rescue *yang* from collapse.

The therapy is given for collapse due to sunstroke.

(2) Puncturing and Bleeding

Points: Renzhong (GV26), Baihui (GV20), Shenmen (HT7) and Shixuan (Ex-UE11)

Technique: Even needling technique is applied by filiform needles on Renzhong (GV26), Baihui (GV20) and Shenmen (HT7) and the bleeding method applied on Shixuan (Ex-UE11) for loss of consciousness due to sunstroke.

[REMARKS]

1. When sunstroke happens, the patient should be moved to a cool place, well ventilated, and measures taken to reduce the body temperature, i.e., cold compress, alcohol bath and taking cold drinks.

2. For a severe case with circulatory failure and loss of consciousness with dehydration, combined therapy with Chinese and Western medicine should be adopted.

STOPPING SMOKING

[INTRODUCTION]

There are no records in ancient Chinese literature related to stopping smoking. Tobacco is a kind of poisoning material, and long-term smoking may lead to imbalance of *yin* and *yang*, abnormal ascending and descending of *qi* and the disturbance of *qi* and blood circulation in the body, resulting in various pathological changes. In recent years, in the field of acupuncture and moxibustion, auricular therapy is commonly applied for stopping smoking and the main points are Lung, Mouth, Heart, Ear-Shenmen and Endocrine.

[CLINICAL EXPERIENCE]

1. CONVENTIONAL ACUPUNCTURE

(1) Puncturing Tianwei Point

Point: Tianwei [the tender point between Lieque (LU7) and Yangxi (LI5)]

Technique: After the point is located precisely, the needles are inserted perpendicularly on bilateral points, 3 mm deep, with strong stimulation and retained for 15 minutes. Four treatments make up one course. The effective treatment rate is 80%.

(2) Puncturing Feishu (BL13)

Points: Feishu (BL13), Xinshu (BL15), Neiguan (PC6), Chize (LU5), Lieque (LU7), Hegu (LI4) and Sanyinjiao (SP6).

Technique: Quick needling technique is applied on Back-Shu points without retaining the needles and strong stimulation applied on the rest points with needles retained for 30 minutes. The treatment is given once a day and 10 treatments make up one course.

2. AURICULAR THERAPY

(1) Seed-Pressing Method with Semen Vaccaria

Points: Lung, Heart, Sympathetic, Ear-Shenmen and Mouth

Technique: Semen Vaccaria is fixed on the tender points with plaster. The points are stimulated with pressing three to five times a day and are pressed for several minutes especially during a craving period. Seven days make up a course and there is a two- or three-day interval between courses. Generally, it needs three to five courses.

(2) Electric Acupuncture

Points: Ear-Shenmen, No.1 area for stopping smoking (a tender point between Lung and Trachea) and No.2 area for stopping smoking (a tender point around the Adrenal).

Technique: One-*cun* filiform needles (Size No.28) are use to puncture bilateral points simultaneously, and electric stimulation is given right after the arrival of *qi*, with continuous wave, 200 times/min frequency. The intensity is determined according to the patient's tolerance. The stimulation lasts for 30 minutes in each treatment, once every other day. Three treatments make up one course.

(3) Combination of Body Points and Auricular Therapy

Points: Body Points: Lieque (LU7), Yangchi (TE4), Neiguan

(PC6), and Shenmen (HT7). Auricular Points: Lung, Triple Energizer, Mouth and Ear-Shenmen.

Technique: Use filiform needles to puncture body points bilaterally with strong stimulation and retain needles for 20 minutes. Ten treatments make up one course. Simultaneously, needle-embedding therapy is applied on one side auricular points in each treatment, retaining the needles for three to five days. The same therapy is then applied on the other side auricular points. After this 10-day cycle, there is a five-day break before the next treatment. Generally, a result is obtained after three months of continuous treatment.

3. MEDICINAL APPLICATION ON ACU-POINTS

Points: Tianwei point [located between Lieque (LU7) and Yangxi (LI5)] and Hegu (LI4)

Technique: Dingxiang (Flos Caryophylli), Rougui (Cortex Cinnamomi) and monosodium glutamate (MSG), an equal dosage for each, are prepared. The first two herbs are ground and screened by No.100 sifter. The black ointment model, six times the dosage of each herb, is melted and mixed with the powder of Dingxiang (Flos Caryophylli). Then MSG is added when the temperature drops to 60°C. The herbal paste is evenly mixed and put on a piece of paper, size 1.5×1.5 *cun* and each herb plaster weighs 1 gm. The herbal plaster is compressed on bilateral Tianwei points and Hegu (LI4) for 24 hours.

[REMARKS]

1. Certain therapeutic result is received in the treatment of stopping smoking by acupuncture and moxibustion, but the subjective effort of a patient must be required.

2. After acupuncture treatment, smokers may commonly feel the taste of a cigarette becoming bitter, and continuous treatment can inhibit smoking desire. The effect is received for some patients after one to two weeks of treatment, but it needs one to three months for heavy smokers.

SIMPLE OBESITY

[INTRODUCTION]

Except obesity due to disturbance of the endocrine or other diseases, most cases refer to simple obesity. Chinese medicine views that obesity is closely related to the spleen and stomach. It is mainly caused by over-eating greasy, sweat and spicy food which transforms into heat and produces fire, leading to hyperactivity of *yang* in the Middle Energizer, excessive heat in the stomach, over-eating and excessive appetite and hyper-nutrition, finally leading to obesity. Alternatively, it is caused by damp due to spleen deficiency, retention of phlegm and damp in muscles and skin, or by *yang* deficiency of the spleen and kidney and retention of damp, manifested by edema and obesity. Excessive stomach fire is treated by reducing stomach fire by auricular points, i.e., Stomach, Hunger Point and Sympathetic. Retention of damp is treated by strengthening spleen to eliminate damp by auricular points, i.e., Spleen, Stomach, Triple Energizer and Endocrine. *Yang* deficiency of the spleen and stomach is treated by warming them by the auricular points, i.e., Kidney, Spleen, Ear-Shenmen, Endocrine and Sub-cortex.

[CLINICAL EXPERIENCE]

1. ELECTRIC ACUPUNCTURE

(1) Selecting Points on the Upper Limbs

Points: Liangqiu (ST34) and Gongsun (SP 4)

Technique: The patient adopts a lying position. Reducing technique with the lifting, thrusting and rotating method is applied after the arrival of *qi* to produce strong stimulation. Then two groups of wires are attached on the bilateral points, stimulating with continuous wave for 30 minutes. The treatment is given once a day for obesity due to retention of damp caused by spleen deficiency.

(2) Selecting Points on the Abdomen

Points: Tianshu (ST25) and Daheng (SP15)

Technique: With the patient in a lying position, use two-*cun* filiform needles to puncture the points bilaterally obliquely and deeply. Electric stimulation is applied after the arrival of *qi* and lasts for 30 minutes. The treatment is given once a day for excess fat, especially on the abdomen.

2. MOXIBUSTION

Points: Main points: Yangchi (TE4) and Sanjiaoshu (BL22). Supplementary points: Diji (SP8), Mingmen (GV4), Sanyinjiao (SP6) and Dazhui (GV14).

Technique: Indirect moxibustion with ginger is applied on each of the chief and supplementary points respectively with big moxa cones. In each treatment, five to six cones are required until the skin turns to red, while skin burning should be avoid. The treatment is given once a day and one month of treatment makes up one course. It is designed for obesity due to *yang* deficiency of the spleen and kidney.

3. AURICULAR THERAPY

(1) Seed-Pressing Method with Semen Vaccaria

Points: Endocrine, Ear-Shenmen, Stomach, Mouth, Lung, Large Intestine, Cardia and Hunger

Technique: Detect tender points as the treatment points around one side's ear points; put Semen Vaccaria on the points and press the seeds until the patient feels soreness, heaviness, numbness or pain, indicating the arrival of *qi*. Three to five days later, the same therapy is applied on the other ear. The treatment is given continuously for 20 days. During the days of seed retention, the patient is advised to press the points with the index finger and thumb three times, each time for five minutes. Generally, the appetite is reduced.

(2) Needle-embedding Method

Points: Ear-Shenmen, Stomach, Large Intestine, Endocrine, Lung, Heart Triple Energizers and Hunger Point.

Technique: In each treatment, after routine sterilization, the needles are embedded on one to two selected points, and fixed with plaster. The fixed place is massaged gently for 30 to 50 seconds until the patient feels distention without pain. The same massage is applied for 30 minutes before meals. The needles are removed in three to four days, then the same method is applied on the other points.

(3) Magnetic Ball-pressing Method

Points: Mouth area and Diaphragm area

Technique: Weak magnetic balls are fixed on the points bilaterally. The points are pressed two or three times a day and continuously for half a month. The next treatment is given after a two-day interval.

4. COMBINATION OF BODY POINTS AND AURICULAR POINTS

Points: Acupoints: Pishu (BL20) and Fenglong (ST40) for excessive phlegm damp in the interior; Tianshu (ST25), Yanglingquan (GB34) and Neiting (ST44) for excessive stomach fire; Shenshu (BL23), Pishu (BL20), Sanyinjiao (SP6) and Taixi (KI3) for deficiency of the spleen and kidney; Ququan (LR8) for obesity after delivery; and Shenshu (BL23) and Sanyinjiao (SP6) for juvenile obesity. The auricular points: Spleen, Endocrine, Kidney, Stomach, Large Intestine, Triple Energizers and Lung.

Technique: Body points are punctured once a day with reducing or reinforcing technique by the lifting, thrusting and rotating needling methods based on reducing for excess and reinforcing for deficiency. Retain the needles for 30 minutes. The needle-embedding method is applied on auricular points. In each treatment, the needles are embedded on one to two selected points bilaterally, pressed twice a day, each time for one minute. The needles are changed once every three to five days. One month of treatment forms one course. The same therapy is repeated one week later.

5. COMBINATION OF AURICULAR POINTS AND MEDICINE

Points: Group 1: Stomach and Endocrine. Group 2: Spleen, Lung and Triple Energizers

Technique: After routine sterilization of points, intradermal needles are embedded and fixed by plaster, twice a week. Four times make up one course. Points of Group 1 are applied in the first course of treatment and Group 2 in the second. Simultaneously, Miraculous Powder of Saposhnikovia is taken orally, twice a day. Or a decoction is prepared, twice decocting for each dose and taken twice with warm water.

[REMARKS]

1. Around 70-80% of patients can reduce weight with different results by simple auricular therapy, and the remarkable therapeutic results are obtained in one to two weeks in most cases.

2. The appetite of most patients is reduced during the treatment, and hunger and appetite are reduced especially by pressing the auricular points for half-an-hour before meals.

COSMESIS

[INTRODUCTION]

Cosmesis by acupuncture is achieved by needling acupoints to promote the circulation of *qi* and blood on the face, benefiting local wrinkle removal and preventing aging, and also treating acne, pigmented spots, blepharochalasis, black spots and butterfly spots. According to the theories of Chinese medicine, the lustrousness and smoothness of skin is closely related to the functions of Zangfu organs, the emotions, six exogenous pathogenic factors and diet, such as *qi* deficiency of the spleen and lung, dysfunctions of the spleen in dominating muscles and lung in dominating skin and hair, and failure of *qi* and blood flowing up to the face. All of those result in facial aging. Overeating greasy and sweat-inducing food leads to upward steaming of damp heat in the spleen and stomach or lung and blood heat attacking the face, resulting in acne. The spleen deficiency fails to produce essential material, resulting in a deficiency of *qi* and blood and lack of nourishment in the muscle and skin. Finally, damp heat steams up to the face and pigmented spots occur. Clinically, different points are selected based on different syndromes.

[CLINICAL EXPERIENCE]

1. CONVENTIONAL ACUPUNCTURE

(1) Removing Facial Wrinkles

Points: Yangbai (GB14) for wrinkles on the forehead, Jingmen (BL1) and Tongziliao (GB1) for the eye region, and Juliao (ST3), Sibai (ST2), Quanliao (SI18) and Yingxiang (LI20) for the cheek.

Technique: Puncture Yangbai (GB14) horizontally with one-*cun* filiform needles (Size: Nos. 34-36), with the tip toward the forehead or the lateral side of the head, Jingming (BL1) perpendicularly 0.2 *cun* deep and Tongziliao (GB1) transversely to Taiyang (Ex-HN5) successively. Puncture Juliao (ST3), Sibai (ST2) and Quanliao (SI18) successively 0.3 to 0.5 *cun* deep and Yingxiang (LI20) subcutaneously with the tip toward the cheek. The supplementary points are selected based on the different figures of the patients. For obesity with weak muscles, Ligou (LR5), Taichong (LR3), Yinlingquan (SP9), Gongsun (SP4), Pishu (BL20) and Ganshu (BL18) are added; for weak constitution, Zusanli (ST36), Taixi (KI3), Houxi (SI3) and Hegu (LI4) are added; and for the normal figure, Waiguan (TE6) and Zusanli (ST36) are added.

(2) Prescription for Removing Pigmented Spots

Points: Main points: Yingxiang (LI20), Sibai (ST2), Xiaguan (ST7) and Jiache (ST6). Supplementary points: For stagnation of the liver *qi*, Neiguan (PC6) and Taichong (LR3) are added; for deficiency of the spleen and stomach, Zusanli (ST36) and Gongsun (SP4) are added; and for insufficiency of *qi* and blood, Zusanli (ST36) and Qihai (CV6) are added.

Technique: Routine treatment is applied once a day or once every other day, and 10 treatments form one course.

2. AURICULAR THERAPY

Points: Endocrine, Ear-Shenmen, Cheek, Adrenal and Lung

Technique: After routine sterilization, intradermal needles are inserted on the auricular points bilaterally and fixed by plasters. The treatment is given once every three to five days and five treatments form one course. It deals with freckles.

3. PRICKING METHOD

Points: Dazhui (GV14), Shenzhu (GV12), Shendao (GV11) and Zhiyang (GV9)

Technique: Two to three points are selected in each treatment and pricked by a thick filiform needle to get a few drops of blood or the cupping method follows pricking. The treatment is given once or twice each week, and is for treating pigmented spots.

4. HOT-RED NEEDLING

Points: The local area of freckle

Technique: After strict sterilization, the needle with a hot and red tip is used to prick the local area swiftly and the point is pressed forcefully after pricking. Rubbing is forbidden to prevent bleeding. Forceful and quick pressing may minimize pain. Some cases are cured after only one treatment. The therapy is applied not only for freckles but also for pigmented spots.

5. ELECTRIC-THERMAL NEEDLING

Points: The center and surrounding area of pigmented spots

Technique: 200 mA to 250 mA electric current is delivered via the electric-thermal needle until the needle turns red, then the red-body needle is swiftly inserted in the center and the surrounding area of the spot, avoiding penetrating the base of it, about 1 to 5 mm deep. Continuous pricking without retaining the needle is applied. The therapy is applied once every seven to 10 days, avoiding any wetting of the local area to prevent infection for two days after needling. Generally, a case with a small infected area is cured by only one treatment, but two to five treatments are needed for a larger area.

[REMARKS]

1. Keeping the skin clean, avoiding misusing cosmetics and applying facial massage correctly in normal frequency will bring benefits in a healthy complex.

2.   Pay attention to diet, undertake strengthening physical exercises, keep a good mood and health and improve self-culture qualities during acupuncture treatment of cosmesis.

CHAPTER TWO
GYNECOLOGY

IRREGULAR MENSTRUATION

[INTRODUCTION]

Irregular menstruation refers to any abnormal changes in the menstrual cycle, quantity and quality, as well as the color of the flow. Moreover, other symptoms may present. Commonly seen cases are antedated and postdated menstruation and irregular menstrual cycle. Modern medicine holds that it is the result of dysfunction of the endocrine and nervous system. Traditional Chinese medicine believes the disease is related with the liver, spleen and kidney. 1) Antedated menstruation is often induced by emotional disturbance, mostly worry and excess mental activity, which disturbs the smooth flow of liver *qi*, thus producing fire after a long period of *qi* stagnation; otherwise, it may result from heat in the uterus or dysfunction of the Chong and Ren meridians due to *qi* deficiency leading to abnormal flow of blood. 2) Postdated menstruation is mostly related to dysfunction of Chong and Ren meridians due to accumulation of cold in the uterus, or the sea of blood cannot be filled up in the due time. 3) Irregular menstrual cycle is often due to indulgence in sexual activity, grand multi-parity or deficiency of spleen and stomach consuming the functions of the liver and kidney, leading to dysfunction of the Chong and Ren meridians. The treatment is to strengthen spleen *qi*, regulate liver *qi*, tonify kidney essence, and adjust the functions of Chong and Ren. Points are mainly selected from the Ren meridian and Taiyin meridian of Foot, such as Qihai (CV6), Guanyuan (CV4), Sanyinjiao (SP6), Xuehai (SP10), Taichong (LR3), Taixi (KI3) and Zusanli (ST36). Antedated menstruation can be treated well with acupuncture by applying the reducing method; moxibustion is not given in this case. Acupuncture and moxibustion are both recommended in postdated menstruation and irregular menstruation by reinforcement for the deficiency syndrome, and reduction for the excess syndrome.

[CLINICAL EXPERIENCE]

1.   CONVENTIONAL ACUPUNCTURE

(1) Combination of Xi-cleft Points and Front-mu Points
   Points: Tianshu (ST25) and Shuiquan (KI5)
   Technique: Puncture perpendicularly 0.5-1 *cun* on Tianshu (ST25), and 0.3-0.5 *cun* perpendicularly on Shuiquan (KI5). As the crossing point of stomach, kidney and Chong meridian, also the Front-mu point of the large intestine, Tianshu (ST25) has strong effect on regulating *qi* and blood. Shuiquan (KI5), Xi-cleft point of kidney, is good at clearing heat, nourishing *yin*, strengthening *qi* and blood, and meanwhile regulating menstruation and stopping pain. The combination of the two points may strengthen the effect of Xi-cleft and Front-mu points, thus playing a better role in the treatment of menstruation disorder. For deficiency syndrome, the reinforcing method and moxibustion are suggested, and the needling and reducing method are suitable for excess syndrome. To strengthen the therapeutic result, other points, such as Guanyuan (CV4), Qihai (CV6), Xuehai (SP10), Diji (SP8), Zhongji (CV3) and Sanyinjiao (SP6), can be taken as secondary points.

(2) Selecting Points According to Differentiation of Syndromes
   Points: Main points: Qihai (CV6), Sanyinjiao (SP6) and Guanyuan (CV4). Supplementary points: Taichong (LR3), Taixi (KI3), Xuehai (SP10), Guilai (ST29), Diji (SP4), Shenshu (BL23), Jiaoxin (KI8), Pishu (BL20), Zusanli (ST36) and Ganshu (BL18).
   Technique: Qihai (CV6), Sanyinjiao (SP6) and Guanyuan (CV4) are punctured with the routine method. The purpose is to adjust the functions of the liver, spleen and kidney as well as Sanjiao. For antedated menstruation, points like Taichong (LR3) and Taixi (KI3) can be added. Xuehai (SP10), Guilai (ST29) and Diji (SP8) are recommended for postdated menstruation, with moxibustion on the abdomen at Guilai (ST29). Perform the reinforcing method on Shenshu (BL23), Pishu

(BL20), Jiaoxin (KI8) and Zusanli (ST36), and the reducing method on Ganshu (BL18) for irregular menstruation. Needles are retained for 30 minutes. Treatment is applied once daily, 10 times forming one course.

2. MOXIBUSTION

Points: Guanyuan (CV4)

Technique: Three to five moxa cones are applied on Guanyuan (CV4) with ginger as insulation. The moxa cone in a soybean size should be kept burning until the ginger color changes to brown. Treatment is applied once in two days from the end of the menstrual circle, 10 times making up one course. The second treatment starts from the end of the next period of menstruation. The above method is indicated mostly for deficiency of *qi* and blood.

3. AURICULAR THERAPY

Points: Kidney, Liver, Spleen, Ovary, Endocrine, Uterus, Intertragus and Brain Point.

Technique: Locate 4-6 points with the ear detector or probe, puncture with the filiform needle or press with vaccaria seeds. The treatment may be given once daily or once every other day, 10 times forming one course. Auricular therapy was performed on 30 cases, of which 18 were cured, 11 were improved and one had no effect.

4. SCALP ACUPUNCTURE

Points: Reproductive areas bilaterally.

Technique: Apply the quick rotating method for one or two minutes after insertion of the needles, keeping the frequency at 100-150 times minute. Afterwards, connect the electric stimulator to the needles for 20 minutes. Treatment is given once daily, 10 sessions forming one course.

5. PRICKING METHOD

Points: Take one point between Yaoyangguan (GV3) and Yaoshu (GV2), the lower the better.

Technique: Prick with a three-edged needle about 0.1-0.15 cm deep, and then protect the skin with sterilized gauze, applying the above treatment once a month and continuously for three months.

6. MEDICINAL APPLICATION ON ACU-POINTS

Points: Shenque (CV8) and Zigong (Extra)

Technique: Prepare Frankincense (Gummi Olibanum) 15 g, Myrrh (Myrrha) 15 g, Peony Root (Rx. Paeoniae Lactiflorae) 15 g, Ox Knee (Rx. Achranthis Bidentatae) 15 g, Scarlet Root (Rx. Salviae Miltiorrhizae) 15 g, Hawthorn Fruit (Fr. Crataegi) 15 g, and Costus Root (Rx. Saussureae seu Vladimiriae) 15 g. Pestle the above medicine into powder and mixed them with the powder of Safflower Flower (Fl. Carthami Tinctorii) 1 g. Put the paste, a mixture of 30 g medicine powder with ginger juice or yellow rice wine, on the points, cover them with gauze and fix the gauze with adhesive plaster. The medicine is changed after two days, and five treatments form one course.

7. MAGNETIC THERAPY

Points: Guanyuan (CV4) and Sanyinjiao (SP6)

Technique: Stick a 500-1500 gauss magnetic plaster on such point for 30-60 minutes, once a day. Five sessions make up one treatment course.

[REMARKS]

1.   Normally the disease is treated five to seven days before the period for about five to seven times continuously. The second treatment starts five to seven days before the next menstrual period.

2.   Avoid taking cold and spicy food, and stay away from mental stimulation.

AMENORRHEA

[INTRODUCTION]

The delay of the onset of menstruation in a girl over 18 years of age, or continuous suppression of menstruation for three months is called amenorrhea. The former is known as primary amenorrhea and the latter as secondary amenorrhea. The disease is mostly related with mental stimulation, pathological change of the pituitary, ovary and endocrine system, as well as underdevelopment of the uterus, or injury. Traditional Chinese medicine classifies amenorrhea into two categories: deficiency and excess. Deficiency syndrome is often caused by insufficiency of *qi* and blood due to dysfunction of the liver and kidney or weakness of the spleen and stomach. Excess syndrome is often related with invasion of cold to the uterus, or *qi* and blood stagnation due to emotional disturbance. Otherwise, it can be caused by damp and phlegm which block the circulation of blood in the Chong and Ren meridians. Treatment is to strengthen the spleen and kidney, nourish blood, regulate menstruation, smooth the circulation of liver *qi*, eliminate damp, and activate *qi* and blood. Points are mainly selected from Ren meridian and Three *Yin* Meridians of Foot, for instance, Zhongji (CV3), Guanyuan (CV4), Xuehai (SP10), Sanyinjiao (SP6), Shenshu (BL23), Pishu (BL20), Ganshu (BL18), Zusanli (ST36), etc. The reinforcing method and moxibustion are applied for deficiency syndrome, and the reducing method for excess syndrome.

[CLINICAL EXPERIENCE]

1. CONVENTIONAL ACUPUNCTURE

(1) Puncture on Single Point
Point: Changqiang (GV1)

Technique: Locate the point in the depression at the midpoint of the coccyx and anus, puncture 1 *cun* deep with the strong-stimulation reducing method and manipulate the needles once every five minutes while they are retained. Each treatment lasts for 20 minutes, and three treatments are taken as one course.

(2) Taking "Four Gate" Points as the Key Points
Points: Hegu (LI4) and Taichong (LR3). Supplementary points: Xuehai (SP10), Sanyinjiao (SP6) and Zhongji (CV3)

Technique: Apply quick needling technique on Hegu (LI4),

Taichong (LR3) and Xuehai (SP10) and retain needles on Sanyinjiao (SP6) and Zhongji (CV3), manipulating the needles twice and each time for one minute. Treatment is given once daily, seven sessions forming one course. Chinese Angelica Ointment for Regulating Blood can be prescribed after the onset of menstruation to strengthen the therapeutic result.

(3) Puncturing in Proper Order

Points: Xuehai (SP10), Zusanli (ST36) and Yongquan (KI1)

Technique: The first step is to puncture Xuehai (SP10) for about 2 *cun* deep, then take Zusanli (ST36) and puncture 1.5 *cun*. After the arrival of *qi* on Zusanli (ST36), select Yongquan (KI1) and puncture 1.0 *cun*. All of the needles are retained for 30 minutes, manipulating them every 10 minutes. Apply the treatment once daily, and 10 times form a course. The above method has the function of *qi* promotion in the meridians and collaterals.

(4) Selecting Points According to Differentiation of Syndromes

Points: ① Hegu (LI4), Qihai (CV6), Xuehai (SP10) and Sanyinjiao (SP9). ② Baihui (GV20), Fengchi (GB20), Shenmen (HT7), Sanyinjiao (SP9), Zhongji (CV3), Qimen (LR14), Taichong (LR3) and Zhongzhu (TE3). ③ Qihai (CV6), Zusanli (ST36) and Sanyinjiao (SP9)

Technique: The first group of points is indicated for spleen deficiency and excessive dampness. For treatment, even movement is often performed. The second group of points is good at treating liver fire produced by *qi* stagnation, and the reducing method is recommended. The third group of points is better for the weakened spleen and stomach, with the reinforcing method and moxibustion often selected, 10 sessions forming one course. The method has been proved clinically effective.

2. MOXIBUSTION

Points: Guanyuan (CV4) and Guilai (ST29)

Technique: Grind some white pepper into powder, adding wheat flour and making a coin size cake with water 0.3 cm thick. Clove Flower-bud (Fl. Caryophylli) and Inner Bark of Saigon Cinnamon (Cx. Cinnamomi Cassiae) are placed in the middle of the cake. Three to six moxa cones are applied on each point. The treatment is given once daily or every other day, three to five treatments forming one course. Moxibustion is indicated for amenorrhea due to accumulation of cold in the uterus.

3. AURICULAR THERAPY

Points: Ear Shenmen, Uterus, Ovary, Endocrine, Subcortex, Liver, Kidney.

Technique: Needles are retained for 15 minutes, and treatment is given once every other day, 10 sessions constituting a course. Semen Vaccaria can be used instead of needles.

4. CUTANEOUS PUNCTURE

Points: Du meridian and Urinary Bladder meridian at the lumbar sacral region, the Three *Yin* Meridians of the Foot at inguinal groove and lower limb.

Technique: Moderate stimulation is applied on these areas. The treatment is given once daily and 10 days form one course.

5. ELECTRIC ACUPUNCTURE

Points: ① Guilai (ST29) and Sanyinjiao (SP6). ② Zhongji (CV3) and Diji (SP8). ③ Qugu (CV2) and Xuehai (SP10)

Technique: After arrival of the needling sensation, connect one of the pair points with electricity for about 20 minutes, keeping the frequency at 2-5 times/second. Different point groups are taken alternately. The treatment is given once a day and 10 times make up one course.

6. HYDRO-ACUPUNCTURE

Points: ① Shuidao (ST28) and Sanyinjiao (SP9). ② Zigong (Extra) and Xuehai (SP10)

Technique: Inject progesterone or stilbestrol to one of the pair points, 0.5 ml at each point, changing the points every other day. Seven days form one treatment course, and there is a five-day break between courses. Therapeutic effects normally appear after two or three courses.

7. COMBINED TREATMENT

Points: Shenshu (BL23), Yinjiao (CV7) and Sanyinjiao (SP6); for deficiency syndrome, Guanyuan (CV4) and Zusanli (ST36) are added; for excess syndrome, Zhongji (CV3), Diji (SP8) and Xuehai (SP10) are added.

Technique: Apply routine needling technique on the above points, reinforcing for deficiency and reducing for excess syndrome. Treatment is given once daily for 30 minutes each time. In cases where the patient has pain in the lumbar and abdomen regions, perform acupuncture at Baliao (BL31, 32, 33, 34) or cupping on the lower abdomen. Main massage therapies are pressing, rubbing (or kneading), pointing, seizing and grabbing. The pressing and kneading methods are applied for two or three minutes at Geshu (BL17), Ganshu (BL18), Pishu (BL20), Shenshu (BL23) and Baliao (BL31, 32, 33, 34); the pointing method at Qihai (CV6) and Guanyuan (CV4); the kneading method five or six times on the abdomen; the grabbing on the muscles of the abdomen and shaking several times. Afterwards, Zusanli (ST36), Diji (SP8) and Sanyinjiao (SP6) for five to six minutes. This treatment was given to 15 patients, six of whom were cured and only one achieved no effect.

[REMARKS]

1. A satisfactory result is often reached by acupuncture or massage for patients whose amenorrhea is related with emotional factors. Medical reports show the high-estrogen-level treatment is more effective.

2. A physical test is necessary to find out the causative factors for secondary amenorrhea.

DYSMENORRHEA

[INTRODUCTION]

Dysmenorrhea is classified into two categories: deficiency and excess. Cold invading during the menstruation period may result in blood stagnation. Retention of blood stasis in the uterus causing obstruction in the meridians and collaterals is the main reason for the pain. Other causative factors leading to excess syndrome are seven emotions that give rise to stagnation of *qi*. Constitutional deficiency or deficiency of *qi* and blood due to dysfunction of liver and kidney may result in emptiness in the sea of blood, malnutrition of the uterus causing pain. Generally speaking, excess syndrome is characterized by pain starting from before or during the period; post-menstrual pain is often classified as deficiency syndrome. The treatment for excess syndrome is to regulate menstruation and relieve pain and smooth the flow of blood in the Chong and Ren meridians. Points are mainly chosen from Ren and Foot Taiyin meridians such as, Zhongji (CV3), Ciliao (BL32), Diji (SP8), etc. The reinforcing method is selected in acupuncture treatment; and moxibustion is recommended. The treatment for deficiency syndrome is to tonify *qi* and blood and strengthen the functions of the liver and kidney. Points are mainly selected from Ren, Du and Foot Shaoyin and Foot Yangming meridians, such as Mingmen (GV 4), Shenshu (BL23), Guanyuan (CV4), Zusanli (ST36), Taixi (KI3), Shuiquan (KI5), etc. The reinforcing method is combined with moxa.

[CLINICAL EXPERIENCE]

1. CONVENTIONAL ACUPUNCTURE

(1) The Method of the 17th Vertebrae

Points: All those below the 17th vertebrae (below lumbar 5th)

Technique: Puncture from 1 to 1.5 *cun*, and keep the needles for 30 minutes. There is normally immediate pain relief for most patients after needling, and remarkable effects have been achieved. If dysmenorrhea results from blood stasis, menstruation will appear 30 minutes after treatment. That is to say, the method above is not only good at pain killing but is also effective in regulating menstrual flow.

(2) Needling the Three Cai Points

Points: ① The three cai points of the heaven, people and earth: Baihui (GV20), Yongquan (KI1) and Xuanji (CV21). ② The three cai points of the upper, middle and lower parts: Dabao (SP21), Tianshu (ST25) and Diji (SP8).

Technique: The two groups of points can be used alternately. The method is particularly good at regulating *qi* and blood in the whole body. Thus it is performed when the patient is in severe pain and nothing else helps.

(3) Puncturing the Single Point
Point: Sanyinjiao (SP6)

Technique: Needle on this point perpendicularly for a patient with pain during the menstrual cycle. Further differentiation must be given for those whose pain cannot be relieved after retaining the needle for 30 minutes.

(4) Puncturing Back-Shu Points
Points: Main points are Sanjiaoshu (BL24), Shenshu (BL23) and Ciliao (BL32). For stagnation of *qi* and blood, Ganshu (BL18) and Qihaishu (BL24) are added; for retention of damp cold, Pishu (BL20) and Guanyuanshu (BL26) are added; as for deficiency of *qi* and blood, Pishu (BL20) and Weishu (BL21) are added.

Technique: Generally apply the lifting and thrusting method. The radiating sensation from the main points must reach the lower abdomen. Needles are supposed to be retained for 15 minutes. A warming needle is used for five to 10 minutes on Shenshu (BL23) and Ciliao (BL32).

(5) Stimulating Chengshan (BL57)
Point: Chengshan (BL57) bilaterally

Technique: The patient takes a prone position, and a six-*cun* needle is selected to stimulate Chengshan (BL57) on both sides, carefully rotating the needle into the point until a strong sensation is felt. Treatment is given for 15 to 30 minutes. Among 13 patients, 11 gained immediate pain relief, and two improved.

2.   MOXIBUSTION

(1) Warming Moxa with a Moxa Stick
Points: Painful area on the abdomen

Technique: The patient lies on his back with knees flexed. Holding an ignited moxa stick, the doctor stands at his side and keeps the stick moving up and down along the abdominal region for 30 to 60 minutes until the patient feels the abdominal pain has been relieved or has disappeared. Warming moxa is often given two or three days before the menstrual period, each time for 15 to 30 minutes, once a day. The above method is very effective at relieving symptoms and pain. Warming moxa is advised for deficiency and cold syndromes.

(2) Circular Moving with a Moxa Stick

Points: Zhiyin (BL67) on both sides

Technique: Hold an ignited moxa stick moving around Zhiyin (BL67) for about 15 to 20 minutes. One course of treatment starts 3 days before the menstrual period until the period finished. The above method is good at treating dysmenorrhea due to cold accumulated in uterus.

(3) Warming Needle

Points: Chenjiang (CV24) and Dazhui (GV14)

Technique: Use even movement on Chenjiang (CV24) and warming needle on Dazhui (GV14). Treatment is given continuously for three months, three days before the menstrual period begins until it is finished.

3. ELECTRIC ACUPUNCTURE

Points: Main points: Zhongji (CV3), Guanyuan (CV4), Xuehai (SP10) and Sanyinjiao (SP6). Supplementary points: Zusanli (ST36), Diji (SP8), Taichong (LR3), Shangqiu (SP5) and Hegu (LI4).

Technique: Connect treatment equipment G6805 with the needles and keep the frequency at three to five times per second, applying infra-red radiation on Qugu (CV2). Treatment is given once a day for 30 minutes each time. Among 45 patients, 35 were cured, eight achieved some effect and two had none.

4. AURICULAR THERAPY

Points: Uterus, Endocrine, Sub-cortex and sympathetic nerve.

Technique: Retain the needles for 15 to 30 minutes and manipulate with the rotating method to strengthen stimulation. Three to five days make up one course of treatment. The above method was chosen to treat 30 patients with primary dysmenorrhea, being very effective in 21 cases and achieving improvement in the other nine.

5.   LASER THERAPY

Points: Sanyinjiao (SP6), and Zigong (Extra), an ear point.

Technique: Apply model GE77 He-Ne Laser Therapy Apparatus on the above two points. Through light guide fiber, the output power reduced from 2.5 mw to 1.5 mw. The treatment starts 10 days before the onset of the menstrual period, once every other day for five minutes, taking points from the same side. Five or six treatments constitute one course. Among 68 patients, the treatment was effective for 35, while 21 were improved and 12 had no effect.

6.   MEDICINAL APPLICATION ON ACU-POINTS

Points: Shenque (CV8) and Zigong (Extra)

Technique: Prepare Frankincense (Gummi Olibanum) 15 g; Myrrh (Myrrha) 15 g; Peony Root (Rx. Paeoniae Lactiflorae) 15 g; Ox Knee (Rx. Achranthis Bidentatae) 15 g; Scarlet Root (Rx. Salviae Miltiorrhizae) 15 g; Hawthorn Fruit (Fr. Crataegi) 15 g; and Costus Root (Rx. Saussureae seu Vladimiriae) 15 g Pestle the above medicine into powder and mix with one g of borneol. Put the paste, a mixture of 30 g medicine powder with ginger juice or yellow rice wine, on the points, cover with gauze and fix with adhesive plaster. The medicine is changed every other day, and five treatments make up one course.

[REMARKS]

1.   Acupuncture treatment is effective for pain relief for primary dysmenorrhea, but the therapeutic effect cannot be guaranteed in treating secondary dysmenorrhea.

2.   Treatment starts three to five days before the onset of menstruation until the period ends. The symptom of pain can be relieved for most of patients after three months of continuous treatment.

3.   Avoid cold and spicy food, and stay away from mental stimulation.

UTERINE BLEEDING

[INTRODUCTION]

This category refers to vaginal hemorrhage in modern medicine caused by functional uterine bleeding, or inflammation of the reproductive organ and cancer. In traditional Chinese medicine, the disease is related with dysfunction of the liver, spleen and kidney, injury on the Chong and Ren meridians causing the failure of blood control. Indulgence in sexual activity consumes kidney essence, and the function of the kidney becomes that of storing and never excreting, so that when the Chong and Ren meridians are injured, the blood cannot be controlled and will run out of the uterus at the wrong time. Other causative factors may be emotional disturbance influencing the smooth flow of liver *qi* causing *qi* and blood stagnation, the accumulated heat forcing the blood circulating out of the normal route. If improper food intake or excessive worrying injures the spleen, its normal function in controlling blood is often disturbed. So the treatment principle is to strengthen spleen function, tonify the kidney, remove stagnation, and clear heat and regulate the Chong and Ren meridians. Points are mainly taken from Ren meridian, with Taiyin, Jueyin and Shaoyin meridians of the foot as the main points, such as Guanyuan (CV4), Xuehai (SP10), Sanyinjiao (SP6), Yinbai (SP1), Zhongji (CV3), Yinlingquan (SP9), Hegu (LI4) and Taichong (LR3). Apply the reinforcing method for deficiency, and the reducing method for excess syndrome.

[CLINICAL EXPERIENCE]

1. CONVENTIONAL ACUPUNCTURE

(1) Puncturing Experience Point

Points: Duanhong point (on the dorsum of hand, 1 *cun* below the 2nd and 3rd metacarpalphalangeal joint, i.e., on the web.)

Technique: Insert the needle 0.5 *cun* deep, and then apply two minutes manipulation with lifting, thrusting and rotating. During retention of the needles, manipulation must be given from time to time.

Treatment can be given once a day for 20 minutes each time. The method above can reduce the volume of blood.

(2) Stimulating Reaction Spots

Points: The positive reaction spots on lumbar region.

Technique: On the lumbar region, the places where soreness, distention, heaviness and pain are present are recognized as positive reaction spots. Two to six points are taken on those areas along the side of the spinal column, inserting the needles about 1-1.5 *cun* deep. Lifting, thrusting and scraping methods are performed. All the needles can be preserved on the points for 30 to 60 minutes, with manipulation given once every 10 to 20 minutes. If treatment is applied while severe bleeding takes place, manipulation must be continued until the bleeding is brought under control. Meanwhile, keep the needles there for another 30 to 60 minutes. After withdrawing the needles, the cupping method is followed on those positive reaction spots along the side of the spinal column. Cupping is applied once daily, for 10 minutes each time. Ten sessions make up one course of treatment.

(3) Puncturing on Xi-cleft Points

Points: Diji (SP 8) and Xuehai (SP 10)

Technique: Insert the needle on Diji (SP 8) and direct the needling sensation down to the medial malleolus. Withdraw the needle under the connective tissue after retaining it on Diji (SP 8) for 10 minutes, and thrust the needle downward for about one *cun* along the running course of the spleen meridian; stick the handle on a piece of adhesive plaster so as to keep the stimulation on the point for 24 hours. If the above method is not effective, the manipulation can be given on Xuehai (SP 10), but the embedding of the needle is placed in the opposite direction from Diji (SP 8).

2. MOXIBUSTION

(1) Warming Moxa with a Moxa Stick

Point: Yinbai (SP 1)

Technique: Ignite one piece of moxa stick and hold it over Yinbai (SP 1) on the medial side of the big toe until the skin turns red. The treatment lasts 15-20 minutes and can be applied three to five times each day. To strengthen the therapeutic effect, two more treatments are suggested.

(2) Moxibustion Applied on the Apinal Column

Points: The 14th vertebrae

Technique: The vertebra at the level of the umbilicus is known as the 14th vertebra. Five cones of grain-like moxa are stuck to the skin surface to stop bleeding. The treatment is given one or two times a day, 10 times being one course.

(3) Indirect Moxa with Insulation

Points: Shenque (CV 8)

Technique: Fill the umbilicus with fried refined salt and put a piece of ginger, 0.2 cm thick and in the size of a five-cent coin, onto the salt, followed by five to seven moxa cones as big as a date. The treatment is applied once a day or once every other day. Three to five sessions form one course.

3. SCALP ACUPUNCTURE

Points: Reproduction area bilaterally

Technique: Rotate the needles rapidly for one or two minutes after insertion, retain them for one or two hours and manipulate them once every five minutes. Electrical stimulation is also recommended, which can be applied for 30 minutes, with a frequency of about 120 times/minute. Treatment may be applied once a day, 10 times considered as one course.

4. BLEEDING METHOD

Points: Yinbai (SP1) and Dadun (LR1)

Technique: Select the place 1.5 cm distal to Yinbai (SP1) and Dadun (LR1), Jing-well points, and bandage tightly with a piece of cloth, pricking above points and causing two or three drops of blood. Stop the bleeding with a sterilized cotton ball. Treatment is performed once daily or once every other day, and a cure should be achieved after one to three treatments. Generally speaking, the bleeding method is more suited for uterine bleeding to derangement of heat and blood or stagnation of *qi* and blood.

5. ELECTRIC ACUPUNCTURE

Points: Guanyuan (CV4), Zhongji (CV3), Zigong (Ex-CA1), Changqiang (GV1) and Dachangshu (BL 25)

Technique: Penetration is performed from Guanyuan (CV4) to Zhongji (CV3), quickly thrusting the needle in and inserting as deep as 2.5-3 *cun*, puncturing obliquely downward and inward on the point Zigong (Ex-CA1) until obvious needling sensation is felt. Connect the electric stimulator on the point and stimulation should be maintained for 20-30 minutes, keeping a frequency of 100 times/minute. Strong tension and a withdrawing sensation can be felt along the vagina and anus. Quick needling is performed on Changqiang (GV1) and Dachangshu (BL 25). The treatment is applied once daily, 10 sessions making up one course.

6. AURICULAR THERAPY

Points: Uterus, Sub-cortex, Endocrine and Ovary

Technique: Strong stimulation is taken at each point, and the needles are retained for 15 minutes. Treatment may start three days before the due time of the menstrual period until the period has completely finished. If the therapeutic results are not satisfactory, continued treatment should be given for two or three months. In some patients, menstruation may temporarily disappear in the following month.

7. COMBINED TREATMENT

Points: Jiaoxin (KI 8) and Heyang (BL 55)

Technique: Taking Jiaoxin (KI 8) or Heyang (BL 55) bilaterally each time, treatment is applied once daily or once every other day. The principle is to take Jiaoxin (KI 8) and Heyang (BL 55) of the left or right side alternately. After two months of continuous treatment, another two months of treatment should be followed to strengthen the therapeutic result. During acupuncture treatment, moxibustion is also performed on the handle of the needles.

[REMARKS]

1. Further diagnosis and physical examination are suggested for

menopausal women with repeated bleeding.

2. Emergency measures must be used during severe bleeding and collapse.

3. The patient should avoid raw, cold food and overwork.

CLIMACTERIUM

[INTRODUCTION]

According to traditional Chinese medicine, before and after the menopause, woman may suffer from a group of symptoms, caused by the continued exhaustion of "Tian Gui" or kidney *qi*, consumption of the essence and blood and impairment of the Chong and Ren meridians, resulting in dysfunction of the Zangfu organs and imbalance of *yin* and *yang*. For instance, the meridians and collaterals may lack warmth if kidney *yin* or *yang* is not sufficient. In other conditions the disease may relate to liver fire caused by stagnated liver *qi*, or dysfunction of the spleen *qi* in transportation and transformation. The principle of treatment is to tonify kidney *qi*, regulate Chong and Ren meridians while smoothing liver *qi*, pacifying liver *yang*, calming down the mind, and strengthening spleen function. Points like Taixi (KI 3), Zusanli (ST 36), Sanyinjiao (SP 6), Neiguan (PC 6), Taichong (LV 3), Shenshu (BL 23) and Ganshu (BL 18) are chosen from Foot Jueyin meridian, Foot Shaoyin meridian, Chong and Ren meridians as the main points.

[CLINICAL EXPERIENCE]

1. CONVENTIONAL ACUPUNCTURE

(1) Shallow Insertion

Points: Fenglong (ST 40) and Shimen (CV 5)

Technique: Insert the needle 0.6 *cun* deep on Fenglong (ST 40) and 0.5 *cun* on Shimen (CV 5) to stop bleeding. Apply the treatment once daily and retain the needles for 30 minutes in each treatment.

The above method is advised for climacterium due to spleen deficiency with accumulation of damp phlegm. Ten treatments form one course.

(2) Puncturing on Meridian Points

Points: Tianshu (ST 25), Zhongwan (CV 12) and Qihai (CV6)

Technique: Put the needles in the above three points about 0.5 *cun* deep, and apply moxibustion on the needles at the places of Tianshu (ST 25) and Qihai (CV6). Apply the treatment once daily and retain the needles for 30 minutes in each treatment. The above method is advised for climacterium due to stagnation of *qi* and blood.

(3) Selecting Points According to Differentiation

Points: Main points: Shenshu (BL 23), Taixi (KI 3), Guanyuan (CV4), Mingmen (BV 4) and Sanyinjiao (SP 6). Supplementary points: Taichong (LV 3), Shenmen (HT 7) and Zusanli (ST 36).

Technique: The reinforcing method is applied on the main points, and moxibustion can be added on Guanyuan (CV4) and Mingmen (BV 4). In cases of hyperactivity of liver *yang*, even movement is suggested on the point Taichong (LV 3). Add Shenmen (HT 7) to calm down the mind, and the reinforcing method on Zusanli (ST 36) to strengthen spleen function. Treatment can be applied once daily, each time for 20 minutes. Ten sessions constitute one course of treatment.

2.   AURICULAR THERAPY

Points: Uterus, Ovary, Endocrine, Ear Shenmen, Sympathetic Nerve and Sub-cortex. For over-excitement and insomnia, Ear Shenmen, Heart and Sub-cortex are needed; Heart and Small Intestine are suggested for palpitation; the groove for lowering blood pressure is good for those suffering from hypertension; and in case of a red complexion, the sympathetic nerve, cheek and lung can be selected.

Technique: Selecting four to six points each time according to differentiation of the syndromes, mild stimulation is performed. Manipulate the needle several times during retention. The course of treatment is comparably long, about 20 times, and treatment is given once a day. For patients suffering from irritability, the bloodletting method or embedding needles can be used on the ear.

[REMARKS]

1. The patient must understand that the menopausal period is a biological process facing all women, so worrying and excessive nervousness are not good for their health.

2. Maintaining a good mood and joining in some sports may benefit their life.

3. Greasy and spicy food must be avoided in the diet.

LEUKORRHEA DISEASE

[INTRODUCTION]

In modern medicine, vaginitis, cervicitis and pelvic inflammation are classified as leukorrhea disease. The main causative factors are deficiency of spleen *qi* and liver *qi* stagnation, which lead to flowing of damp heat to the lower part of the body, or insufficiency resulting from kidney deficiency. Other reasons include pathogenic damp attacking the uterus after menstruation or delivery, which impair the Ren and Dai meridians. The principle of treatment is to tonify the spleen and kidney, strengthen the function of Ren and Dai meridians. Points are mainly selected from Ren, Foot Taiyin and Foot Shaoyin meridians such as Daimai (GB 26), Guanyuan (CV 4), Zhongji (CV3), Sanyinjiao (SP 6), Yinlingquan (SP 9) and Zusanli (ST 36). For damp heat, apply the reducing method and avoid moxa; and combine reducing and moxibustion for patients with cold and damp. For kidney deficiency, the reinforcing method must be combined with moxa.

[CLINICAL EXPERIENCE]

1. CONVENTIONAL ACUPUNCTURE

(1) Puncturing the Four Flower Points

Points: Danshu (BL 19) and Geshu (BL17) (the four flower points)

Technique: Apply the reducing method for heat (morbid leukorrhea); and adopt the combining reinforcing method with moxibustion for deficiency syndrome (watery, dilute and white leukorrhea). The needles should be retained for 20 minutes. The treatment is given once a day, 10 sessions forming one course. The description in *Standards of Diagnosis and Treatment* says that the four flower points have incredible effect in treating leukorrhea disease. In recent years other points are also prescribed according to the symptoms and signs. For example, Guanyuan (CV 4) and Sanyinjiao (SP 6) are added for irregular menstruation; Neiguan (PC 6) and Shenmen (PC 7) for palpitation; Shenshu (BL 23), Daimai (GB 26) and Zusanli (ST 36) for weakness of the four limbs.

(2) Taking One Point

Points: Huantiao (GB 30) bilateral

Technique: Continuously apply strong stimulation on Huantiao (GB 30). Only when electric stimulation radiates downward to the heel, can a therapeutic effect be expected. Retain the needles for 20-30 minutes. Manipulation should be applied from time to time. Treatment is given once daily, and 10 sessions make up one course.

(3) Selecting Extra Points

Points: The point is situated posterior to Sanyinjiao (SP 6)

Technique: The patient should lie down on his back and naturally stretch out the lower limbs. The needle is inserted obliquely upward forming an angle of 30° to the skin surface. While the needle is completely in the skin, thrust it further horizontally some 1-1.5 *cun*. Retain the needle for 20-30 minutes. The treatment is given once daily for 10 days. The overall effective cure rate is 90.1%.

(4) Taking Eight Liao Points as Main Points

Points: Main points: Shangliao (BL31), Ciliao (BL 32), Zhongliao (BL 33) and Xialiao (BL 34). Supplementary points: Sanyinjiao (SP 6), Zusanli (ST 36), Zhongwan (CV12), Pishu (BL 20), Neiguan (PC 6) and Tanzhong (CV 17).

Technique: Select one or two pairs of *liao* points, putting the needle in about 0.5-1.2 *cun*. Continue lifting, thrusting and rotating the needle for one or two minutes. After withdrawal, sit cups on the place for 10-15 minutes. Select two or three secondary points based on differentiation, keeping the needles on the points for 20 minutes. Treatment is applied once daily, and 10 treatments make up one course.

2. MOXIBUSTION

Points: Mingmen (GV 4), Shenque (CV 8) and Zhongji (CV 3)

Technique: Apply warming moxa with a moxa stick until the skin is slightly congested. The warming method is performed for 15 minutes on each point. Treatment can be given once daily or once every other day, 10 sessions making up one course. This method is indicated for kidney *qi* deficiency with impairment at the lower body.

3. AURICULAR THERAPY

Points: For spleen deficiency, Spleen, Lung and Uterus; for damp heat, Spleen, Adrenal, Uterus, Pelvic and Sanjiao; and for kidney deficiency, Kidney, Endocrine, Uterus and Ovary.

Technique: Insert a 0.5-*cun* filiform needle on the cartilage of the selected point after sterilization, and retain it for 30-60 minutes; or embed the needle on the ear at the same points. Treatment should be given alternately on both sides of the ear, once daily or once every other day. Moxibustion should be applied on the handle of the needle for both spleen and kidney deficiency. Sterilize the points carefully with a dry cotton ball and press the hole of needle after withdrawal. Afterwards, clean the ear with 75% alcohol. In 21 cases, two were cured in one treatment, 16 cases were cured after two to five treatments, another two were cured after five treatments, and one case failed in a follow-up survey.

4. HYDRO-ACUPUNCTURE

Points: Daimai (GB 26) and Sanyinjiao (SP 6)

Technique:

1) Take 2 ml of Herba Andrographis Paniculatae and inject 0.5 ml on each point. Treatment is applied once every other day, 10 sessions making up one course.

2) The same procedure can be given with 2 ml of placental tissue fluid.

3) Take 4 ml injection of Radix Salviae Miltiorrhizae or compound prescription of Radix Angelicae Sinensis and inject 1 ml on each point. Treatment can be given once daily, 10 sessions constituting one course.

4) Take 4 ml of injection of berberine and inject 1 ml on each point. Treatment can be given once a day or once every other day, 10 sessions making up one course.

All of these four methods are effective in the treatment of leukorrhea disease, and any of them can be selected.

5. LASER THERAPY

Point: Uterine neck

Technique: First of all, empty the bladder and expose the uterine neck. After routine gynecological sterilization, apply cauterization with carbon dioxide laser, focusing on the area of the uterine neck, and make a round circle from outside gradually moving inward. The area for cauterization should be 1-2 mm larger than the eroded area; the depth may vary from 1-6 mm according to the state of the disease. Generally speaking, leukorrhea disease can be cured in one treatment.

6. WRIST-ANKLE ACUPUNCTURE

Points: The two points in the lower limbs (3-finger breadth above the tip of medial malleolus, posterior to tibia)

Technique: Insert the needle obliquely at an angle of 30° to the skin surface, and then puncture horizontally along the subcutaneous range for about 1.4 *cun*. Retain the needle for 20-30 minutes. The treatment is applied once a day. In 22 deficiency cases, 15 patients were cured, six improved and one saw no improvement.

7. COMBINED TREATMENT

(1) Combining Acupuncture with Moxibustion

Point: Zhongji (CV 3)

Technique: The reinforcing method is advised for heat syndrome and excess syndrome, while retaining the needle on Zhongji (CV 3) for 15 minutes. The reducing method is suggested for cold syndrome and deficiency syndrome. Moxibustion should be added for 20-30 minutes. According to clinical experience, only one point Zhongji (CV 3) is enough in the treatment of leukorrhea with good therapeutic effect. The reason is that Zhongji (CV 3) is the crossing point of the Ren meridian with the three *yin* meridians of the foot, so that applying proper technique on this point may exert good therapeutic effect in varying circumstances, such as clearing damp heat or cold, regulating liver *qi*, nourishing *yin* and strengthening the spleen and kidney.

(2) Combining Acupuncture with Cupping

Points: Main points: Ciliao (BL 32). Supplementary points: Mingmen (GV 4), Ligou (LR 5) and Sanyinjiao (SP 6).

Technique: The patient lies on his abdomen. Select a 2-2.5 *cun* filiform needle, and insert it obliquely downward from Ciliao (BL 32). The needling sensation is expected to radiate to the lower abdominal region or the perineum. Apply even movement for patients with damp and cold, retaining the needle for 30 minutes. Meanwhile, Mingmen (GV 4) should be used with moxa, and manipulation is given twice during needle retention. As for the treatment of damp heat, the reducing method with lifting, thrusting and rotating must be adopted. The cupping method is recommended on the needles for 15 minutes, and secondary points Ligou (LR 5) and Sanyinjiao (SP 6) should be combined. The above method can be applied once daily, five treatments making up one course. In 36 cases, 27 were cured and nine improved.

[REMARKS]

1. Acupuncture is good at treating leukorrhea disease. Usually after two or three sessions, a therapeutic effect can be expected.

2. For women over 40, when leukorrhea is morbid or watery with foul smell, the gynecological or oncological department should undertake a further examination.

3. Continence as regards sexual activity, good menstrual hygiene and keeping the vulva clean are important.

EPILEPSY DURING PREGNANCY

[INTRODUCTION]

At the late stage of pregnancy, sometimes during delivery or after delivery, the patient may suddenly fall down to the ground and lose consciousness. Other symptoms are convulsion of the limbs with the jaw closed, staring eyes, frothy salivation and intermittent attacks of unconsciousness. This is known as "epilepsy during pregnancy" or "eclampsia." Before the onset of eclampsia symptoms, such as headache, dizziness, blurred vision, abdominal discomfort, stuffiness in chest and scanty urination may be present, and this is named "re-eclampsia" in modern medicine. In this period, hypertension, edema, albuminuria and some other bodily signs may be apparent. The onset of eclampsia is closely related with insufficiency of blood supply to the liver wood. During pregnancy, when blood accumulates in the uterus in order to feed the fetus, there will be lack of blood supply for the liver wood, so that internal liver wind may be stirred up. The other causative reason is spleen deficiency, which fails to transport body fluid for disposal. Epilepsy is induced by the block of damp phlegm. The principle of treatment is to pacify liver *yang*, stop the convulsion and dispel wind, strengthen spleen and eliminate phlegm. The points are selected from spleen meridian of foot Taiyin, stomach meridian of foot Yangming, liver meridian of foot Jueyin as well as Du meridian, such as Baihui (GV20), Dahui (GV14), Shenting (GV24), Yintang (Ex-HN3), Zusanli (ST36), Fenglong (ST40), Sanyinjiao (SP 6) and Taichong (LR 3). Even movement is suggested. The needles are retained for 20 minutes. Treatment is given once daily, 10 sessions constituting one course.

[CLINICAL EXPERIENCE]

1.　CONVENTIONAL ACUPUNCTURE

(1) Selecting Yuan-primary Point and Point of Marrow
Points: Juegu (GB 39) and Taixi (KI 3)

Technique: Insert the needle obliquely on Juegu (GB39), applying the even method. Reinforce Taixi (KI 3) and retain the needles for 30 minutes. Treatment is given once daily, 10 sessions making up one course. Selecting Juegu (GB39), the meeting place of marrow, can pacify liver *yang* and eliminate wind; Yuan-primary point Taixi (KI 3) can tonify essence and marrow, so it is good at treating the root cause of the disease.

(2) Taking Extra Point

Points: Extra point Sishencong (Ex-HN1)

Technique: Apply the even method on Sishencong (Ex-HN1) with frequent rotating, 120 times/minute, for one to two minutes. The needles are retained for one to two hours, and are manipulated once every 10 minutes. The above method can calm the mind. Shenting (GV24) is recommended to wake up the spirit.

(3) Puncturing the Four Gate Points

Points: Hegu (LI 4) and Taichong (LR3)

Technique: The even method is applied on all the four points Hegu (LI 4) and Taichong (LR3) bilateral. The needles are retained for 60 minutes, and manipulation can be given several times during this period. Treatment can be given daily or in several hours. In order to strengthen the therapeutic effect, points like Yintang (Ex-HN3), Renzhong (GV26), Neiguan (PC 6) can be added, rotating the needles for one or two minutes with the even method. Quickly withdraw the needles.

(4) Needling Three **Cai** *Points*

Points: Renzhong (GV26), Qihai (CV6) and Yongquan (KI 1)

Technique: Quick needling is applied on the above three points—that is, quickly withdrawing the needles after the arrival of *qi*. Treatment is given once or twice a day. Because Renzhong (GV 26) is located in the upper part of the body, Qihai (CV6) in the middle and Yongquan (KI 1) on the foot, they are named as the three *cai* of the heaven, people and earth.

2. MOXIBUSTION

Points: ① Zhongwan (CV12). ② Huiyin (CV1) and Sanyinjiao

(SP6)

Technique: If group one is selected, 50 cones of moxa the size of big Chinese date are used. The indication is for epilepsy after delivery. Immediate effect can be expected. For group two, warming moxa with a moxa stick is applied. Treatment is given once or twice a day, 10 minutes on each point. An interval of 6-8 hours must be kept between treatments.

3. MEDICINAL APPLICATION ON ACU-POINTS

Points: Shenque (CV8) and Guanyuan (CV4)

Technique: A cream is made from 120 g talc (Talcum-hash). Grind it into fine powder, pestle 30 g of talc into a paste and put it on the point, cover them with gauze and fix the gauze with plaster. When the paste is getting dry, change to another one. This method is considered effective for eclampsia.

4. AURICULAR THERAPY

Treatment is performed in different stages:

(1) Pre-eclampsia

Points: Uterus, Sympathetic Nerve, Endocrine, groove for lowering blood pressure, Forehead and Brain.

Technique: Detect sensitive point and stimulate with a 0.5-*cun* filiform needle to provide strong stimulation for one or two minutes. This method may be given once or twice a day, 10 sessions making up one course.

(2) During Seizure

Points: Ear Shenmen, Sympathetic Nerve, Liver, Uterus, groove for lowering blood pressure, lowering blood pressure point, vein on the back of the ear, Heart and Brain.

Technique: Prick and cause bleeding on the groove for lowering blood pressure or the vein on the back of the ear. Select two to four points from the group and reduce them with strong manipulation.

(3) Remission Stage

Points: Ear-Shenmen, Sympathetic Nerve, Adrenal, Brain, Heart, Kidney and Forehead.

Technique: Embed needles or vaccaria seed (Vaccaria Semen) on the points.

5. WRIST-ANKLE ACUPUNCTURE

Points: Hand$_1$ and Hand$_3$

Technique: Select the above points from both sides, put the needles in horizontally, retain them for one or two hours. In 216 patients with hypertension due to toxemia of pregnancy, 81 remarkably improved, 36 gained good effect, 46 slightly improved and 53 witnessed no effect.

[REMARKS]

1. Eclampsia is an acute disease, and acupuncture is only considered as a supplementary treatment in emergency departments.

2. During the seizure stage, the patient should lie down quietly without any disturbance to avoid a sudden coma, which may hurt the patient or cause suffocation.

MALPOSITIONING OF FETUS

[INTRODUCTION]

After 30 weeks of pregnancy, if the fetus is found to be in an abnormal position due to plurigravida with abdominal muscular relaxation, this is understood to be malpositioning of the fetus. Because most of the time the patient has no subjective symptoms, and definite diagnosis, such as pelvic presentation, horizontal position or oblique position, can only be obtained through gynecological examination. Traditional Chinese medicine believes malpositioning of the fetus is related with *qi* and blood deficiency, weakness in rotating the fetus or stagnation of *qi* and blood, so that the position of fetus cannot be changed. The principal of treatment is to regulate *qi*, promote *qi* and blood circulation. Points are mainly selected from Taiyang and Taiyin meridians of foot, such as Zhiyin (BL67) and Sanyinjiao (SP6), with the even movement or reinforcing method. Treatment is applied once or twice a day, retaining the needles for 30 minutes. Ten treatments constitute one course.

[CLINICAL EXPERIENCE]

1.   CONVENTIONAL ACUPUNCTURE

(1) Selecting Single Point
Point: Zhiyin (BL67)
Technique: The patient may relax herself on an armchair or bed with her belt undone. Apply quick needling technique and puncture on both sides of Zhiyin (BL67) with a one-*cun* needle. Put the needle horizontally along the skin surface 0.2-0.3 *cun* deep. The reinforcing method is recommended. Keep the needles in place for 30-60 minutes.

(2) Selecting Bilateral Points
Points: Sanyinjiao (SP6) and Zhiyin (BL67)
Technique: Select Sanyinjiao (SP6) and Zhiyin (BL67) on both sides of the body. The needle inserted in Sanyinjiao (SP6) should be 0.8-1 *cun* deep, sending the sensation upward along the running course of the meridian. The needle inserted into Zhiyin (BL 67) should be 0.3 *cun* deep. Manipulation is performed every 10 minutes during the needle retention. Treatment is given once daily, three times forming a course. In 70 cases, 61 were cured and nine had no effect.

2.   MOXIBUSTION

Moxibustion with a Moxa Stick
Point: Zhiyin (BL67)
Technique: Hold the moxa stick over point Zhiyin (BL67) on both sides of the body. Treatment is applied one to three times a day, each time for 15-30 minutes. In 69 cases, 66 were effective and three had no effect (total effective rate being 95.7%).

3.   AURICULAR THERAPY

Points: Uterus, Sympathetic Nerve, Sub-cortex, Liver, Spleen and Abdomen

Technique: Embed Semen Vaccaria alternately on both sides of the ear, changing new seeds after three to four days. Stimulate the points three times a day, each time for 15 minutes. Of 169 cases, 138 were successfully treated, of whom 111 cases were cured with the first treatment; 17 cases were cured after two treatments, and 10 patients after three treatments. A study found the curative rate for women under 7-8 months pregnancy was over 91.67%, falling to 79.54% for the eight and ninth months, and 25% for those over nine months.

4. LASER THERAPY

Point: Zhiyin (BL67)

Technique: Laser therapy is applied on Zhiyin (BL67) at both sides of the body, five to eight minutes for each side. (The wavelength is 6328 A, power 5 mW and electric current 6-8 mA). Treatment is given once daily, three to five times forming one course. A total of 41 cases out of 46 patients were successfully treated with this method.

[REMARKS]

1. Acupuncture has good therapeutic effect for a malpositioned fetus because it is much safer and more convenient comparing with other therapies. The effective rate is above 80%. Pluripara has better effect than primipara. The best treatment result is expected for women during the 7th month of pregnancy; from the 8th month on, the therapeutic effect declines.

2. Comparing different therapies, moxa has better effect than electric therapy, warming needle, laser therapy and the bleeding method.

3. As there are many causative factors that may lead to the onset of the disease, such as contracted pelvis and deformity of uterus, it is advisable for patients to be handled by the gynecological department.

4. After acupuncture treatment the patient is advised to lie down in the genupectoral position.

5. Laboratory observation on 41 cases of patients showed that applying of moxa on Zhiyin (BL67) may improve the excretion of cortex from adrenal gland, and stimulate the movement of the fetus in the uterus, which will help the correction of its position.

PROTRACTED LABOR

[INTRODUCTION]

Protracted labor is mostly due to abnormality in the obstetric canal or malposition of the fetus, which may also be related with overreaction of primipara or premature labor causing too much bleeding. Constitutional deficiency and weakness of uterine contraction or stagnation of *qi* and blood may all cause the disease. The treatment principle is to nourish *qi* and blood, remove stagnation in the meridians and collaterals. The points are mainly selected from Hand Yangming and Foot Taiyin meridians, such as Hegu (LI4), Sanyinjiao (SP6) and Zhiyin (BL67). The even movement method is advised in the treatment.

[CLINICAL EXPERIENCE]

1.   CONVENTIONAL ACUPUNCTURE

(1) *Puncturing Single Point*

Point: Jianjing (GB21)

Technique: Puncture bilateral Jianjing (GB21) with the reducing method, 1 *cun* deep, with strong stimulation for one to two minutes. Retain the needles for five minutes. The same method is given repeatedly three times. Electric therapy can be advised, the frequency being 30 Hz, for five to 10 minutes. Applying this method can improve the duration of labor, with delivery mostly occurring in six to 10 hours.

(2) *Taking Four Gate Points*

Points: Hegu (LI4), Taichong (LR3) and Sanyinjiao (SP6)

Technique: Puncture perpendicularly 0.5 *cun* with the reducing method on Hegu (LI4). The reducing method is performed on Sanyinjiao (SP6); and the even movement method is selected on Taichong (LR3) for 0.5 *cun*. Retain the needles for 10-20 minutes.

(3) *Puncturing Odd Points*

Points: Duyin (on the second toe, on the midpoint of transverse crease of digital joint)

Technique: Select a one-*cun* filiform needle and puncture 0.3-0.5

cun perpendicularly, reducing with strong stimulation. Hanging moxa may be used for 10-15 minutes. It is better if Hegu (LI4) and Sanyinjiao (SP6) are both used, reinforcing for the former point and reducing for the latter.

(4) Selecting the Eight Liao Points

Points: Shangliao (BL31), Ciliao (BL32), Zhongliao (BL33) and Xialiao (BL34)

Technique: Puncture perpendicularly on above points and manipulate them for one to two minutes. The needles are retained for 60 minutes, with manipulation given once every 10 minutes. This is advised for the flowing down of amniotic fluid and relieving pain. Reinforcing Hegu (LI4) and reducing Sanyinjiao (SP6) is advised.

2. MOXIBUSTION

Points: ① Hegu (LI4) and Sanyinjiao (SP6). ② Shangliao (BL31) and Ciliao (BL32). ③ Zhiyin (BL67) and extra point Duyin

Technique: Hanging moxa is used on one of the groups; and moxibustion is given continuously until labor is over.

3. AURICULAR THERAPY

(1) Needling on the Points

Points: Lumber Vertebrae, Kidney, Sub-cortex, and Adrenal

Technique: When the uterine orifice is opened to 4 cm, strong stimulation can be performed to accelerate the labor procedure or manipulation is given once every three minutes.

(2) Injection

Points: Uterus, Shemen and Sympathetic Nerve

Technique: Two units of oxytocin is injected on each point.

4. MEDICINAL APPLICATION ON ACU-POINTS

Points: Yongquan (KI1) and Shenque (CV8)

Technique: Apply a paste of Castor leaf (Folium Ricini) on the above points, or prepare a medical cake consisting of two pieces of Croton Seed (Fructus Crotonis—Ba Dou) and 0.3 g Navel Gland Secretions of the Musk Deer (Secretio Moschus Moschiferi—She Xiang)

and put it on one of the two points. Apply the medicine before labor and remove immediately afterwards.

[REMARKS]

1.   Acupuncture treatment is mostly effective in the treatment of contraction weakness, non-stenosis of the pelvis, cephalopelvic disproportion and abnormality of the birth canal.

2.   The patient is advised to relax, take proper food and do some exercises so as to improve energy for labor.

3.   It is understood that a combination of distal and local points may produce better therapeutic effect than simply using local or distal points. For example, a better effect will be achieved by combining Hegu (LI4) and Sanyinjiao (SP6) with Zhibian (BL54) rather than using Hegu (LI4) and Sanyinjiao (SP6) or simply Zhibian (BL54).

INDUCED ABORTION

[INTRODUCTION]

Artificial stopping of pregnancy is called induced abortion. If it is done with acupuncture, it is considered safer and more effective if the operation is performed within the third month of pregnancy.

[CLINICAL EXPERIENCE]

1.   CONVENTIONAL ACUPUNCTURE

(1) Taking Points by Groups

Points: ① Hegu (LI4) and Sanyinjiao (SP6). ② Changqiang (GV1) and Yinlingquan (SP9)

Technique: Mild stimulation is performed on Hegu (LI4) with the reinforcing method. Strong stimulation is given on Sanyinjiao (SP6), puncturing upward from Sanyinjiao (SP6), and a good therapeutic effect can be expected if the needling sensation radiates to the abdominal region. Thrust obliquely upward on Changqiang (GV1) for about 3 *cun* when the needling sensation is expected to reach the lumbar region, and on Yinlingquan (SP9), where the sensation must reach the inguinal groove. The needles are retained for 30 minutes, with manipulation given once every five minutes. Treatment is performed twice daily, continuously for two or three days. The two groups of points should be used alternately.

(2) Puncturing Mainly on the Back-Shu Points

Points: Shenshu (BL23), Dachangshu (BL25) and Weizhong (BL40)

Technique: On Shenshu (BL23), the tip of the needle should be thrust obliquely downward, forming an angle of 45°. The needle is inserted about 1-1.5 *cun* deep. Puncture perpendicularly on Dachangshu (BL25) for 1.5-3 *cun* deep, performing the lifting and thrusting method combined with scrapping technique. The rotating method is suggested on Weizhong (BL40), the needle being inserted perpendicularly to a depth of 0.5 to 0.8 *cun*. Lift the needles out of the points after continuous manipulation for five to 10 minutes.

(3) Combining Local and Distal Points

Points: ① Distal points: Hegu (LI4), Sanyinjiao (SP6) and Zusanli (ST36). ② Local points: Zhibian (BL54), Ququan (LR8) and Henggu (KI11). ③ Combining local and distal points: Zhibian (BL54), Hegu (LI4) and Sanyinjiao (SP6)

Technique: Reinforce Hegu (LI4) and Zusanli (ST36), and reduce Sanyinjiao (SP6) and Zhibian (BL54). When Ququan (LR8) and Henggu (KI11) are punctured, the needling sensation is expected to radiate to the external genitalia or the abdominal region. The needles are retained for 20-30 minutes. Electrical therapy is sometimes selected to strengthen the therapeutic effect. A few patients also use powder of Inner Bark of Saigon Cinnamon (Cx Cinnamomi Cassiae) mixed with Camphor to fill up the umbilicus, which is covered with Plaster for Rheumatic Pain, and warmed by a moxa stick. A total of 219 patients selected this method for ocyodinic and induction of labor; 109 out of 134 patients received treatment for ocyodinic labor and achieved good results, while it appeared effective for 56 out of 85 patients who selected this method for induction. The three groups of points have been used alternately in the treatment. Comparatively speaking, the third group, which combined local points with distal points, is more effective.

(4) Penetrating Method

Points: Penetrating from Neiguan (PC6) to Sanyangluo (TE8)

Technique: After routine sterilization, quickly thrust a three-*cun* filiform needle on Neiguan (PC6), rotate the needle into the point and forming a 45-degree angle toward the direction of Sanyangluo (TE8). The tip of the needle must reach the point, but keep the needle inside the skin, the strength of stimulation relying on the patient. The above method may be used to prevent a comprehensive response after induction of labor, which is performed before, during and after the operation. The rotating method is applied on each side of the points for one minute, the amplitude limited to within 180°.

2.   ELECTRIC ACUPUNCTURE

Points: Renzhong (GV20) and Chengjiang (CV24)

Technique: Take a one-*cun* No.30 filiform needle and insert it obliquely, forming a 15-degree angle to the skin surface. Upon the arrival of a needling sensation like soreness, distention and numbness, connect the needles with an electric stimulator, Chengjiang (CV24) connected with the positive side, and Renzhong (GV20) with the negative side. The electric therapy should last for 15-30 minutes. During induction, the volume of current can be increased until the tissues are removed. Cut down the electricity and withdraw the needles when the operation is finished. In 106 cases, dilation was not needed after needling in 85 of them; 101 patients felt satisfied with this method, and only five suffered pain. Because Renzhong (GV20) comes from the Du meridian and Chengjiang (CV24) from the Ren meridian, so they may balance *yin* and *yang*.

3.   AURICULAR THERAPY

Points: Uterus, Ovary, Endocrine, Shenmen and exciting point

Technique: Insert the needle onto the cartilage after routine sterilization, apply strong stimulation with the reducing method, and rotate the needle for three to five minutes. During needle retention, normally 30 minutes, manipulation is given once every 10 minutes.

Treatment is applied from two or three times a day, four to six sessions forming one course of treatment.

4. COMBINED TREATMENT

Point Application with Electric Therapy

Points: Shenque (CV8), Hegu (LI4) and Sanyinjiao (SP6)

Technique: Grind 60-90 g of castor leaves (Folium Ricini) and fry them with wine. Use it to cover Shenque (CV8), changing to another paste when it becomes cold. Simultaneously, needle Hegu (LI4) and Sanyinjiao (SP6), and connect the needles with an electric stimulator for 20 minutes. Treatment is performed twice a day; continuous treatment is given for three to five days. In 10 cases of induction, nine had successful delivery within six to 24 hours.

[REMARKS]

1. As the therapeutic effect of acupuncture treatment is not definite, it is often taken as a supplementary treatment method.

2. We would like to recommend complicated acupuncture treatment. As it is realized that needling may promote the contraction of the uterus and enlarge the uterine neck, combining acupuncture with injection of glucose and posterior pituitary hormone in the uterine cavity may achieve complete abortion. The therapeutic effect is more reliable for long-term pregnancy.

3. Abortion performed with acupuncture is safer for women less than three months pregnant. If treatment has been given for over 10 times, twice daily, but there is no therapeutic effect, uterine curettage should be carried out.

RETENTION OF PLACENTA

[INTRODUCTION]

The causative factors for retention of the placenta vary, but are mostly due to exhaustion during delivery. Other reasons include stagnation of *qi* and blood due to wind-cold invasion, enlargement of the placenta and deficiency of primary *qi*. The treatment principle is to eliminate wind-cold, activate blood and tonify *qi*. Points are mainly selected from the Ren meridian, Taiyang and Taiyin meridians of the foot, such as Jiangjing (GB21), Zhongji (CV3), Kunlun (BL60), Hegu (LI4) and Sanyinjiao (SP6). The reducing method is performed for excess syndrome, and reinforcing is selected for deficiency syndrome.

[CLINICAL EXPERIENCE]

1. CONVENTIONAL ACUPUNCTURE

(1) *Puncturing on Single Point*
Point: Zhiyin (BL67)
Technique: Puncture 0.1-0.2 *cun* deep on Zhiyin (BL67), gradually increasing the volume of stimulation from moderate to high. Retain the needles for five to 10 minutes.

(2) *Puncturing on Yuan-primary Point*
Point: Hegu (LI4)
Technique: Immediately after delivery, needle on both sides of Hegu (LI4) with strong stimulation. The needles are retained for 20 minutes, manipulation given every three minutes.

(3) *Taking Group Points*
Points: ① Hegu (LI4) and Sanyinjiao (SP6). ② Zhongji (CV3) and Kunlun (BL60). ③ Zhiyin (BL67) and extra point Duyin.
Technique: The three groups of points are selected in turn, each time one group of points, using the reducing method with strong stimulation. A warming needle or a moxa stick can be given to those with blood stagnation for 10 to 30 minutes.

2. MOXIBUSTION

(1) *Moxa Cone*
Points: Zhiyin (BL67) or extra point Duyin
Technique: Set a moxa cone in the size of a rice grain on Zhiyin (BL67) or extra point Duyin; direct moxibustion without scarring is suggested. Each time three to five cones are used.

(2) *Indirect Moxibustion with Salt*

Point: Shenque (CV8)

Technique: Cover the point with a thin layer of fried salt, twist moxa wool into a moxa cone as big as a green bean, place it onto the point and ignite it. Normally, three cones are used, but up to seven can be applied in case there is severe vaginal bleeding. During the process, bulging is often found on the abdomen, which is caused by uterine contraction. The border of uterus is clearly seen at the place two-finger breadth above the umbilicus shortly after the placenta is going to be squeezed out. When bleeding is severe due to the placental retention, hypophyseal hormones or ergot injection can be prescribed. During the process of moxibustion, if there is too much heat produced which is above the tolerance of the patient, it is proper to change the moxa cone to a place close by. In 108 cases out of 126 patients, the placenta was removed without applying any other medication; only 18 cases needed an injection of hypophyseal hormones or ergot.

3. ELECTRIC ACUPUNCTURE

Points: Hegu (LI4) and Sanyinjiao (SP6)

Technique: Perform the reinforcing method on Hegu (LI4), the needle inserted perpendicularly. Reducing is applied on Sanyinjiao (SP6), and electric therapy added on the points after the arrival of *qi* (the frequency is kept to 20 times/second).

4. AURICULAR THERAPY

Points: Uterus, Endocrine, Adrenal, Sympathetic Nerve, Abdomen and Lumbar.

Technique: The perpendicular method is performed with a filiform needle on the above points, and strong stimulation is advised. The needles are retained for 20 minutes, manipulation being given every five minutes.

[REMARKS]

1. Acupuncture is effective in the treatment of this disease.

2. If bleeding is severe, leading to hemorrhagic shock, comprehensive treatment combining TCM and Western medicine should be adopted.

POSTPARTUM SYNCOPE

[INTRODUCTION]

Postpartum syncope, which refers to the group of symptoms, such as dizziness, blurred vision, vomiting and even coma, takes place after delivery. The main causative factors are constitutional weakness, excessive bleeding from labor, both *yin* and nutrient blood being deficient, and the floating out of blood that draws away *qi* and energy from the body.

[CLINICAL EXPERIENCE]

1. CONVENTIONAL ACUPUNCTURE

(1) Puncturing Single Point
Point: Renzhong (GV26)
Technique: The reinforcing method is given with the needle punctured perpendicularly on the point, rotating for one minute, and retaining it for 10 minutes. The therapeutic effect comes immediately after treatment, usually after two or three minutes. To prevent the recurrence of shock, 10% sodium bromide or 50% glucose can be given as an intravenous injection.

(2) Combining Main Points with Secondary Points
Points: Baihui (GV20) and Zusanli (ST36) are taken as the main points; Zhongwan (CV12) is selected for vomiting; and Neiguan (PC6) for palpitation.

Technique: Reinforcing is given on the main points and the needles are retained for 30 minutes with occasional manipulation. Scondary points are selected according to symptoms and signs.

(3) Penetrating Method

Point: Penetrating from extra point Yuyao to Sizhukong (TE23)

Technique: Puncture obliquely from Yuyao and then thrust the needle toward the direction of Sizhukong (TE23). The needle can be inserted from 1-1.5 *cun* deep, and strong stimulation is suggested. A good therapeutic effect is expected.

2. MOXIBUSTION

(1) Moxa Cone

Point: Shenque (CV8)

Technique: Cover the point with fried salt, and set a moxa cone in the size of a Chinese date on it. Continuous treatment is given until the patient's abdomen becomes warm and the patient wakes up.

(2) Moxa Stick

Point: Qihai (CV6)

Technique: The patient lies on her back with knees flexed. Hanging moxa is performed on Qihai (CV6) for 30-60 minutes until the patient wakes up.

3. CHINESE MASSAGE

Chinese massage is performed along the abdomen [Guanyuan (CV4), Zhongji (CV3), Guilai (ST29) and other points] for about 15 minutes clockwise. This method may stimulate the uterine contraction and stop bleeding. Meanwhile finger pressure can be applied for two minutes on each point, such as Renzhong (GV26), Suliao (GV25), Xuehai (SP9), Zusanli (ST36), Sanyinjiao (SP6) and Kunlun (BL60).

4. AURICULAR THERAPY

Points: Shenmen, Adrenal, Endocrine, Sympathetic Nerve, Heart, Kidney, Liver and Spleen.

Technique: Take three to five points each time and puncture with the filiform needle. Strong stimulation is given for one to two minutes. Retain the needles for 30 minutes with some manipulation.

[REMARKS]

1.   Acupuncture has good therapeutic effect in the treatment of postpartum syncope, especially moxibustion. For example, a large amount of moxa can be applied on Baihu (GV20), Guanyuan (CV4) and other points.

2.   Emergency treatment with TCM and Western medicine is suggested in case of severe shock.

POSTPARTUM TORMINA

[INTRODUCTION]

The onset of the disease is caused by *qi* and blood stagnation, and stagnation is the reason for the pain. Loss of blood during delivery, retention of placenta, invasion of wind-cold and stagnation of food may all result in the disease. For deficiency syndrome, the principle of treatment is to tonify *qi* and blood and dispel cold; and for excess syndrome, it is to remove stagnation of *qi*. Points are mainly selected from Ren meridian and three *yin* meridians of the foot, such as Guanyuan (CV4), Qihai (CV6), Zhongwan (CV12), Zusanli (ST36), Taichong (LR3), Taixi (KI3) and Tianshu (ST25). Generally reinforcing is used for the deficiency syndrome.

[CLINICAL EXPERICENCE]

1.   CONVENTIONAL ACUPUNCTURE

(1) Puncture Single Point

Points: Sanyinjiao (SP6)

Technique: Insert the needle into the point with the rotating method. Retain the needle for a period between 30 minutes and 24 hours. In 92 cases, 90 patients gained pain relief after the first treatment and the other two cases were treated with point block therapy.

(2) Taking Points Mainly from Ren Meridian

Points: Zhongji (CV3) or Guanyuan (CV4)

Technique: Puncture Zhongji (CV3) or Guanyuan (CV4) as deep as 1.5-2 *cun*, rotating the needle with even movement. The needles are retained for 30-60 minutes.

(3) Taking Group Points

Points: ① Zhongji (CV3) and Sanyinjiao (SP6). ② Guanyuan (CV4) and Zusanli (ST36). ③ Zhongji (CV3) and Zusanli (ST36). ④ Zhongji (CV3) or Guanyuan (CV4).

Technique: Select one group of points and perform strong stimulation on Zhongji (CV3) and Sanyinjiao (SP6). Other points are punctured as usual. Keep the needles on all of the points for more than 60 minutes.

2. MOXIBUSTION

(1) Indirect Moxa with Ginger

Points: Zhongji (CV3) and extra point Zigong

Technique: Moxibustion is applied with a piece of ginger 0.2 cm thick and in the size of a coin, with a moxa cone in the size of a five-cent coin on it. The warmth produced should penetrate down to the abdomen until the patient feels comfortable. Ten daily treatments make up one course.

(2) Moxa Stick

Points: Qihai (CV6), Guilai (ST29) and Qichong (ST30)

Technique: Hanging moxa is applied on each point, each time for 15-20 minutes. The treatment is given once or twice a day, 10 sessions forming one course.

3. AURICULAR THERAPY

Points: Endocrine, Ovary, Sub-cortex, Abdomen and lumbosacral region.

Technique: Puncture perpendicularly with a filiform needle; the reducing method is applied for excess syndrome, reinforcing for deficiency. The needles are retained for 20-30 minutes. Alternatively, embed seeds on the points, five treatments forming one course.

4. INTRA-DERMAL NEEDLING

Points: Sanyinjiao (SP6), Yaoyangguan (GV3), Shangxian (the point is located between the 5th lumbar vertebral and sacral vertebral) and Ah-shi points.

Technique: Intra-dermal needling is applied where there is tenderness on Sanyinjiao (SP6), Yaoyangguan (CV3) and Shangxian. After treatment, among 40 cases, the tenderness disappeared in 23 patients, pain was relieved in 11, and only 6 patients saw no improvement (total effective rate 85%). The therapeutic effect is closely related with the setting of the needles on the points. For those with severe illness, the needles should be retained for a longer time, and the period should vary from five minutes up to 36 hours.

[REMARKS]

1.   Moxibustion is more effective in cases where the points are selected properly. Normally, the pain is relieved or disappears after one or two treatments.

2.   If abdominal pain cannot be relieved, the function of uterus fails to be restored, and there is retention of lochia, one must consider whether there is blood stasis or partial placental adhesion remaining in the abdominal cavity. A further examination is suggested.

POSTPARTUM RETENTION OF URINE

[INTRODUCTION]

The disease is caused by paralysis of the bladder sphincter according to modern medicine. Traditional Chinese medicine believes that the exhaustion of *qi* and blood during labor may lead to dysfunction of lung in regulating the water passage, and resulting in retention of urine in the bladder; or the consumption of spleen and kidney during labor may damage the functions of the kidney, influence *qi* activity in the urinary bladder and disturb the normal function of the spleen in water transportation and transformation, thus leading to urination disturbance after delivery. The principle of treatment is to smooth the circulation of *qi* and water, warm up and tonify the lung and kidney, promote the function of the spleen and resolve dampness. Because the excretion of urine relies on the *qi* activity of the urinary bladder, and this, in turn, is related with the coordination of the lung, spleen and kidney and Sanjiao, so the points are selected from the crossing points of the above meridians with Du and Ren meridians, Back-Shu points, and lower He-sea points, such as Qugu (CV2), Sanyinjiao (SP6), Zhongji (CV3), Guanyuan (CV4), Shenshu (BL 23), Pangguangshu (BL28), Xiaochangshu (BL27), Yinlingquan (SP9) and Zusanli (ST36). The even method is mostly applied.

[CLINICAL EXPERIENCE]

1. CONVENTIONAL ACUPUNCTURE

(1) *Penetrating Method*

Points: Zhongji (CV3) penetrating to Qugu (CV2), and Shenshu (BL23) penetrating to Mingmen (GV4).

Technique: First of all puncture perpendicularly 1-1.5 *cun* on Zhongji (CV3). After the arrival of *qi*, thrust the needle toward the direction of Qugu (CV2), and adopt the reducing method. Withdraw the needle after 10-20 minutes, then insert it into Shenshu (BL23) until the needling sensation arrives, then further thrust the needle toward the direction of Mingmen (GV4); the reducing method with rotating is used. Treatment is applied from one to two times daily, five sessions forming one course.

(2) *Combining the Back-Shu and Front-Fu Points*

Points: Shenshu (BL23), Pangguangshu (BL28), Zhongji (CV3) and Jingmen (GB25)

Technique: Puncture perpendicularly on Zhongji (CV3), apply the reducing method by thrusting and rotating the needles until the needling sensation reaches the perineum. Then puncture perpendicularly on Jingmen (GB25) for about 0.3-0.5 *cun*. Retain the needles on Zhongji (CV3) and Jingmen (GB25) for about 10 minutes; manipulation of the needles is suggested. Quick needling is applied on Shenshu (BL23) and Pangguangshu (BL28). In the treatment, the Front-Mu and Back-Shu points of the kidney and urinary bladder are selected to strengthen the function of the kidneys in receiving *qi*, and the urinary bladder in its *qi* activity. In this way, the circulation of water can be improved.

2. MOXIBUSTION

Points: Shenque (CV8)

Technique: Fill the point with baked salt and cover it with a scallion cake, 0.3 cm thick. A moxa cone in the size of a soybean is ignited on the top of the cake until a burning sensation is felt. Usually five to seven cones are used. When the warmth of moxa penetrates the abdomen, the sensation of urine may appear. To strengthen the therapeutic effect, moxibustion should be performed once every other day.

3. FINGER NEEDLING METHOD

Points: The midpoint between umbilicus and symphysis pubis

Technique: Press hard with the middle finger of the right hand on the point, the left hand assisting the right hand, and press down to the spinal cord in most cases. The performance should be within the limitations of the patient (except obese women). After three to five minutes operation, urination should occur.

4. ELECTRIC ACUPUNCTURE

Points: Penetrating from Weibao [2 *cun* below Weidao (GB28)] to Zhongji (CV3), or Zhongji (CV3) to Qugu (CV2).

Technique: Take one group of points and perform with the reducing method, more rotating than thrusting, for about two or three minutes. Then connect the needles with an electric stimulator for 10-20 minutes. Treatment can be applied once or twice a day. This method is especially good for those patients who have tried catheterization many times without effect.

5. COMBINED TREATMENT

(1) Acupuncture and Acupoint Injection

Points: Guanyuan (CV4), Zhongji (CV3), Sanyinjiao (SP6) and

Zusanli (ST36)

Technique: Moxa stick is used on Guanyuan (CV4) and Zhongji (CV3) for half an hour. Meanwhile, puncture Sanyinjiao (SP6) bilateral and retain the needles for 20 minutes. An injection of 2 ml (0.5 mg) of neostigmine is applied on Zusanli (ST36) bilaterally.

(2) Acupuncture and Moxibustion Technique (Setting the Mountain on Fire)

Points: Baihui (GV20), Zhongji (CV3), Weibao which is 2 *cun* below Weidao (GB28), Zhigou (TE6), Chize (LU5), Qihai (CV6), Zusanli (ST36) and Sanyinjiao (SP6).

Technique: Moxibustion is applied on Baihui (GV20) for five minutes. With special acupuncture technique-setting the mountain on fire, the needle is inserted from Zhongji (CV3) and Weibao, which is 2 *cun* below Weidao (GB 28), 2.5 *cun* deep until the sensation of urine is felt. Needling followed moxa is performed on the rest of the points, retaining the needles for three to five minutes. Acupuncture and moxibustion technique is performed twice a day with an interval of three to four hours.

[REMARKS]

1. For patients who have suffered from urination disturbance after labor mostly may suffer from infection in the urinary tract due to catheterization. Acupuncture treatment is very effective in this circumstance.

2. Patients are advised to relax and maintain a comfortable position. A warm compress can relieve the tension and pain in the abdomen.

LACTATION INSUFFICIENCY

[INTRODUCTION]

Lactation insufficiency is mostly related with *qi* and blood deficiency due to weak body constitution. Sometimes it is caused by stagnation of liver *qi*. In the former case, the breast is soft without distention and pain; in the latter case, the breast is hard with distending pain, and fever may also be present. The principle of treatment is to tonify *qi* and blood, regulate liver *qi*, and promote secretion of milk. Points are mainly selected from the Foot Yangming meridian, such as Rugen (ST18), Tanzhong (CV17), Shaoze (SI1), Zusanli (ST36) and Qimen (LR14). The reinforcing method with moxibustion is performed for deficiency syndrome, and the reducing method is advised for excess syndrome.

[CLINICAL EXPERIENCE]

1. CONVENTIONAL ACUPUNCTURE

(1) Puncturing Experience Points

Points: Rugen (ST18), Shaoze (SI1), Tanzhong (CV17)

Technique: The needle is inserted toward the direction of the breasts from Tanzhong (CV17), and inserted downward from Rugen (ST18) for about 1.5-2.0 *cun*. Shaoze (SI1) is punctured 0.2 *cun* deep. The needles are retained for 30 minutes, and manipulation is given once every five minutes. After withdrawal of the needles, milk may flow. This is an effective ancient treatment.

(2) Puncturing Special Points

Points: Ruquan, which is 0.5 *cun* anterior to Jiquan (HT1), posterior to the musculus pectoralis major, anterior to the transverse crease of the axilla. Secondary points: Shaoze (SI1) and Tanzhong (CV17)

Technique: Apply bird-pecking needling technique on Ruquan; the even method is performed on Shaoze (SI1) and Tanzhong (CV17). The best needling sensation is numbness and distention in the chest. Retain the needles for 20 minutes, manipulation being performed once every five minutes. Treatment is given once a day.

(3) Puncturing Ah-shi Points

Points: The three Ah-shi points (3 *cun* anterior, posterior and lateral to the nipple), Tanzhong (CV17) and Neiguan (PC6).

Technique: Puncture from the Ah-shi points obliquely toward the direction of the nipple. The needle can be inserted as deep as 0.8-1 *cun*; the reducing method with strong stimulation is performed.

The needles can be retained for 20 minutes, manipulation being given once every five minutes. Perform the routine needling method on Tanzhong (CV17) and Neiguan (PC6). The reinforcing method is recommended for excess syndrome; and the reducing method is advised for deficiency syndrome. The needles are retained for 20 minutes, manipulation being given once every five minutes. Treatment is given once a day.

2. MOXIBUSTION

Points: Tanzhong (CV17), Rugen (ST18) and Zusanli (ST36)

Technique: Indirect moxibustion with ginger insulation is performed on each point. Three to five cones of moxa are used, each in the size of a Chinese date. Treatment is given once a day.

3. AURICULAR ACUPUNCTURE

Points: Sensitive points on the chest region and mammary gland.

Technique: Insert 0.5-cm-long filiform needles on the points. The patient may feel severe pain, but it will disappear within a second. The depth of the needle should be enough to fix it on the point, and they should be retained for 10-15 minutes. Treatment may be given once a day; both sides of the ear are used.

4. COMBINED TREATMENT

(1) Combination of Needling with Cupping

Points: Xinshu (BL15)

Technique: The patient adopts a sitting position with the head slightly down, and should be relaxed. Insert the needle perpendicularly 0.3-0.5 *cun* deep and apply rotating and scraping technique until distention and soreness are felt. Lift the needle under the skin surface, and thrust it in again, making a 30-degree angle toward the spinal cord and Shenshu (BL23), 0.8-1.2 *cun* deep. The quick needling method is performed. The same technique is used on both sides of the points. After withdrawal of the needle, cupping is performed for 10-15 minutes. The treatment is given once or twice a day, and the therapeutic effect can be achieved after two to four treatments.

(2) Acupuncture and Moxibustion Technique (in groups)

Points: Shaoze (SI1), Tanzhong (CV17), Rugen (ST18), Jiquan (HT1), Zusanli (ST36) and Hegu (LI4)

Technique: The first treatment needling is performed on Shaoze (SI1), while moxa is used on Tanzhong (CV17). In the second treatment, needling is performed on Jiquan (HT1), and moxa is used on Rugen (ST18). Normally, treatment may start from the 3rd day after delivery, with the above treatment performed each once a day. In some cases, the therapeutic effect can be more effective if Zusanli (ST36) and Hegu (LI4) are used once.

[REMARKS]

1. Acupuncture treatment is effective for the disease. The first treatment should be no later than the 2nd day after delivery. At least, treatment should start within one week after delivery. Generally speaking, the earlier the treatment the better the therapeutic effect.

2. During treatment, the patient must be totally relaxed, and pay more attention to diet. Nutrition can be taken as tea after cooking in water with jujube fruit (Fr. Ziziphi Jujubae), mulberry parasite (Rm. Loranthi seu Visci) and spatholobus stem (Caulis Spatholobi), and soup cooked with pig feet or crucian carp is good at tonifying *qi* and blood so as to promote the excretion of milk.

3. If for any case, lactifuge is necessary, Jianjing (GB21), Guangming (GB37), Zusanli (ST36) and Zulinqi (GB41) can be punctured with the reducing method, retaining the needles for 30 minutes while manipulating them once every 10 minutes. When withdrawing the needles, shake the handle and take them out slowly, keeping the point hole open. Treatment can be performed once daily until the patient is cured. The conclusion is that acupuncture is not only good at promoting milk flow, but is also capable of returning milk. As a supplementary method, oral administration of decoction barley sprout (Fr. Hordei Vulgaris Germinantus) is recommended. To prevent the onset of mastitis, external application of mirabilite (Ntrii Sulfas) would be good for the patient. Besides, there are points called returning milk points—the midpoint of the 4th thoracic verte-

brae is named as point 1; the midpoint of the 5th thoracic vertebrae is named as point 2; and the midpoint of the 6th thoracic vertebrae is named as point 3. The reducing method is performed with perpendicular technique on those points.

PROLAPSE OF UTERUS

[INTRODUCTION]

The onset of the disease is related with deficiency of *qi* in middle *jiao*, or deficiency of kidney *qi* resulting in dysfunction of the Chong, Ren and Dai meridians. Clinically, prolapse of uterus is divided into three categories: I. Uterine cervix prolapsed below the level of ischial spine but above the vaginal orifice; II. Uterine cervix and part of uterine body prolapsed out of the vaginal orifice; and III. Uterine body completely prolapsed out of the vaginal orifice. The principle of treatment is to strengthen the spleen and kidney, strengthen the function of the Chong meridian and raise the uterus. Points are mainly selected from Ren and Du meridians, as well as the three *yin* meridians of the foot, such as, Baihui (GV20), Qihai (CV6), Guanyuan (CV4), Weidao (GB28), Zhaohai (KI 6), Taixi (KI 3), Taichong (LI 3) and Sanyinjiao (SP 6). Retain the needles for a long time; and the reinforcing method is combined with moxa.

[CLINICAL EXPERIENCE]

1. CONVENTIONAL ACUPUNCTURE

(1) Combination of Local and Distal Points

Points: Weibao [6 *cun* lateral to Guanyuan (CV4)], extra point Zigong and Sanyinjiao (SP6)

Technique: Apply the rotating method on Weibao with large amplitude until the patient feels contraction at the uterus. Insert the needle obliquely from extra point Zigong toward the direction of the pubic symphysis, and continue in until the patient feels soreness and a contracting sensation at the perineum. Insert the needle obliquely from Sanyinjiao (SP6) toward the direction of the perineum. The best therapeutic effect is expected if the needling sensation reaches the perineum. Retain the needles for 30-60 minutes. Treatment can be applied two or three times a week, two to three weeks forming one course.

(2) Thick Needle

Points: Baihui (GV20), Qichong (ST30), Weidao (GB28), Sanyinjiao (Sp6) and Huanshangxue (2 *cun* above 0.5 *cun* lateral to the midway between the coccyx and great trochanter)

Technique: Select a six-*cun* needle (Size No.26), puncture 4-6 *cun* deep on Weidao (GB28), Huanshangxue (2 *cun* above 0.5 *cun* lateral to the midway point between the coccyx and great trochanter) and Qichong (ST30) and lift and thrust the needle toward the direction of the uterus. Sparrow-pecking needling technique may produce a kind of electrical shock, which goes to the perineum or lateral side of the abdomen. An upward lifting sensation of the uterus after needling is expected. The acupuncture method is also applied on Baihui (GV20) and Sanyinjiao (SP6). Take points from one side of the body and change to the other one in the next treatment. Treatment is given once a day and 10 sessions form one course. Before treatment, the patient should empty the urinary bladder. Rotating and retaining the needle is not suggested. The appropriate stimulation is determined according to the patient's constitution and sensitivity to the needles.

(3) Long Needle

Points: Weidao (GB28), extra point Weibao and Weigong (one *cun* below Weibao)

Technique: One of the above points is selected each time. Strong stimulation is required on the perineum and lower abdomen, inserting the needle downward to the deep layer of fat and toward the direction of the pubic symphysis. Points like Qugu (CV2), Sanyinjiao (SP6), Yinlingquan (SP9) and Zusanli (ST36) can be combined. Treatment is given once a day, 10 sessions making up one course. Most of the time, the needles are not retained.

2. MOXIBUSTION

(1) Indirect Moxa with Ginger

Points: Beihui (GV20), Guanyuan (CV4), Qihai (CV6), Shenque (CV8), Daimai (GB26), Zusanli (ST36), Sanyinjiao (SP6) and Yinlingquan (SP9).

Technique: Select three to five points each time, putting a moxa cone on a piece of fresh ginger; three to seven cones of moxa are placed on each point. Treatment is applied once every other day. Five treatments are considered as one course.

(2) Indirect Moxa with Salt

Point: Shenque (CV8)

Technique: Entirely fill the umbilicus with fine salt, a moxa cone in the size of a soybean above it; five to seven moxa cones are used on each point. Treatment is applied once every other day, five treatments making up one course.

(3) Steaming

Point: External genitalia

Technique: Prepare black plums (Fructus Mume) 60 g; magnolia vine fruit (Fructus Schisandrae) 10 g; and pomegranate rind (Pericarpium Granati) 10 g. After boiling them in hot water for 30 minutes, place the decoction in a box and use it to steam the area of the external genitalia and also wash the area until the decoction cools down. Each dose is used repeatedly two or three times daily.

(4) Warming Moxa with Moxa Stick

Points: Baihui (GV20), Qihai (CV6), Guanyuan (CV4), Zusanli (ST36), Sanyinjiao (SP6), the region of the perineum, Shenque (CV8), Daimai (GB26), Shenshu (KI3), Shangliao (BL31), Ciliao (BL32), Zhongliao (BL33), Xialiao (BL34) and Zaohai (KI6).

Technique: Select three to five points each time, with the treatment applied for 10 to 20 minutes on each point. Seven to 10 treatments are considered as one course. A three-day interval is advised between two treatments.

(5) Topical Application of Drugs

Point: Baihui (GV20)

Technique: Grind one piece of caster seed (Semen Ricini) into a paste and stick it on Baihui (GV20). A hot compress is recommended. The treatment may be applied three times a day, 30 minutes each time. Change to a new paste after two days. Six days are regarded as one treatment course.

3.   ELECTRIC ACUPUNCTURE

Points: Zigong (EX-CAI), Guanyuan (CV4) and Weidao (GB28)

Technique: Puncture perpendicularly the above points, apply the lifting and thrusting method and then connect power, low frequency three to five HZ on Zigong (EX-CAI) and Weidao (GB28). Treatment is applied once a day, 10 sessions forming one course.

4.   HYDRO-ACUPUNCTURE

Points: Pishu (BL20), Ganshu (BL18), extra point Tituo and Weibao

Technique: A 5% Chinese Angelicae injection is used on the above points, 0.5-1 ml to each point. Treatment is applied once every other day, 10 treatments forming one course.

5.   CATGUT-EMBEDDING METHOD

Point: Tigong point

Technique: Select a lumbar puncture needle (Size No.20) and thrust it into the point, embedding 1.5-2.0 cm long No.0 surgical catgut into the point. Treatment can be given once every 10-15 days. If it is necessary, an injection of 1-2 ml of Radix Angelicae Sinensis or Flos Carthami simultaneously with catgut embedding may strengthen the therapeutic effect.

6.   LASER THERAPY

Points: Dahe (KI12), Guilai (ST29), Qihai (CV6), Guanyuan (CV4), Zusanli (ST36), Sanyinjiao (SP6) and Baihui (GV20).

Technique: Apply laser therapy to three to five points each time. Treatment can be given once a day and should last five minutes each time. Ten sessions form one course.

7. SCALP ACUPUNCTURE

Points: Foot Motor and Sensory Area, Reproduction Area bilaterally

Technique: Apply scalp acupuncture with the quick rotating method until distention and a hot sensation are felt in the local region. Treatment may be applied once every other day, 10 sessions making up one course.

[REMARKS]

1. A good therapeutic effect can be expected, especially when the Bolus for Reinforcing Middle Jiao and Replenishing *qi* (Buzhong-yiqi Wan) is also prescribed for the patient.

2. It is important that, before the operation, the patient must urinate fully and the prolapsed uterus should be pushed back into the vagina. Fitting the buttock higher during treatment is also necessary.

3. After treatment, the patient may exercise one or two times in the genupectoral position, each time for 30 minutes.

4. Elevator exercise is necessary, which should be done twice a day, each time 10-15 minutes.

STERILITY

[INTRODUCTION]

Primary sterility refers to the condition in which a woman fails to become pregnant without any contraception after a couple live together for three years, and secondary sterility refers to the condition in which a woman fails to become pregnant again without any contraception three years after the last labor or abortion. The mechanism of pregnancy is that kidney *qi* is abundant, essence blood is excessive, Ren and Chong meridians are flourishing, and the menstruation is regular; then a sperm and an egg can join together. If the *qi* and blood are disordered due to kidney deficiency, liver stagnation or phlegm damp, pregnancy will be difficult. The treatment used various modes, with excess and deficiency syndrome. For deficiency syndrome, the treatment principle is to warm the kidney, fill the essence and benefit Chong and Ren meridians; for excess syndrome, it is to pacify the liver, relieve stagnation and resolve phlegm and damp for the purpose of harmonizing *qi* and blood, regulating menstruation, making contraception possible. The points of Ren Meridian, Yangming Meridian of Hand and Foot, Three Yin Meridians of Foot are selected as main points, such as Qihai (CV6), Guanyuan (CV4), Taichong (LR3), Zusanli (ST36), Sanyinjiao (SP6), Taixi (KI3) and Fenglong (ST40), with reinforcement for deficiency and reduction for excess.

[CLINICAL EXPERIENCE]

1.   CONVENTIONAL ACUPUNCTURE

(1) Combination of Main Point and Supplementary Point

Points: Main points: Zhongji (CV3) and Sanyinjiao (SP6). Supplementary point: Dahe (KI12).

Technique: Start the treatment on the 12th day in the menstrual cycle. It is given once a day on three successive days, and even technique on each point.

(2) Deep Puncturing

Points: Zhongji (CV3), Guilai (ST29), Zigong (extra) and Sanyinjiao (SP6).

Technique: Puncture the points on the abdomen 3 to 4 *cun* deep, and Sanyinjiao (SP6) 2 *cun* deep with even technique by lifting, thrusting, rotating of the needles on all the points so as to produce needling sensation on the abdomen and perineum. Retain the needle for 15 minutes while manipulating the needle occasionally the treatment is given once a day, 10 times forming one course.

(3) Selection of Points According to Differentiation of Syndrome

Points: Main points: Zhongji (CV3), Guanyuan (CV4), Zigong (extra) and Guilai (ST29). Supplementary points: for *qi* and blood deficiency, add Zusanli (ST36), Zhongwan (CV12); for stagnation of liver *qi*, add Ganshu (BL18), Neiguan (PC6) and Taichong (LR3); for obstruction of phlegm and damp, add Fenglong (ST40), Yinlingquan

(SP9) and Sanyinjiao (SP6); for obstruction of uterus by blood stasis, add Geshu (BL17), Quehai (SP10) and Shuidao (ST28).

Technique: Puncture the main points in every treatment with even technique to create needling sensation to the uterus and perineum. Retain the needle for 30 minutes, manipulating it once every five minutes. Select other points according to differentiation of syndrome with reinforcement for deficiency and reduction for excess; and retain the needle for 30 minutes. Treatment is given once a day, 10 times forming one course.

2. MOXIBUSTION

(1) Direct Moxibustion

Points: Main points: Guanyuan (CV4) and Zhongji (CV3). Supplementary points: Zusanli (ST36) and Sanyinjiao (SP6).

Technique: Select one of the main points and one of the supplementary points in turn, putting 10 moxa cones in the size of a soya bean in succession on the points, once a day. Seven times make up one course.

(2) Moxibustion with Salt

Point: Shenque (CV8).

Technique: Fill the umbilicus with fried fine salt, and put a moxa cone as big as a soya bean on it. Ignite five to 10 cones continuously, once a day or every other day, five to seven times forming one course. If blisters appear on the local area after moxibustion, prick them with a sterilized syringe needle, and apply gentian violet and gauze on the skin to avoid infection.

(3) Moxibustion with Ginger

Points: Shenshu (BL23), Ganshu (BL18), Pishu (BL20) and Gaohuangshu (BL43).

Technique: Select two pairs of points every time in turn and apply moxibustion with ginger on them. Use five to 10 cones as big as a kernel of the date on each point, once a day. Seven times make up one course.

(4) Triangular Moxibustion

Points: Take the length of the patient's mouth as the basic unit, three units as one side of a triangle with the umbilicus as one angle, then the other two angles are the points for moxibustion.

Technique: Apply 11 cones as big as grain with direct moxibustion or moxa stick on each point. Start the treatment on the first day of the period, 10 times altogether, in three successive months.

(5) Moxibustion on the Extra Points

Points: Baomen [2 *cun* left to Guanyuan (CV4)] and Zihu (2.5 *cun* right to Guanyuan).

Technique: Apply 21 cones as big as grain on each point, once a day, 10 times forming one course. This method is indicated for woman unable to conceive for the first time or for a long time after the previous labor.

3. BLEEDING METHOD

Points: Yaoyangguan (GV3), Quze (PC3) and Yinlingquan (SP9).

Technique: Prick these points to let out three drops of blood from each once a day. This method is indicated for sterility due to stagnation of liver *qi* or blood stagnation.

4. ELECTRIC ACUPUNCTURE

Points: Zhongji (CV3), Guanyuan (CV4), Zigong (extra) and Sanyinjiao (SP6).

Technique: After puncturing the points perpendicularly, connect the abdominal points with an electric machine for 30 minutes, once a day, three treatments forming one course. Usually, one should start the treatment on the14th day of the period, or one month after pneumoperitoneography or peritoneoscopy for amenorrhea. One course of treatment is given every month.

5. CATGUT-EMBEDDING METHOD

Point: Sanyinjiao (SP6).

Technique: Embed catgut thread into Sanyinjiao (SP6) of both sides on the12th day after menstruation, and once a month. This method was applied in 24 cases where there had been no ovulation, and 22 were followed up, of which 18 had achieved ovulation, 16 became pregnant, and four were ineffective. Research shows that cat-gut embedding on Sanyinjiao can not only induce ovulation, but also treat polycycstic ovary syndrome because it has similar action to clomiphene in inducing ovulation but without other side effects and the risk of over-stimulation.

6. COMBINED TREATMENT

(1) Combination of Acupuncture and Moxibustion Treatment

Points: Yinjiao (CV7), Shiguan (KI18), Guanyuan (CV4), Baomen (extra) and Zihu (Extra).

Technique: According to *About Hundreds of Diseases*: Yinjiao (CV7) and Shiguan (KI18) can be used for sterility. So puncture these two points with mild stimulation and heavy moxibustion, and retain the needle for 30 minutes, once every other day. The patients should also carry out moxibustion by themselves on Guanyuan (CV4), Baomen (extra) and Zihu (extra) until the skin becomes hot and congested, before sleeping every night. Ten treatments form one course.

(2) Combination of Acupuncture and Moxibustion Treatment (Warming the Uterus and Breeding a Fetus)

Points: Guanyuan (CV4) and Jiaoxin (KI8).

Technique: Puncture Guanyuan (CV4) and Jiaoxin (KI8) with reinforcement by rotating the needle, retain it for 20 minutes, and then make moxibustion by moxa stick until warmth is felt on the lower abdomen. The treatment should be given once a day, 10 times forming one course. Because these two points are able to regulate the Chong and Ren meridians, tonify the spleen and kidney, activate blood to remove the obstruction and clear the lower *jiao*. Acupuncture can warm the uterus and produce a fetus.

[REMARKS]

1. Acupuncture has a certain effect on sterility, but it is of better effect if combined with acupuncture and herbal medicine.

2. Research into the mechanism of improvement of ovulation with acupuncture by puncturing Zhongji (CV3), Xuehai (SP10) and

Dahe (KI12) on a rabbit found that between two and four hours later the peak of luteotropic hormone was achieved, along with increased progesterone, and ovulation was directly observed. These changes may be caused by release of follicule-stimulation hormone and prolan B luteinizing hormone by the anterior pituitary when the hypothalamus-pituitary system are excited through stimulating a certain mechanism.

PRURITUS VULVAE

[INTRODUCTION]

The condition involving an itching sensation on the external genitalia and vaginal tract, or more severely, unendurable itching and pain, restlessness, sometimes itching and pain around the anus or morbid leucorrhoea of different degree in woman, is called pruritus vulvae. In modern medicine, pruritus vulvae can be often found in trichomonas vaginitis, colpomycosis and leukoplakia vulvae. This problem can be caused by overeating greasy and sweet food, leading to spleen deficiency, excessive damp, producing heat and flowing to the liver meridian and lower *jiao*; or by old age and weak constitution, resulting in deficiency of the liver and kidney, insufficiency of essence blood, failure of nourishment to the genitalia; or by prolonged illness, giving rise to deficiency of *yin* blood, lacking of nourishment in the external genitalia. The treatment principle is to clear heat and damp, pacify the liver and strengthen the spleen, nourish *yin*, moisten dryness, and stop itching and pain. The points are mainly selected from Ren Meridian, Foot-Shaoyang, the three *yin* meridians of the foot, such as Guanyuan (CV4), Zhongji (CV3), Xuehai (SP10), Yingu (KI10), Ququan (CV2), Dadun (LR1) and Daimai (GB26) with reinforcement for deficiency, and reduction for excess, and the needles are retained for 30 minutes, once a day. Ten treatments form one course.

[CLINICAL EXPERIENCE]

1. CONVENTIONAL ACUPUNCTURE

(1) Use of Eight Liao Points Only

Points: Shangliao (BL31), Ciliao (BL32), Zhongliao (BL33) and Xialiao (BL34)

Technique: Puncture all the points perpendicularly with reducing technique by rotating the needle forcefully in order to make a traveling sensation to the perineum. Retain the needle for 30 minutes during which it should be manipulated a few times. Treatment is given once a day, 10 times forming one course.

(2) Puncturing a New Point

Point: Xiazhibianque [The patient lies laterally with the lower leg straight, the upper leg bent forming an angle of 130° on the popliteal fossa. Move the trunk forward a little bit, then take the line connecting the iliac spine and the middle of the greater trochanter as one side, drawing a equilateral triangle. The point is the junction of the other two sides. Because this point is just located below Zhibian (BL54), it is called lower Zhibian (Xiazhibianxue)].

Technique: Use a 3.5-5 *cun* needle (Size No.28), puncture it perpendicularly into the point with the body of the needle forward (to the abdomen) at an angle of 10° to cause the needling sensation to reach the lower abdomen, external genitalia, and perineum. Retain the needle for one to two minutes and then take it out. Severe after-sensation may result from long needle retention. Treatment is given once a day, or once every other day. Ten times form one course.

(3) Puncturing the Nearby Points

Points: Yinlian (LR11), Qugu (CV2) and Huiyin (CV1).

Technique: Puncture all the points with moderate stimulation by rotating the needle and causing traveling sensation to the external genitalia, once a day.

(4) Combination of Main Points and Supplementary Points

Points: Main points: Zhongji (CV3) and Huiyin (CV1). Supplementary points: Qichong (ST30), Yinlingquan (SP9), Zhaohai (KI6) and Taichong (LR3).

Technique: Insert the needle quickly, lift, thrust and rotate the needle with small amplitude (no lifting and thrusting on the perineum). Retain the needle for 30 minutes after the arrival *qi*. Give the treatment twice a week, 10 times forming one course. The needle sensation of abdominal points refers to the external genitalia, and it is better to be able to feel warm and hot on the perineum during needle retention.

(5) Single Puncture

Points: Guanyuan (CV4), Dachangshu (BL25), Taichong (LR3) and Rangu (KI2).

Technique: Puncture Guanyuan (CV4) and Dachangshu (BL25) perpendicularly with lifting, thrusting and rotating the needle to send the needling sensation to the external genitalia and then immediately remove the needle (single puncture). Retain the needle on Rangu (KI2) for 20 minutes, manipulating it four times. Treatment is given once a day, 10 times forming one course.

2. MOXIBUSTION

Point: Dadun (LR1).

Technique: Apply direct moxibustion with three to five moxa cones as big as grain, once a day or once every other day. Five treatments form one course. Alternatively, apply moxa stick on the points of both sides 10 to 15 minutes each.

3. AURICULAR THERAPY

Points: Shenmen, Genitalia, Lung, Uterus, Pelvic Cavity, Ovary, Endocrine, Liver and Kidney

Technique: Puncture three to five points each time with moderately strong stimulation, retaining the needle for 30 minutes. Treatment is given once a day, five to 10 times in each one course. Alternatively, fix the seeds on the ear points.

4. LASER THERAPY

Points: ① Zhongji (CV3), Yinlian (LR11), Yinlingquan (SP9), Ligou (LR5), Ququan (LR8), Sanyinjiao (SP6) and Huiyin (CV1). ② Ear point: Zigong, Endocrine, Pelvic Cavity and Ovary.

Technique: Apply a He-Ne laser needle 3 to 25 mv, on three to five body points, or two to four ear points with radiation on each point for five minutes, once a day, 10 times forming one course.

5. ELECTRO-THERMAL NEEDLING

Point: The affected area.

Technique: Direct the thermal effect onto the affected area with electro-thermal needle. The problem is treated by thermal radiation from the interior to the exterior and from the deep to the shallow region. The best electric currency is 70 to 80 mA, 37-39° C. Needle the point transversely, 0.3 cm deep for the case with thickening, retaining the needle for 20 minutes. Treatment is given once a day, 10 times in one course. This method is indicated for leukoplakia vulvae.

6. COMBINED TREATMENT

(1) Electric Acupuncture Plus Moxibustion

Points: ① Guanyuan (CV4), Qugu (CV2), Yinfu (1 *cun* inferior, and 1 *cun* lateral to clitoris) and Sanyinjiao (SP6). ② Zuogushangxue (2 *cun* and a little lateral to the midpoint of the line connecting the greater trochanter and the tip of the coccyx) and Ciliao (BL32). ③ Guanyuan (CV4), Qugu (CV2), Yinlian (LR11) and Biguan (ST31).

Technique: Puncture the three groups of points in turn and needle Yinfu with a three-*cun* needle obliquely downward, Guanyuan (CV4) and Sanyinjiao (SP6) with reinforcement, Ciliao (BL32) with reduction, other points with even technique. Connect Zuogushangxue and Ciliao (BL32) with an electric machine for 20 to 30 minutes with continuous wave. Then put a moxa apparatus with 2 moxa sticks, 1.5 *cun* long, inside on the external genitalia for 30 minutes. Treatment is given once a day, 10 times forming one course.

(2) Moxibustion Plus Auricular Therapy

Point: Zusanli (ST36), Sanyinjiao (SP6) and affected area. Ear points: Shenmen, external genitalia area, Sub-cortex and Endocrine.

Technique: Apply moxibustion on Zusanli (ST36) of both sides,

Sanyinjiao (SP6) of both sides for 10 minutes on each point, and on the external genitalia for 20 to 30 minutes. Treatment is given once a day, 10 times making up one course. Fix the Wanbuliuxing seeds on the ear points once every other day, using the two ears in turn. Ten sessions form one course.

7. BLEEDING METHOD

Point: Weizhong (BL40).

Technique: Prick Weizhong (BL40) of both sides and cause bleeding, with three to five drops of blood, in order to reduce heat and toxin from the blood system. This method is indicated for pruritus vulvae of damp-heat type and is given once every other day. Five treatments form one course.

[REMARKS]

1. Pay attention to the hygiene of the external genitalia, and often wash and change underwear.

2. It is applicable to eat light food, rather than pungent, hot, greasy and sweet food, such as seafood, snacks, mint and coriander.

VOMITING DURING PREGNANCY

[INTRODUCTION]

The condition in which nausea, vomiting, dizziness and anorexia appear, or even vomiting occurs immediately after a meal, at an early stage of pregnancy, is called vomiting during pregnancy, or "morning sickness." Such symptoms as nausea, preference for a sour taste, being very choosy about food, or occasional vomiting with phlegm and saliva in the morning are considered as a normal reaction of early pregnancy, and they will disappear in time. Western medicine sees this problem as related with mental, nervous and endocrine factors. TCM holds that because of the halt in menstruation after the pregnancy begins, the blood cannot be discharged, so the turbid *qi* in the blood will flow up adversely with fire of the liver and stomach, or because of obstruction of phlegm-damp in the middle *jiao* due to spleen deficiency, stomach *qi* fails to descend. The treatment principle is to harmonize the middle *jiao*, benefit *qi*, cause the descent of the adverse *qi* and stop vomiting. The points of the Hand Yangming, Foot Yangming, Spleen Meridian and Ren Meridian are mainly used, such as Neiguan (PC6), Gongsun (SP4), Tanzhong (CV17), Hegu (LI4) and Zusanli (ST36), and punctured with even technique.

[CLINICAL EXPERIENCE]

1. CONVENTIONAL ACUPUNCTURE

(1) Penetrating Puncture

Point: Penetrating from Neiguan (PC6) to Waiguan (TE5).

Technique: Puncture the points with a 1.5-*cun* needle and even technique with moderate stimulation. Retain the needle for 30 minutes, giving the treatment once or twice a day. Ten times form one course. For poor appetite, add Zusanli (ST36) with reinforcing technique. The manipulation should not be strong for fear of affecting the fetus.

(2) Selecting of Points According to Differentiation of Syndrome

Points: ① Zusanli (ST36), Taichong (LR3) and Zhongwan (CV12). ② Taichong (LR3), Zusanli (ST36) and Yanglingquan (GB34). ③ Fenglong (ST40), Zusanli (ST36) and Neiguan (PC6).

Technique: For stomach deficiency, Zusanli (ST36) and Taichong (LR3) are the main points, supplemented by Zhongwan (CV12) and Neiguan (PC6), all punctured with reinforcement; for liver heat, Taichong (LR3) and Zusanli (ST36) are the main points, supplemented by Yanglingquan (GB34); for phlegm type, Fenglong (ST40) and Zusanli (ST36) are the main points, supplemented by Neiguan (PC6). Retain the needles for 30 to 40 minutes, manipulating the needles two or three times and giving the treatment twice a day with six to eight hours of intervals. Change the treatment to once a day after the condition is alleviated. In 39 cases of morning sickness that were treated, 33 proved effective after five to seven days of treatment; only one was totally ineffective.

2. MOXIBUSTION

(1) Moxibustion with Medicinal Moxa Stick

Points: Zhongwan (CV12), Tiantu (CV22), Juque (CV14), Zusanli (ST36) and Neiguan (PC6).

Technique: First grind 30 g of the rhizome of Chinese atractylodes into fine powder, twisting moxa leaves into moxa wool, and mixing them together. Make a medicinal moxa stick, 20-25 cm in length, and 1.2 cm in diameter. Select three to five points in each treatment, igniting the moxa stick and applying mild warming technique for 10 to 20 minutes, once to three times a day. Five times make up one course.

(2) Moxibustion with Moxa Cones

Point: Jianshi (PC5)

Technique: Apply moxibustion with ginger, preferably a fresh one, and 0.3 cm in thickness. Altogether, 30 cones in the size of rice should be used, once a day. Five times make up one course. This method is indicated for the condition of retching and vomiting with porridge, soup and medicine.

3. AURICULAR THERAPY

Points: Stomach, Diaphragm, Esophagus, Mouth, Cardia, Heart, Shenmen, Chest, Sanjiao, Sub-cortex and Sympathetic.

Technique: Every day, select three to five points, puncture them with reinforcing technique and retain the needle for 30 minutes. Treatment is given once a day, 10 times forming one course. Alternatively, apply an embedding needle in the ear points.

4. HYDRO-ACUPUNCTURE

(1) Injection of Vitamin

Points: Tiantu (CV22), Neiguan (PC6) and Zhongwan (CV12)

Technique: Inject 0.5 ml of mixed fluid containing vitamin B_1 100 mg/2 ml and vitamin B_6 50 mg/2 ml into each point, once a day, five times constituting one course. This method is indicated for all kinds of morning sickness.

(2) Closing Method

Point: Positive point (2 to 4 cm lateral from the fifth to the ninth thoracic vertebra)

Technique: First find out the positive point. While inserting the needle 2 to 2.5 cm deep according to the fatness of the patient, pay attention to the response of the patient and see whether there are bubbles or blood in the syringe in order to be able to decide that there has been no injury to the lung and pleura. Then slowly inject 0.5 to 1% procaine 10 to 20 ml. After withdrawing the needle, massage the local area, and then ask the patient to lie down and rest.

5. CUTANEOUS PUNCTURE

Points: Around both sides of eyelid, arcus superciliaris, forehead, both sides of temporal regions, anterior of the auricle, nape and sacral region.

Technique: Apply a cutaneous needle on the above areas. In accordance with the different areas, make circular, transverse or longitudinal stimulation with four to five lines (circles) on each area. For the obstructive sensation in the throat, also stimulate the skin around the thyroid cartilage. To increase the therapeutic effect, the patient needs to cough moderately during the application to shake the throat and trachea.

6. CATGUT-EMBEDDING METHOD

Points: Neiguan (PC6) and Zusanli (ST36),
Technique: Embed the catgut thread into these two points.

[REMARKS]

1. Selection of points in acupuncture treatment should be made based on the term of the pregnancy. For a pregnancy of less than five months, it is better to select Zhongwan (CV12), Youmen (KI21) and Jianli (CV11) with some other points on the four extremities. For a pregnancy of more than five months, it is better to select points on the four extremities for fear of hurting the fetus.

2. According to clinical reports, acupuncture has no adverse influence on the fetus, but it should be carefully used for the woman with a history of habitual abortion, or it can be replaced by other

methods.

3. When you apply the methods introduced in the chapter, the stimulation must be gentle to avoid hurting the fetus and less points used as well.

CHAPTER THREE
PEDIATRICS

ACUTE INFANTILE CONVULSION

[INTRODUCTION]

An acute infantile convulsion is a disease marked by twitching of the four limbs, mouth closed, opisthotonos and semi-consciousness. Because of its rapid onset, urgent and severe condition, it is called acute infantile convulsion. It is more common among children under the age of five. It can be caused by weak constitution, further complicated by seasonal pathogenic factors attacking the interior of the body along the meridian, leading to failure of yang *qi* to disperse, accumulation of excessive heat, and disturbance of liver wind; or by irregular intake of food and milk, injury to the spleen and stomach, resulting in abnormal transformation and transportation of water and food essence, retention of water changing into phlegm that produces heat and wind; or by sudden great fear and fright. The treatment principle is to eliminate the pathogenic factors, clear the heat, resolve the phlegm, calm down the mind, and open the orifice with the points of Du Meridian, Hand Yangming, Foot Jueyin as the main points, such as Hegu (LI4), Taichong (LR3), Yanglingquan (GB34), Shuigou (GV26), Zhongwan (CV12), Fenglong (ST40), Laogong (PC8) and Shenmen (HT7), using swift and shallow needling technique without retention of needle, with reducing technique or bleeding technique by three-edged needle, but no moxibustion. Central nervous system inflammation, for example, epidemic encephalitis, encephalitis B, toxic bacillary dysentery can be treated by reference to this chapter.

[CLINICAL EXPERIENCE]

1. CONVENTIONAL ACUPUNCTURE

(1) Reducing Du Meridian

Points: Main points: Fengfu (GV16), Shendao (GV11), Dagui (GV14), Zhongshu (GV7) and Jizhong (GV6). Supplementary points: Fengchi (GB20) and Fenglong (ST40).

Technique: Prick the points of Du Meridian without retention of needles in order to remove the pathogenic factors and stop convulsion. For the case caused by phlegm and heat, add Fengchi (GB20) and Fenglong (ST40) to resolve phlegm and reduce wind.

(2) Penetrating Puncture

Points: Houxi (SI3) to Laogong (PC8) and Zusanli (ST36)

Techniques: Insert a two-*cun*, No.30 stainless filiform needle from Houxi (SI3), then obliquely toward Laogong (PC8) with strong stimulation. After the arrival of *qi*, manipulate the needle for two minutes, and then take it out. Also apply strong simulation on Zusanli (ST36), taking out the needle after the sensation is achieved. In case of intractable persistent convulsion, the needle can be retained for 20 to 30 minutes.

(3) Puncturing He-sea Point

Points: Main points: Quchi (LI11) and Hegu (LI4). Supplementary points: Yintang (Extra) and Renzhong (Extra)

Technique: Needle Quchi (LI11) and Hegu (LI4) bilaterally with reducing technique and strong stimulation, without retention of needle. Prick the supplementary points by the filiform needle or apply the bleeding method by a three-edged needle, drawing a drop of blood as big as a bean.

(4) Combination of Points of the Upper and Lower Part of the Body

Points: Renzhong (GV26), Changqiang (GV1), Shixuan (extra), Dazhui (GV14), Zhongwan (CV12), Zusanli (ST36), Yanglingquan (GB34), Kunlun (BL60), Qiuxu (GB40), Quchi (LI11) and Jiexi (ST41).

Technique: First prick Shixuan (extra) by a three-edged needle to cause bleeding so as to clear heat and detoxify, and dredge the meridian *qi* of the upper *jiao*; puncture Renzhong (GV26) with reducing technique, which is a key point to relieve the convulsion, to clear the brain and stop the attack; needle Kunlun (BL60) and Yanglingquan (GB34) to strengthen the effect; further puncture Changqiang (GV1) to lower the upward perverted *qi*, smooth Du Meridian and make the clear *yin* and *yang* rise and turbid *qi* decline. This is the beginning point of the Du Meridian that originates in the uterus, travels upward along the vertebra and enters the brain together with Renzhong (GV26). The other points are needled with the routine method. This method is indicated for acute convulsion caused by an attack of external wind heat and damage of *yin* by a high fever.

(5) *Three-Region Points Puncture*

Points: Renzhong (GV26), Shaoshang (LI1) and Yongquan (KI1)

Technique: Prick the upper, middle and lower regions of each point by a filiform needle to a depth of 0.1 to 0.2 *cun* and immediately withdraw the needle after the arrival of *qi*, so as to regulate *qi* activity of the whole body, as was mentioned in the *Song of Point Selection for Intractable Diseases*, namely, "for infantile convulsion, use Shaoshang (LI1), and reduce Renzhong (GV26) and Yongquan (KI1), but not deeply."

2. BLEEDING METHOD

Points: Shaoshang (LI1), Shangyang (LU11), Renzhong (GV26), Waiguan (TE5) and Yanglingquan (GB34).

Technique: Prick the first three points with a three-edged needle to cause a little bleeding, and then observe the condition of the patient. If the convulsion doesn't stop, quickly puncture the remaining points. Remove the needle immediately after the arrival of *qi*. This method is suitable for convulsion due to a high fever. After the manipulation is finished, the upward perverted *qi* can be lowered, the fever reduced and convulsion stopped.

3. AURICULAR THERAPY

Points: Shenmen, Central Rim, Heart, Liver, Kidney, Brain,

Forehead, Ear Apex and Sub-cortex.

Technique: Apply strong stimulation on the ear points by a fili-form needle, manipulating it for one minute before removal. Select two to four points each time, or connect with electricity for three minutes.

[REMARKS]

Acute infantile convulsion is a common obstetrical disease, because children have incomplete development of the nervous system, and easily become overexcited due to various kinds of stimulation. As a result, many diseases may lead to convulsion. Acupuncture treatment can stop the convulsion and spasm to relieve the urgent condition. After that, the etiology of the condition should be ascertained and corresponding measures taken.

CHRONIC INFANTILE CONVULSION

[INTRODUCTION]

Chronic infantile convulsion is a disease marked by convulsion, emaciation and diarrhea. It more often occurs in children aged under five after a prolonged illness or severe disease, or possibly developed from acute convulsion without proper treatment. It may be caused by dysfunction of the spleen and stomach, and exhaustion of *yang* of the middle *jiao*, or by the over-action of liver wood on earth and interior disturbance of deficient wind. The treatment principle is to strengthen the spleen, tonify the kidney, pacify the liver and reduce wind. The main points include those from the Ren Meridian and Foot Yangming, such as Ganshu (BL18), Pishu (BL20), Shenshu (BL23), Weishu (BL21), Zhongwan (CV12), Zusanli (ST36), Tianshu (ST25), Qihai (CV6), Taichong (LR3) and Yintang (extra). Reinforcing technique is used and moxibustion may be applied if necessary. The child patient with a sequel of meningitis can be treated by referring to this chapter.

[CLINICAL EXPERIENCE]

1. CONVENTIONAL ACUPUNCTURE

(1) Mainly Using the Points of Du Meridian

Points: Main points: Renzhong (GV26), Dazhui (GB14), Shenzhu (BL10) and Jinsuo (GV8). Supplementary points: Houxi (SI3), Yanglingquan (GB34), Hegu (LI4), Taichong (LR3) and Anmian (extra).

Technique: First, take the points of the Du meridian, perform "sparrow-pecking" moxibustion on Renzhong (GV26), and prick the remaining points with strong stimulation and without retention of the needle. If the therapeutic effect is not obviously seen, use the supplementary points with the pricking method and no retention of the needle.

(2) Selection of Points According to Differentiation of Syndrome

Points: Baihui (GV20), Neiguan (PC6), Quchi (LI11), Yanglingquan (GB34), Juegu (GB39) and Zusanli (ST36); for mental excitement, add Shenmen (HT7), Fengfu (GV16), Sanyinjiao (SP6) and Anmian (extra); for dementia, add Dazhui (GV14), Yamen (GV15) and Fengchi (GB20); for aphasia, add Yamen (GV15), Lianquan (CV24), Guanchong (TE1) and Hegu (LI4); for difficult swallowing, add Tiantu (CV22), Hegu (LI4) and Jiache (ST6); for trembling, add Shousanli (LI10), Jianshi (PC5), Hegu (LI4), Yinlingquan (SP9), Dazhui (GV14) and Anmian (extra).

Technique: This method is indicated for a child patient with a sequel of encephalitis for calming down the mind, and removing the obstruction from the meridians and collaterals. For a mild condition, use the main prescription; for those with accompanied symptoms, select a different prescription. Reducing technique is used on all the points.

2. MOXIBUSTION

(1) Moxibustion with Moxa Stick

Points: Dazhui (GV14), Pishu (BL20), Weishu (BL21), Guanyuan (CV4), Qihai (CV6) and Zusanli (ST36).

Technique: Apply wild-warming technique on each point for five minutes daily, 10 times making up one course.

(2) Moxibustion with Moxa Cone

Points: Dazhui (GV14), Tianshu (ST25), Guanyuan (CV4) and Shenque (CV8).

Technique: Apply three cones on Dazhui (GV14), five on Tianshu (ST25), five on Guanyuan (CV4) and three on Shenque (CV8) with non-scarring method. The treatment is applied once a day and 10 days in succession.

(3) Moxibustion on Shenque (CV8)

Point: Shenque (CV8).

Technique: Burn moxa leaves into ash and place on the point Shenque (CV8); or place a slice of garlic and moxa leaves respectively over the point. The treatment is performed with 20 to 30 cones daily.

3.   AURICULAR THERAPY

Points: Shenmen, Heart, Liver, Occiput and Sub-cortex.

Technique: Shallow puncturing or applying Wangbulouxing seeds.

4.   BLEEDING METHOD

Points: Main points: Shixuan (extra), Sifeng (extra) with the bleeding method, Pishu (BL20), Shenshu (BL23) and Zusanli (ST36). Supplementary points: for fever, use Dazhui (GV14) and Quchi (LI11) with the bleeding method, and Waiguan (TE5) with the reducing method; for sleepiness, use Daling (PC7) and Shenmen (HT7) with the reinforcing method, for clonic convulsions, use Ganshu (BL18) and Taichong (LR3) with the reducing method.

Technique: Bleeding technique is used by a three-edged needle or a No.26, 1 *cun* needle, selecting the points as required by the circumstances of the case.

[REMARKS]

1.   Reducing technique is used for chronic convulsion, reinforcing to strengthen the root condition. After the convulsion is stopped,

the spleen and stomach are mainly regulated in order to benefit the productive source of *qi* and blood.

2. In most cases, needling can stop the convulsion, but after that, the causative factors should be identified to prevent recurrence.

INFANTILE FEVER

[INTRODUCTION]

Fever is one of the common clinical symptoms in obstetrics. It is more often caused by an attack of exogenous pathogenic wind, and secondly, by improper intake of food and milk with retention of food in the interior. For fever due to exogenous factors, it is better to use the points of Du Meridian, Hand Yangming and Hand Taiyang, such as Dazhui (GV14), Waiguan (TE5), Shaoshang (LU11) and Hegu (LI4), with reducing technique in needling or bleeding technique; for fever due to retention of food, it is better to use the points of Hand Shaoyang, Hand and Foot Yangming, such as Shangyang (LI1), Guanchong (TE1), Zusanli (ST36), Zhongwan (CV12) and Xuanji (CV21), with reducing technique in needling or bleeding technique. Those obstetrical diseases like upper respiratory tract infection, acute tonsillitis, epidemic flu, pneumonia, indigestion, dysentery, salmonella infection may bring about fever.

[CLINICAL EXPERIENCE]

1. CONVENTIONAL ACUPUNCTURE

(1) Puncturing Du Meridian

Points: Dazhui (GB14), Taodao (GV13), Shenzhu (BL10) and points under the spinous process of T3, 4, 5, 6, altogether 7 points.

Technique: Puncture the points of Du Meridian from Dazhui (GV14) and points between each intervertebral space, altogether seven points. After sterilizing, pinch up the skin gently, stimulating it strongly to cause bleeding without retention of the needle.

(2) Puncturing the Exteriorly-Interiorly Related Meridians
Points: Shaoshang (LU11), Hegu (LI4) and Quchi (LI11).

Technique: Prick Shaoshang (LU11) to cause bleeding, puncture Hegu (LI4) and Quchi (LI1) 0.5 to 1.5 *cun* deep and quickly rotate the needle with strong stimulation. There should be no retention of the needle for children under the age of two. Retain the needles for five to 15 minutes for those above two years of age, manipulating them once. Treatment may be given one to three times a day according to the change of body temperature. It will be considered ineffective if fever cannot be reduced by then. This method has been used for 911 cases of fever, and the effective rate is 72.9%. The body temperature will be lowered with one treatment in some children. Needling can be applied again for recurrence of fever, and is effective in most cases, but at least there should be an interval of 90 minutes to two hours between treatments. For diarrhea, add Zusanli (ST36); and for nausea and vomiting, add Neiguan (PC6).

(3) Selection of Points According to Differentiation of Syndrome
Points: Fengchi (GB20), Dazhui (GV14) (both are punctured first), Quchi (LI11) and Hegu (LI4). For a high fever, use Shixuan (extra), Erjian (ear apex) (applying the bleeding method on both points with four to five bloods out on each); for convulsion, use Baihui (GV20) and Yintang (extra); for vomiting, use Zhongwan (CV12), Tianshu (ST25), Qihai (CV6) and Shangjuxu (ST37); for pain of throat, use Shaoshang (LU11) and Yamen (GV15); for asthma and cough with sputum, use Feishu (BL13), Tiantu (CV22), Chize (LU5) and Fenglong (ST40); for whooping cough, use Feishu (BL13), Sifeng (extra) and Taiyuan (LU9); for mumps, use Jiaosun (TE20) and Ah-shi points; and for listlessness and weak constitution, use Guanyuan (CV4).

Technique: Use a No.22 needle and quickly insert it into the point, then withdraw it immediately after the arrival of *qi*. At the same time, shake the needle hole and let it bleed. If no bleeding occurs, press and squeeze the point and make it bleed with two or three drops of blood. In addition to the main points, use two or three supplementary points, and perform the treatment twice a day.

2. BLEEDING AND CUPPING

Points: Shixuan points (extra) on the hand and foot, Zanzhu (BL2) and Dazhui (GV14).

Technique: Quickly needle Shixuan on the hand and foot and Zanzhu (BL2) to cause bleeding; prick Dazhui (GV14) to cause bleeding, and then apply cupping on it for 10 minutes. This method is good for a prolonged high fever (higher than 39°C).

3. AURICULAR THERAPY

(1) Embedding Seeds on the Ear

Points: Main points: Shenmen, Sympathetic, Lung and Ear Apex. Supplementary points: Trachea, Tonsil, Throat, Spleen and Large Intestine.

Technique: Use the ear point detector to identify the sensitive points mentioned above on the corresponding areas on the auricle, then press them for a few seconds, applying Wanbuliuxing seeds on three to six points bilaterally each time. Tell the parents to press the seeds several times every day.

(2) Bleeding Method on Ear Apex

Points: Ear Apex and Reducing Fever Point.

Technique: First, massage the auricle to make it congested. After applying routine sterilization on it with 70% alcohol, puncture the ear apex by a No.4 syringe needle, then change to the back of the ear and puncture downward 0.2 to 0.3 *cun* along the auricle to the reducing fever point to cause three to five drops of blood to come out.

[REMARKS]

With a view of clinical practice, needling with reducing technique and bleeding technique by a three-edged needle can reduce body temperature so as to relieve the acute condition of children. But because of the pure *yin* and pure *yang* in children's bodies, and the rapid change of the condition, the child's reaction should be carefully observed. If the temperature cannot be lowered after one or two treatments, use a combination of TCM and Western medicine.

WHOOPING COUGH

[INTRODUCTION]

Whooping cough is an acute infectious disease caused by hemophilus pertusis, and is more common in winter and spring. It is marked by paroxysmal onset and continuous cough, accompanied by aspiratory roaring. Some time after the attack, it may stop for a while, but then reoccur for a number of times each day, so that it is called "paroxysmal cough." Because of its long duration and difficulty to be cured, it is also called "whooping cough." Traditional Chinese medicine thinks that this problem is caused by invasion of pathogenic wind heat, leading to dysfunction of the lung to dominate the descending and dispersing, obstruction of turbid phlegm in the *qi* passage and failure of lung *qi* to descend. The treatment principle is to relieve the exterior syndrome, clear lung heat, resolve phlegm and stop the cough. The points of Hand Taiyin, Hand Yangmin, and corresponding Back-shu points are mainly selected, such as, Lieque (LU7), Hegu (LI4), Fengmen (BL12), Feishu (BL13) and Gaohuangshu (BL43), with reducing technique in the attack stage and reinforcing technique in the remission stage.

[CLINICAL EXPERIENCE]

1. CONVENTIONAL ACUPUNCTURE

(1) Puncturing Sifeng Point

Points: Sifeng (extra) bilaterally.

Technique: Puncture the point two or three mm deep with a one-*cun* needle, then immediately take it out, drawing off some yellowish white sticky fluid. Treatment is given once every other day, three times in one course. Avoid puncturing the small veins to cause bleeding.

(2) Puncturing He-Sea Point

Points: Zusanli (ST36) and Hegu (LI4),

Technique: For prolonged cough with weak constitution, select He-sea point of Yangming Meridian of Hand and Foot, i.e., Zusanli (ST36) and Hegu (LI4). Apply reinforcing first and reducing secondly on Zusanli (ST36), and reduce on Hegu. For fever, add Dazhui (GV14) and Quchi (LI11); for poor appetite, add Neiguan (PC6) and Shangqiu (SP5); for epistaxis, add Taiyuan (LU9) and Jingqu (LU8).

(3) Puncturing the Points on the Back

Points: Main points: Fengmen (BL12), Feishu (BL13) and Dingchuan (Extra). Supplementary points: Yuji (LU10), Shaoshang (LU11), Tiantu (CV22), Fenglong (ST40) and Quchi (LI11).

Technique: Use quick needling technique on the Back-Shu point as deep as 0.2 to 0.4 *cun* once every day or once every other day. Four treatments make up one course with an interval of two to five days between courses. If there is no effect, add supplementary points.

2. MOXIBUSTION

Points: Feishu (BL13), Tiantu (CV22) and Jinsuo (GV8).

Technique: Apply suspended moxibustion on each point for 10 to 15 minutes daily, or whenever there is an onset of coughing, 10 treatments making up one course. This method is very effective for prolonged whooping cough.

3. AURICULAR THERAPY

Points: Brachia, Lung, Pingchuan, Shenmen and Sympathetic.

Technique: Puncture two or three points by a filiform needle with even technique every day, or embed seeds on the ear points for those who are afraid of a needle, intermittently on the two ears, once a day.

4. BLEEDING METHOD

Points: Shaoshang (LU11), Shangyang (LI1), Zhongchong (PC9) and Shaoze (SI1).

Technique: Prick the above points bilaterally by a three-edged needle once a day, five treatments constituting one course. Three courses of treatments may be given.

5. CUPPING

Points: ① Shenzhu (GV12) and Tiantu (CV22). ② Feishu (BL13), Fenglong (ST40) and Lieque (LU7).

Technique: Use the two groups of points in turn, one group a day. Apply reducing first and cupping next on Shenzhu (GV12), and then puncture Tiantu (CV22). Prick Feishu (BL13) a few times, then perform cupping. Adopt even technique on Lieque (LU7), and the reducing method on Fenglong (ST40).

6. HYDRO-ACUPUNCTURE

Point: Chize (LU5) bilaterally.

Technique: Paroxysmal cough is a symptom of the respiratory system, so select bilateral He-sea points of the lung meridian. Make 25 to 50 mg of streptomycin into a 0.5 ml solution, and inject them into the points of both sides as deep as 1 to 1.5 cm, once a day. Five treatments form one course, and there should be two courses at most. There should be an intradermal test carried out before the injection. It has also been found that the injection of chloromycetin on Kechuan point or Feishu (BL13) can also be effective.

7. MEDICINAL APPLICATION ON ACU-POINT

Points: Feishu (BL13), Xinshu (BL15) and Geshu (BL17).

Technique: Prepare processed Baijiezi (dried seeds of Brassica alba) 21 g, Yuanhu 21 g, Gansui (the root of Euphorbia Kansui) 12 g, Xixin (the root of Chinese wild ginger) 12 g, grind them into a fine powder, and store them in a sealed container for use. The above amount of herbs will form five doses. Before application, mix one fifth of above amount of herbs with fresh ginger juice into a paste, adding a little musk. Place the mixture on six pieces of oily paper, and apply on the three pairs of points, fixing them with plasters. On each occasion, the medicinal application should last four to six hours, and is given once every 10 days. The effective rate is over 70%.

[REMARKS]

If fever, shortage of breath, and flapping of the nose are found, pneumonia may have developed; and if coma and convulsion are present, possibly toxic meningitis may have occurred. Both changes of the condition should be carefully observed.

INFANTILE DIARRHEA

[INTRODUCTION]

Infantile diarrhea is a common pediatric disease manifested as frequent bowel movement, loose or watery feces. It may occur in any season, but is more common in summer and autumn. Diarrhea is caused by dysfunction in separating the clear from the turbid due to invasion of exogenous pathogenic summer heat and damp with irregular food intake as the zang-fu organs of children are delicate; or due to prolonged illness with weakness of the spleen and stomach. The principle of treatment is to clear heat and damp, promote digestion, relieve retention of food, strengthen the spleen and warm the kidney. The points of Foot Yangming, Foot Taiyin and Ren Meridian are mainly used, such as Zhongwan (CV12), Tianshu (ST25), Guanyuan (CV4), Zusanli (ST36) and Sanyinjiao (SP6). For damp heat and retention of food, only use acupuncture and no moxibustion; for irregular food intake, puncture the points with reducing technique; and for cold damp of the spleen and stomach, use acupuncture and moxibustion with reinforcing technique.

[CLINICAL EXPERIENCE]

1. CONVENTIONAL ACUPUNCTURE

(1) Regulating Ren and Du Meridian

Points: Changqiang (GV1) and Chengjiang (CV24).

Technique: Insert a 2.5-*cun* (Size No.28) needle quickly into Changqiang (GV1), and then perpendicularly insert the needle 1.5 to 2 *cun* deep between the coccyx and the rectum without any lifting and thrusting. Apply reinforcement by rotating the needle for about one minute and then withdraw it. Press the needle hole with a sterilized cotton ball. Shallowly puncture Chengjiang (CV24) 0.3 *cun* deep, apply reducing by rotating the needle for one minute and then withdraw it, pressing the needle hole to prevent bleeding. The treatment is given once a day, usually one to three times in succession. This method is good to regulate *yin* and *yang*.

(2) Combination of Front-Mu Point and Yuan-Source Point

Points: Tianshu (ST25) and Hegu (LI4).

Technique: Puncture these two points perpendicularly with reinforcing technique. For a mild condition, add Zhongwan (CV12) and Neiting (ST44); for a severe condition, add Guanyuan (CV4) and Zusanli (ST36); for fever, add Taichong (LR3); for vomiting, add Guanyuan (CV4), Changqiang (GV1) and Dachangshu (BL25). This method has been applied in 108 cases of infantile diarrhea, with 107 being cured after an average of three treatments, and only one proving ineffective.

(3) Puncturing the Extra Point

Point: Zhixiexue [extra, 0.5 *cun* inferior to Guanyuan (CV4)].

Technique: Perpendicularly puncture 1 *cun* deep. Moxibustion may also be used for persistent diarrhea. Treatment is normally given once a day, but can be given several times for severe cases.

(4) Penetrating Puncture

Points: Puncture Zusanli (ST36) to Shangjuxu (ST37) by penetrating technique.

Technique: First puncture Zusanli (ST36) perpendicularly 0.5 to 1 *cun* deep and manipulate the needle for one minute with even technique. Then, lift the needle to the subcutaneous region, penetrate from Zusanli (ST36) to Shangjusu (ST37) straight and rotate the needle for one to two minutes to regulate the *qi* movement of the intestine.

2. MOXIBUSTION

(1) Moxibustion with Moxa Cone over the Cake Made of Roudoukou

Points: Tianshu (ST25), Shenque (CV8) and Guanyuan (CV4).

Technique: Mix an equal amount of nutmeng, Evadia rutaecarpa and Chaoxiaohuixiang, grind the mixture into a fine power, and store it in a bottle for future use. While doing moxibustion, take out a certain amount of powder and grind it with fresh onion white into a paste. Make a few cakes as big as a five-cent coin and put them on the points with five moxa cones on top. This treatment is given once a day. It is indicated for diarrhea due to *yang* deficiency of the spleen and the kidney in children.

(2) Mild-Warming Technique

Points: Tianshu (ST25), Guanyuan (CV4), Shenque (CV8), Pishu (BL20) and Shenshu (BL23).

Technique: Apply mild-warming technique on the points with two to three sticks on each point daily until the skin turns slightly red.

(3) Moxibustion by Dengcao

Point: Changqiang (GV1).

Technique: Burn one end of Dengcao with tea oil on it, and apply it on Changqiang (GV1). Usually, the diarrhea may be stopped by one treatment. If not, repeat three to five days later.

3. THREE EDGED-NEEDLE THETAPY

(1) Puncturing the Jing-Well Point

Point: Shangyang (LU11).

Technique: Prick the point a few times with a three edged-needle until there is a little bleeding, once a day, three times making up one course. For vomiting, add Neiguan (PC6); for diarrhea due to cold damp, add Guanyuan (CV4) with moxibustion.

(2) Puncturing the Extra Point

Point: Sifeng (Extra).

Technique: Prick Sifeng (Extra) with a three edged-needle and then squeeze out a small amount of blood or yellowish white fluid, once a day, only applying this method on one hand each time alternately. Two to four treatments form one course. For severe condition, add Neiguan (PC6) and Gongsun (SP4).

4. CUTANEOUS PUNCTURE

Points: Urinary Bladder, Stomach, Spleen and Ren meridians.

Technique: Tap the first line of the UB meridian from Ganshu (BL18) downward to Xiaochangshu (BL27), Ren meridian from Zhongwan (CV12) to Guanyuan (CV4), Stomach Meridian of the Foot Yangming from Liangmen (ST21) to Tianshu (ST25), and Zusanli (ST36) to Jiexi (ST41), and Gall Bladder Meridian of the Foot Taiyin from Yinlingquan (SP9) to Sanyinjiao (SP6). Tap the points with gentle force until the skin turns a little red. For high fever, also tap Quchi

(LI11) and Hegu (LI4) with more heavy force and cause slight bleeding, once a day, five times in one course.

5. HYDRO-ACUPUNCTURE

Points: Tianshu (ST25) and Zusanli (ST36).

Technique: Inject 0.5 ml of Vitamin B1 into each point for five days in succession as one course.

6. CUPPING

Point: Zhongwan (CV12), Qihai (CV6), Ganshu (BL18), Pishu (BL20) and Dachangshu (BL25).

Technique: Use the small-sized cup for children aged above two years, selecting two or three points each time and retaining the cup for five minutes, once a day. This method is more effective for diarrhea due to cold or retention of food.

7. MEDICINAL APPLICATION ON ACU-POINT

Point: Shengque (CV8).

Technique: Grind 15 g of Chinese gall and 10 g of alum together into a very fine powder for future use. Heat 30 g of yellow wax in a pot to make them melt, then add the powder and mix until it becomes even. Let it cool and store for future use. Put one g of ointment on a piece of plaster 4×4 cm, melting it with a mild fire, applying it on Shenque (CV8) once a day. The method has been proved always effective for cold type of diarrhea by ancient and present clinical practice, as it was said in *Recovery of Thousands of Diseases*: "Infantile diarrhea can be stopped by ointment made by mixture of Chinese gall and vinegar."

8. LASER THERAPY

Points: Main points: Shengque (CV8) and Zusanli (ST36). Supplementary point: Zhixie point (Extra).

Technique: First radiate the main points by laser, three to five minutes on every point. But, if there is no obvious result after three treatments, add supplementary points. Five treatments constitute one course. A total of 93 cases of prolonged infantile diarrhea were treated in this way, with 72 cured, 14 improved and seven ineffective (total effective rate 92.5%).

9. COMBINED TREATMENT

Point: Sifeng (Extra).

Technique: Sterilize Sifeng (Extra) of both sides, prick them with a needle 0.1 *cun* deep, and squeeze out yellowish white transparent sticky fluid or cause bleeding. Then, perform massage with the patient in a supine condition. The method is that pinch up the skin of the coccyx by the two thumbs and four fingers, push forward with the thumbs standing, while pulling backward with the other fingers. Stop at the seventh cervical vertebrae. Do this five to seven times every time until the skin along the vertebral column turns red. Puncture Sifeng (Extra) and apply massage once a day, or twice for severe cases. A total of 108 cases of diarrhea due to indigestion were treated in this way, with 102 cured, five improved and only one ineffective.

[REMARKS]

1. During treatment, attention should be paid to diet control. It is better to eat less, but more frequently, in order to take in a certain amount of nutrient and water, but avoiding vomiting.

2. If a child shows signs of irritability, restlessness, frequent vomiting or abdominal distention, deep and long breathing, feeble pulse, extremely cold limbs and convulsions, these may be considered as critical signs of acidosis and water electrolyte imbalance. In this case, a combination of Western medicine and TCM should be adopted immediately.

INFANTILE MALNUTRITION

[INTRODUCTION]

Infantile malnutrition is a chronic disease marked by sallow complexion, emaciation, sparse hair, loss of appetite, distended belly or potbelly, and listlessness. It is found more often in children under the age of five. The pathogenesis of this problem is that such factors like irregular food intake, early conclusion of lactation, poor nutrition after an illness, taking powerful drugs and parasitic disease may result in dysfunction of the spleen and stomach, and exhaustion of body fluid. The failure to digest water and grain means they are retained for a long time so as to produce heat, and lead to malnutrition. The treatment principle is to build up the spleen and promote digestion. The points of the Foot Taiyin and Foot Yangming are used, such as Xiawan (CV13), Zusanli (ST36) and Shangqiu (SP5) with even technique, and Sifeng (Extra) with bleeding technique.

[CLINICAL EXPERIENCE]

1. CONVENTIONAL ACUPUNCTURE

(1) Puncturing Five-Shu Point

Points: Main points: Zusanli (ST36), Dadu (SP2) and Taibai (SP3). Supplementary points: Shenmen (HT7) and Taixi (KI3).

Technique: Zusanli (ST36) is the He-sea point of the stomach, Dadu (SP2) is the Ying-spring point of the spleen, Taibai (SP3) is the Shu-stream point of the spleen, Shenmen (HT7) is the Shu-stream point of heart, and Taixi (KI3) is the Shu-stream point of kidney. Both sides of the points are needled. Only one minute of lifting, thrusting and rotating of the needle should be applied to those less than one year old, without retention of the needle. Reinforcing technique by rotating the needle is used for those above the age of one, with retention of the needle for three to five minutes. It is given once a day, and seven treatments are considered as one course, with a one-week interval.

(2) Combination of Points According to Differentiation of Syndrome

Points: Main points: Sifeng (Extra). For abdominal distention, add Zhongwan (CV12) and Zusanli (ST36); for diarrhea, add Tianshu (ST25), or Dachangshu (BL25); for restlessness and irritability, add Neiguan (PC6) or Daling (PC7).

Technique: Insert a 0.5-*cun* long needle quickly into the point of Sifeng (Extra), rotate the needle three to five times, and then take it out swiftly and squeeze out some yellowish white transparent mucous. Daling (PC7) is punctured 0.2 to 0.3 *cun* deep, the others 0.3 to 0.5 *cun* deep by rotation of the needle and rapid manipulation. It is given once a day. Sifeng (Extra) was used to treat 220 cases, with a 93.18% cure rate.

2. MOXIBUSTION

(1) Moxibustion with Moxa Cone
Point: The depression 3 *cun* above coccyx.

Technique: Put some Vaseline or garlic juice on the point, and apply three cones as big as a date kernel. According to *Compendium of Acupuncture*, it is said that, for infantile malnutrition and emaciation, use moxibustion with three moxa cones on the depression 3 *cun* above the coccyx.

(2) Mild-Warming Technique with Moxa Stick
Points: ① Zhangmen (LR13). ② Shenzhu (GV12), Dazhu (BL12) Zhongwan (CV12) and Zusanli (ST36).

Technique: Apply sparrow-pecking technique with moxa stick on Group One or Two, one day one group, 10 minutes on each point. According to *Collections of Acupuncture and Moxibustion*, it is said that for thin children with weakness in all four limbs and failure of shoulder and back to lift, moxibustion should be used on Zhangmen (LR13).

3. PRICKING METHOD

Point: Where there is a subcutaneous nodule around feng and guan of the thumb.

Technique: Prick the nodule after sterilization with a sterilized sewing needle or a three-edged needle until the fibers are broken. This is given once a day, three times making up one course.

4. CUTTING FAT THERAPY

Point: Yuji (LU10).

Technique: First apply local anesthesia on the point Yuji (LU10), then cut the skin vertically 0.4 to 0.5 cm long and 0.3 cm deep, inserting into the cut and performing massage. There will be a better effect if a needling sensation appears. Remove a little fat as big as a yellow bean, apply stopping bleeding powder on the wound and cover it with sterilized gauze and a bandage. After dressing it, press with the thumb to avoid bleeding. Remove the dressing three days later. First cut the left hand, and seven to 10 days later, cut the skin of the point of the right hand. Usually, the problem can be cured by one treatment. A total of 350 cases were treated, with an effectiveness of 95.8%. Research into the pathogenesis of treatment of infantile malnutrition by cutting Yuji (LU10) suggests that even though the pathogenesis of this problem is completed, weakness of the spleen and stomach is the core of it; in a prolonged condition, other internal organs will be involved, resulting in general failure in the long run. Yuji (LU10) is the Ying-spring point of the Lung Meridian of Hand Taiyin, and cutting this point can stimulate the Lung Meridian of Hand Taiyin and make lung *qi* strong and full. Because the lung connects to hundreds of meridians, if lung *qi* is plentiful, spleen *qi* will be strong so as to achieve the purpose of treating malnutrition.

5. MEDICINAL APPLICATION ON ACU-POINT

Points: Shenque (CV8) and Mingmen (GV4).

Technique: First make up the malnutrition ointment. Mirabilite 19 g, apricot kernel 6 g, Cape jasmine 3 g, scallion stalk seven pieces, seven jujubes (remove the kernel), distiller's grains of the first process 30 g, and Huimian 90 g are mixed together into plaster. Divide them into two parts on two oily papers, and apply them on the points, fixing in place with plaster. Make a new dressing every three days, and usually it will be better after two or three times. Continue the treatment until there is recovery.

6. CHIROPRACTIC TREATMENT

Let the child patient lie face down, exposing the back. The practitioner lifts the point Changqiang (GV1) by two fingers, kneading and releasing skin intermittently upward to Dazhui (GV14). After doing this three times, repeat from Banhuanshu (BL30) to Dazhu (BL11), again three times. The treatment is given once a day, six times forming one course. There should be a gap of five days before the second course commences.

7. COMBINED TREATMENT

Points: Sifeng (Extra), Zusanli (ST36), Pishu (BL20), Weishu (BL21) and Pigen (3.5 *cun* lateral to the first lumber vertebra).

Technique: Prick Sifeng (Extra) with a three-edged needle and squeeze out some yellowish white mucous, then puncture the other points. After the arrival of *qi*, rotate the needle a little without retention. It is given once a day and three successive treatments constitute one course. After one course, the child can take Jian'er Heji prescribed by the author (Dangshen, the rhizome of large-headed atractylode, Chinese yam, Maiya, Shijunzirou, Mairou respectively 60 g, Jineijin 90 g, Sanleng, Ezhu, the root of herbaceous peony, respectively 30 g, ground into powder, and put into bags with 0.6 g each). It is advisable to eat more pork meat and pig liver.

[REMARKS]
1. During treatment, attention should be paid to diet. Do not eat too much oily and greasy food.
2. Stool test should be given to check for worm eggs. If parasites are found in the stool, they should be killed.

INFANTILE PARALYSIS

[INTRODUCTION]
Infantile paralysis, which is also called infantile Wei syndrome, is an infectious disease caused by invasion of epidemic and toxic pathogens. The clinical manifestation at early stage is similar to the common

cold, but is marked by paralysis of limbs, and muscular atrophy and deformed joints in the later stages. This problem falls into category of poliomyelitis in modern medicine, and is more prevalent in summer and autumn, but does appear in other seasons, and is mostly seen in children between the ages of one to five. It can be caused by an attack of wind heat to the lungs, resulting in failure to disseminate body fluid, and depriving tendons and vessels of nourishment; or by accumulation of damp heat in Yangming, resulting in relaxation of tendons, and failure to control the bones and joints; or by deficiency of essence and blood due to prolonged illness, resulting in muscular atrophy. The principle of treatment is to eliminate the pathogens, remove the obstruction from meridians and collaterals, warm and nourish the meridians and collaterals. The points of Yangming Meridian are mainly used, such as Jianyu (LI15), Quchi (LI11), Waiguan (TE5), Hegu (LI4), Houxi (SI3), Dazhui (GV14), Biguan (ST31), Futu (ST32), Huantiao (GB30), Zusanli (ST36), Xuanzhong (GB39) and Kunlun (BL60), with even technique.

[CLINICAL EXPERIENCE]

1. CONVENTIONAL ACUPUNCTURE

(1) Multiple Direction Puncture

Points: Jianyu (LI15), Quchi (LI11), Waiguan (TE5), Hegu (LI4), Huantiao (GB30), Jimen (SP11), Yinmen (BL37), Biguan (GB31), Yanglingquan (GB34) and Jiexi (ST41)

Technique: All the points are punctured with multiple-direction technique. First, the needle is inserted perpendicularly to a certain depth, rotated once or twice, and then lifted to the subcutaneous region. Then it is inserted toward the other directions. When all the five directions (upper, lower, left, right and middle) are finished, the needle should be removed immediately. Because of lack of nourishment of *qi* and blood for a long time, the atrophic limbs cannot endure strong stimulation, so only gentle stimulation should be given. "Multiple-direction puncture" is an acupuncture technique derived from Hegu Puncture.

(2) Penetrating Technique

Points: Main points: Changqiang (GV1) to Mingmen (GV4), Mingmen (GV4) to Zhiyang (GV9), and Zhiyang (GV9) to Dazhui (GV14). Supplementary points: For paralysis of upper limbs, puncture Jianyu (LI15) to Quchi (LI11), and Waiguan (TE5) to Quchi (LI11); for paralysis of lower limb, puncture Weizhong (BL40) to Chengfu (BL36), for aversion of foot, puncture medial malleolus to Sanyinjiao (SP6); for inversion of the foot, puncture external malleolus to Guangming (GB37); and for retroversion of the knee joint, puncture Zusanli (ST36) to Xiyangguan (GB33).

Technique: Insert a 6 to 8 *cun* needle (Size: No.26) into the skin, forming an angle of 15° between the needle body and skin. Quickly manipulate the needle through the skin. When the needle reaches the above points, lift and thrust the needle three to five times, and remove it. The treatment is given once a day, 10 times forming one course, with an interval of three to five days between two courses. The supplementary points are punctured with penetrating technique by a long needle.

(3) Setting the Mountain on Fire

Points: Main points: Biguan (ST31), Liangqiu (ST32), Zusanli (ST36), Neiting (ST44), Shenzhu (GV12), Yaoyangguan (GV3) and Taixi (KI3). Supplementary points: Huantiao (GB30), Fengshi (GB31), Yanglingquan (GB34), Juegu (GB39), Sanyinjiao (SP6), Qiuqu (GB40) and Taichong (LR3).

Technique: Select four to five points each time. For paralysis of the upper limbs, add Shousanli (LI10) and Hegu (LI4); for difficulty of swallowing, add Futu (LI18) and Tiantu (CV22); for paralysis of the abdominal muscle, add Tianshu (ST25) and Guilai (ST29); and for low speech, add Lianquan (CV23), Zhaohai (KI6) and Neiguan (PC6). Use a 1 to 1.5 *cun* needle (Size: Nos.28 to 30) to puncture, inserting it by rotation. After the needling sensation is obtained, twirl the needle downward to 1 *cun* deep, manipulating it with three levels on each point for three minutes with the method of setting the mountain on fire. Remove the needle when it is finished. The treatment is given once a day, 30 times constituting one course, and three courses in all with seven-day intervals.

2. THICK-NEEDLE PUNCTURE

Points: Huantiao (GB30), Fengshi (GB31), Heyang (BL55), Chengshan (BL57), Yanglingquan (GB34), Mingmen (GV4) and Shendao (GV11) to Zhiyang (GV9) by penetrating technique.

Technique: Huantiao (GB30), Fengshi (GB31), Chengshan (BL57) and Yanglingquan (GB34) are punctured with strong stimulation and no retention of needle. For muscular atrophy, the method of curing the muscle by lifting and thrusting is applied because this can reach many branches of meridians and collaterals so as to promote the circulation of *qi* and blood and increase the body temperature. The points of Du Meridians should be stimulated by a thick needle because they govern all the six Yang Meridians and *yang* dominates movement. Then, the six Yin Meridians will be also influenced with *qi* and blood circulating, thus *yin* and *yang* will become balanced. The point Mingmen (GV4) is thought to dominate the twelve meridians, so it is used in the prescription for it can improve the circulation of *qi* and blood.

3. ELECTRIC ACUPUNCTURE

Points: According to the area with motor impairment, select the corresponding vertebral space. For example, paralysis of musculus quadriceps femoris leads to the failure of extending function of knee joint, the spinal segment controlling its movement is between L2 and L4, and the corresponding spinal space is between T10 and L1.

Technique: The patient adopts a supine position. Select the area for puncturing on which routine sterilization is applied, fixing the space between the spinous process of two vertebrae with the left hand, and holding the needle in the right hand. Insert a 1 or 1.5 *cun* needle about 0.5 *cun* deep into the skin, connecting to the electricity with low frequency of less than 30 Hz, every four to five minutes, shutting off the power for two minutes, and then switching on again. The total time used is 20 minutes. The treatment is given once a day, ten times making up one course.

4. MAGNETIC THERAPY

Points: On the upper limbs: Quchi (LI11), Waiguan (TE5) and

Hegu (LI4); on the lower limbs: Huantiao (GB30), Yinmen (BL37) Yanglingquan (GB34) and Xuanzhong (GB39).

Technique: Select the points according to the affected place. ① Shaking magnetic method: Select two to four points for 40 to 60 minutes everyday. ② Magnetic needle method: After the treatment finishes everyday, put 1,000-2,000 g smagnetic slices on the subcutaneous needles, changing them every three days, and using two to four points each time.

5. CUTANEOUS PUNCTURE

Points: For paralysis of upper limbs, use points of Du Meridian (from neck to T4), Yangming Meridian of Hand, Taiyang Meridian of Hand, such as Quchi (LI11), Hegu (LI4) and Waiguan (TE5). For paralysis of lower limbs, use Du Meridian, Urinary Bladder Meridian (lumber and sacral parts), Yangming Meridian of Foot, Taiyin Meridian of Foot, Jueying Meridian of Foot and Shaoyang Meridian of Foot. For paralysis of abdominal muscle, add Yangming Meridian of Foot, Taiyin Meridian of Foot, and Shaoyang Meridian of Foot on the abdomen.

Technique: Tap by the cutaneous needle with moderate or gentle stimulation, once a day, 10 times forming one course.

6. HYDRO-ACUPUNCTURE

Points: Quchi (LI11), Hegu (LI4), Waiguan (TE5), Futu (ST32), Yinmen (BL37), Zusanli (ST36) and Sanyinjiao (SP6).

Technique: Use 10% glucose injection fluid, Vitamin B_1, compound Angelicae fluid, Vitamin B_{12}. The 10% glucose injection should be on the point where the muscle is thick, such as Yinmen (BL37), Zusanli (ST36) or Futu (S32) with 10 ml in each point, and 0.5 to 1 ml in each point for other fluid. Select two to four points every time, once a day or once every other day. A total of 10-20 successive treatments form one course.

7. CATGUT-EMBEDDING METHOD ON THE POINT

Points: The points of Yangming Meridian of Hand and Foot are used as main points with supplementary points on the paralytic muscles. For paralysis of upper limbs, use Dazhui (GV14), Jianyu (LI11), Quchi (LI4) and Waiguan (TE5); for paralysis of lower limbs, use Mingmen (GV4), Huantiao (GB30) and Zusanli (ST36). For the supplementary points, first puncture Yang Meridian, then Yin Meridian; first upper limbs, then lower limbs; first the mild side, then the severe side.

Technique: (1) Use the embedding method on the most superficial points by a triangular needle. After routine sterilization, apply local anesthesia on the area 1.5 to 3 cm lateral to the points, pulling the thread through the triangular needle, penetrating through the point from one anesthesia point and coming out from another anesthesia point. Pull the thread back and forth a few times in order to cause numb and the distending sensation on the point, and cut the thread along the skin without exposing it, and make a dressing. (2) Use the embedding method on the deep points with a puncturing needle. After applying local anesthesia on the points, prick the skin of the points and apply massage on the broken skin with the puncturing needle (with dull tip) to produce stimulation in order to cause numbness and a distending sensation. While withdrawing the syringe, push the needle hole to leave the catgut thread in the points, and then close the cut with forceps. A 1-2 cm thread is used for three to five points each time, once per month. The treatment is usually given two to six times.

[REMARKS]

The time within two months since the onset is the key time for the acupuncture treatment for its high curative rate and less sequels. The therapeutic effect within one year is good, but less improvement is seen for more than two years. The treatment is somewhat effective in some patients with disease of long duration but without severe muscular atrophy if they insist on the acupuncture and massage treatment. Acupuncture is only effective for the condition of long duration, severe deformity of joint and muscular atrophy.

EPIDEMIC PARASITES

[INTRODUCTION]

Epidemic parasites is an acute non-suppurative inflammation of the parotid gland caused by invasion of filterable virus through the respiratory tract, which is commonly called "mumps" and is often seen in winter and spring among children aged five to 15. It will leave life-long immunity after the first attack. In the early stage, it is marked by fever, chills, vomiting and poor appetite; later by redness, swelling and hotness, and pain on the parotid region unilaterally or bilaterally may appear. It can be caused by invasion of wind, febrile and toxic factors to the lung and stomach via the mouth and nose. The treatment principle is to dispel wind and heat, clear the collaterals, subdue the swelling with the points of Hand Shaoyang and Foot Yangming as the main points, such as Yifeng (TE17), Jiache (ST6), Waigan (TE6), Hegu (LI4), Quchi (LI11) and Fenglong (ST40) with reducing technique.

[CLINICAL EXPERIENCE]

1. CONVENTIONAL ACUPUNCTURE

(1) Puncturing Extra Point

Points: Mumps (0.3 *cun* below the ear lobe on the cheek), Jiacha (ST6), Jianjing (GB21) and Hegu (LI4).

Technique: Insert the needle while rotating it with strong stimulation, retaining it for 15 to 30 minutes with manipulation once every three to five minutes. Treatment can be given once a day, or twice in severe cases. This method was used for 27 cases, and all were cured within three days.

(2) Puncturing Jing-Well Point

Points: Shaoshang (LU11) as the main point; and Hegu (LI4) and Yifeng (TE17) as the supplementary points.

Technique: Puncture Shaoshang (LU11) quickly by a one-*cun* needle (Size No.26) and rotate it to enlarge the needle hole until it bleeds. Then puncture other points with reducing technique. Treat it once a day, or twice for severe cases.

(3) Surrounding Technique

Point: Affected area

Technique: Quickly puncture five to six needles around the swollen parotid gland without retention after the arrival of *qi*. Treat once a day, or twice to three times a day if necessary. For fever, add Hegu (LI4) and Quchi (LI11).

(4) Single Needle Method

Point: Puncturing point (The midpoint of the line between the angle of mandible and ear lobe of the affected side)

Technique: Insert the needle obliquely at an angle of 15° to 30° toward the corner of the mouth and to the center of the swollen gland. Insert the needle quickly and manipulate it for two or three minutes, then take it out. In the treatment of 100 cases studied, 95 were completely cured, but five cases accompanied by other problems were not effective.

(5) Puncturing Shousanli (LI10).

Point: Shousanli (LI10).

Technique: Puncture the point of the affected side (bilateral points if both are affected) 1 to 1.5 *cun* deep with moderately strong stimulation. While needling, press the enlarged lymph nodes of the affected side. It was found that, with this treatment, lymph nodes disappeared gradually followed by alleviation of the swollen parotid gland.

2. MOXIBUSTION

Point: Jiaosun (TE20).

Technique: Use the moxa stick or burning moxibustion on the affected side, once a day, and it can be cured by one to three treatments. Burning moxibustion: burn rush with vegetable oil inside and apply moxibustion on Jiaosun (TE20) quickly. Move it away while lit, and it is stopped when there is the sound "pa." According to observation of 1,490 cases in five hospitals, the total curative rate is about 95%, and most cases were cured by one to three treatments.

Explanation: Burning moxibustion is a reducing technique and functions to dispel wind and heat, soften the masses. The reason for the effectiveness of this method in the treatment of the problem is that the effect of the meridian point is combined with " Blowing the fire quickly can make reducing," and the application technique is the key to its effectiveness.

3. ELECTRIC ACUPUNCTURE

Points: Hegu (LI4), Shaoshang (LU11), Jiaosun (TE20) and stimulating point of parasites of the affected side (the upper border of the swollen gland).

Technique: When puncturing the stimulating point of parasites, insert the needle from the upper border of the swollen gland with an angle of 45° and then into the tissue of the swollen parotid gland as deep as 1 to 1.5 *cun*. Afterward, connect the needle with the electric machine, 100 to 200 times per minute in frequency, and retain for 10-15 minutes. The electrical output is dependent on the endurance of the patient. After removing the needle, prick Shaoshang (LU11) of both sides to release five to seven drops of blood from each point, once a day, or twice a day for severe cases. The point of Jiaosun (TE20) is punctured horizontally by penetrating technique toward the back of the ear.

4. AURICULAR THERAPY

Points: Tip of the antitragus, Shenmen, helix1-6, Brain, Cheek, Parotid Gland and Endocrine.

Technique: Use two or three points each time with strong stimulation by a filiform needle, retaining it for 20 to 30 minutes, once or twice a day. Alternatively, press the ear points by Wangbuliuxing seeds until the swelling of the parotid gland disappears.

5. COMBINED TREATMENT

Point: Jiaosun (TE20).

Technique: Sterilize the point with the routine method, and prick one to three times with a three-edged needle gently, squeezing it until there is slight bleeding. The treatment is given once a day on the affected side. Usually pain and swelling will disappear with one to three treatments. In case of fever over 38°, some herbs should be taken, including Banlangen (Chinese herbal medicine for treating cords) 15 g, Gancao (licoric roof) 9 g. Shengma 6 g, Congbai (scallion stalk) two pieces (the dosage is suitable for children under 10). Take one bag of decoction each day. This method is obviously effective for parasites without suppuration and broken skin.

[REMARKS]

1. This problem is an epidemic disease, so patients should be kept quarantined until the swelling of the parotid region completely disappears.

2. Children without parasites in kindergartens and primary schools in an epidemic area can be punctured on the point of Hegu (LI4) with certain prophylactic effect.

INFANTILE ENURESIS

[INTRODUCTION]

Infantile enuresis refers to a condition in which the children above three years of age often have urination during sleeping, but don't notice it until they are awaken. It is also called "bedwetting." TCM holds that this problem may be caused by deficiency of kidney *qi* and deficiency of spleen and lung *qi,* so the treatment principle is to tonify kidney *qi,* regulate and nourish liver and kidney, and warm the lower *jiao.* The points of Ren Meridian, Foot Shaoyin, Hand Taiyin, and Foot Taiyin are selected as the main points, such as Taiyuan (LU9), Guanyuan (CV4), Shenshu (GV23), Sanyinjiao (SP6), Taixi (KI3), Zusanli (ST36) and punctured with reinforcing technique and moxibustion.

[CLINICAL EXPERIENCE]

1. CONVENTIONAL ACUPUNCTURE

(1) Single Point Method

Point: Yongquan (KI1) or Renzhong (GV26).

Technique: Puncture Yongquan (KI1) 0.3 to 0.5 *cun* deep with rotating technique and manipulate it quickly without retention of needle. This method is given once a day, and is indicated for enuresis resulting from deficiency of kidney *yin* and suppression of primary *yang*. Puncture Renzhong (GV26) toward the septum nasi 0.2 to 0.5 *cun* deep with rotating technique, retaining the needle for 30 minutes and manipulating once every 10 minutes. The treatment is given once a day. Renzhong (GV26), a point of Du Meridian, governs *yang* of the whole body, so this method is suitable for enuresis brought about by dysfunction of urinary bladder control.

(2) Foot Puncture (Nocturnal Urination Point)

Point: The midpoint of the transverse crease of the lowest on the sole of the little toe of both sides.

Technique: After routine sterilization, puncture the point by rotating the needle 0.5 *cun* deep. When the tip of the needle touches the bone, twirl the needle with larger amplitude until the child feels severe pain in the foot and distention and also feels hot in the lower abdomen. Retain the needle for 30 minutes, manipulating it once. The treatment is given once a day or once every other day, seven times being considered as one course. This method is good for intractable nocturnal urination.

(3) Puncturing Baihui (GV20) and Sishencong (Extra)

Points: Baihui (GV20) and Sishencong (Extra).

Technique: Puncture Baihui (GV20) and Sishencong (extra) perpendicularly until the tip of needle touches the bone membrane with distention and heaviness. Most cases can be effectively treated by two to three treatments, but some may need up to 30 times.

(4) Combination of Points According to the Promotion of Eight Confluent Point

Point: Lieque (LU7), Zhaohai (KI6), Shenting (GV24) and Benshen (GB13).

Technique: Puncture the four points with reinforcing technique. Needle Shenting (GV24) and Benshen (GB13) transversely along the scalp. Retain the needles for 20 minutes, once a day, five times making up one course. Lieque (LU7) connects with the Ren Meridian, and Zhaohai (KI6) connects with Yinqiao Meridian, so these two points are combined according to the idea of promoting the eight confluent points. Besides, as metal can produce water, Lieque (LU7) is the Luo-connecting point of the Lung Meridian which can tonify kidney qi. Zhaohai (KI6) together with Shenting (GV24) and Benshen (GB13) can strengthen *yang*, suppress *yin*, clear the mind, and build up the brain, and stop the enuresis.

(5) Selecting the Luo-connecting Points of Hand and Foot Shaoyin

Point: Tongli (HT5) and Dazhong (KI4).

Technique: Puncture both points with reinforcing technique and retain the needles for 20 minutes. These two points are effective for cases due to too deep sleep and inability to awaken during the night. It was said in *Statement of Hundreds of Diseases* that for reluctance to speak and sleepiness, use Tongli (HT5) and Dazhong (KI4). The occurrence of enuresis can be caused by deficiency of kidney *qi* and failure of the heart to house the mind, so we may puncture the Luo-connecting points of the heart and kidney in order to tonify the mind.

2. MOXIBUSTION

(1) Non-scarring Moxibustion

Points: Baihui (GV20), Mingmen (GV4), Guanyuan (CV4) and Zhongliao (BL33).

Technique: Use two points every day, applying seven small moxa cones as big as a broad bean on each point. Keep changing the cones when the patient feels burning hot.

(2) Moxibustion with Salt

Point: Shenque (CV8).

Technique: Fill the umbilicus, and the point Shenque (CV8) with fried fine salt level with the umbilicus. Put a moxa cone as big as the broad bean over the point, applying three to seven cones each time.

The treatment is given once every other day, five times forming one course.

3. CUPPING

Point: Guanyuan (CV4) or Zhongji (CV3).

Technique: Apply cupping on one point once a day, and retain the cap for 10 minutes. This method is suitable for children who are afraid of needles.

4. INTRA-DERMAL NEEDLE

Point: ① Changqiang (GV1) and Sanyinjiao (SP6). ② Lieque (LU7) and Sanyinjiao (SP6). ③ Guanyuan (CV4) and Sanyinjiao (SP6). ④ Zhongji (CV3).

Technique: Choose one of the four groups, and embed an intra-dermal needle at 6 pm, fixing them with plaster. The following morning, remove the needle. The treatment is given once a day, five days forming one course.

5. AURICULAR THERAPY

Points: Shenmen, Urethra, Kidney, Urinary Bladder, Sub-cortex, Brain Point and Endocrine.

Technique: Select two or three points and stimulate them with Wangbuliuxing seeds. The child should be told to press the seeds a few times a day, especially before sleeping. This method is suitable for children who are afraid of needles.

6. MEDICINAL APPLICATION ON ACU-POINT

Point: Shenque (CV8).

Technique: Grind Wubeizi 3 g and Heshouwu 3 g together into powder and mix it with vinegar. Apply to the umbilicus, covering it with gauze. This is done before sleeping everyday, and the materials are removed the next morning. It is used three to five times in succession.

7. COMBINED TREATMENT

Points: Baihui (CV20), Neiguan (PC6), Guanyuan (CV4), Zhongji

(CV3) and Taixi (KI3).

Technique: Puncture the points shallowly with reinforcing technique, and apply moxa on Zhongji (CV3) and Guanyuan (CV4) with a moxa box. Retain the needles for 30 minutes, and do moxa for 20 to 30 minutes. This treatment is given once a day. The author has treated enuresis by this method and it is proved always effective. Usually the whole treatment lasted five days.

[REMARKS]

1. It is very effective to treat enuresis by acupuncture, but for the condition caused by organic change, the primary disease should be treated.

2. The recurrence of this disease is very high. After the symptoms are controlled by treatment, one to three more treatments should be carried out to strengthen the therapeutic result.

3. During the treatment, the cooperation of the parents is needed to control the children's water intake, and waken them up at a fixed time so as to cultivate their conscious habit of getting up to urinate. The children should be also encouraged to get rid of any sense of inferiority or shyness.

UNDERDEVELOPMENT OF INFANTILE INTELLIGENCE

[INTRODUCTION]

Underdevelopment of infantile intelligence can be caused by the mother's illness during pregnancy, or heredity factors, or labor injury, or contracting illness in childhood, and is mainly manifested as an intelligence disorder. TCM thinks the problem results from congenital deficiency, leading to weakness of the liver and kidney, and poor nourishment of *qi* and blood; or improper milk feeding after birth, giving rise to general weakness, frequent sickness, and deficiency of

333

essence and marrow. The treatment principle is to tonify the kidney to strengthen the essence, build up the spleen to nourish *qi*. The points of Ren and Du Meridians are used as main points, such as Dazhui (GV14), Jinsuo (GV8), Yaoyangguan (GV3), Fengchi (GB20), Baihui (GV20), Zusanli (ST36), Sanyinjiao (ST36), Hegu (LI4) and Taichong (LR3).

[CLINICAL EXPERIENCE]

1. CONVENTIONAL ACUPUNCTURE

(1) *Method of Tonifying Liver and Kidney*

Points: Main points: Ganshu (GV18), Shenshu (GV23), Taichong (LR3) and Taixi (KI3). Supplementary points: Zusanli (ST36), Sanyinjiao (SP6), Baihui (GV20), Sishencong (Extra), Dazhui (GV14), Lianquan (CV23), Fengchi (GB20), Tianquan (PC2), Hegu (LI4), Neiguan (PC6),Yanglingquan (GB34), Xuanzhong (GB39) and Guanyuan (CV4).

Technique: Puncture the main points every time to tonify the liver and kidney and benefit *yuan*-primary *qi* of the body, and Sanyinjiao (SP6) and Susanli (ST36) to strengthen the spleen and stomach to build up the acquired foundation. Puncture other points according to the condition. Apply reinforcing technique on each point, and immediately take out the needle after the arrival of *qi*. The treatment is given once a day, 30 times making up one course. This method is suitable for five kinds of retardation in children.

(2) *Method of Selecting Points in Group*

Points: ① Renzhong (GV26), Zhigou (TE6), Hegu (LI4), Shuifen (CV9), Yinjiao (CV7), Shuidao (ST28), Zhongji (CV3), Zusanli (ST36) and Sanyinjiao (SP36). ② Fengfu (GV16), Fengchi (GB20), Dazhui (GV16), Mingmen (GV4), Yinmen (BL37), Weizhong (BL40), Chengshan (BL57), Xuanzhong (GB39) and Fuliu (KI7). ③ Tap gently the back Jiaji points with a plum-blossom needle.

Technique: First tap the back Jiaji points (Extra) until the skin turns red, then choose one group of points with quick needling technique, once a day. Among these points, Fengchi (GB20), Fengfu

(GV16) and Renzhong (GV26) are punctured without retention of needle, other points on the limbs with retention of needle. Ten treatments constitute one course with a two-day interval between courses. This method is effective for hydrocephalus.

2. MOXIBUSTION

(1) Moxibustion on the Umbilicus

Points: One point 0.5 *cun* above and the other 0.5 *cun* below the umbilicus.

Technique: Apply three to five moxa cones as big as grain on each point, or mild-warm moxibustion with moxa stick for 10 minutes.

(2) Moxibustion on the Ankle

Points: Two sides of the ankle.

Technique: Apply mild-warm moxibustion with the moxa stick on the medial and lateral aspects of the ankle for 10 minutes respectively. The treatment is given once a day with 10 treatments making up one course. It is used for children with speech retardation.

(3) Moxibustion on the Back-Shu Points

Point: Xinshu (BL15).

Technique: Apply three big moxa cones as big as a date kernel with ginger bilaterally. This is given once a day, with 10 treatments forming one course. The method is indicated for deficiency of heart *qi* and weakness of the tongue root.

3. AURICULAR THERAPY

Point: Kidney, Sub-cortex, Brain Stem, Brain Point, Occiput and Heart.

Technique: Puncture the ear points with reinforcing technique once a day and single technique, 10 times forming one course; or fix Wangbuliuxing seeds on the ear points for three to five days, 10 times being one course.

4. HYDRO-ACUPUNCTURE

Point: ① Yamen (GV15) and Shenshu (BL23). ② Fengchi (GB20) and Zusanli (ST36). ③ Dazhui (GV14) and Neiguan (PC6).

Technique: For simple low intelligence, select these groups in turn; for other complications, such as paralysis, select other points according to the differentiation. Inject acetyl-glutamine 100 mg (one syringe) on the points of head, and compound injection fluid with herbs activating blood circulation (Chinese angelica root injection fluid, safflower injection fluid, the rhizome of chuanxiong injection fluid, codonopsis pilosula injection fluid) on the points of four limbs and trunk with 1 ml on each point. Administer once every other day, 10 times in one course, a 7-10 day interval between courses. This method is indicated for underdevelopment of the brain.

5. CATGUT-EMBEDDING METHOD

Points: Fengchi (GB20), Yamen (GV15), Dazhui (GV14), Taodao (GV13), Xinshu (BL15), Jueyinshu (GV14), Ganshu (BL18), Shenshu (BL23), Mingmen (GV4), Zhishi (BL52), Neiguan (PC6) and Zusanli (ST36).

Technique: Put a piece of catgut thread into the tube needle and inject it into the deep part of the point, using two or three points each time. The selection of points is decided by the real condition of each patient. For speech problems, use Yamen (GV15) and Xinshu (BL15) for emaciation, use Pishu (BL20), Shenshu (BL23) and Zusanli (ST36); for mania, take Neiguan (PC6), Jueyinshu (GV14) and Dazhui (GV14); for low intelligence, use Fengchi (GB20), Mingmen (GV4), Zhishi (BL52) and Taodao (GV13). Apply embedding once every 20-30 days, five times in one course.

6. SCALP ACUPUNCTURE AND BODY ACUPUNCTURE

Points: Main points: Sishencong (extra), Tongli (HT5), Naoqing [2 *cun* above Jiexi (ST40)]. Supplementary points: Hegu (LI4), Neiguan (PC6), Yamen (GV15), Lianquan (CV23), Zusanli (ST36), Sanyinjiao (SP6), Shenshu (BL23), Huantiao (GB30) and Yanglingquan (GB34). Scalp acupuncture: Motor area, speech area and sensory area.

Technique: Puncture Sishencong (Extra) every time, Tongli

(HT5), Naoqingin intermittently; and two to three supplementary points every time. The treatment is given once a day, 10 times in one course, with a three-day interval between courses. There are three methods of needling Sishencong (Extra): ① The needles are punctured respectively from Sishencong (Extra) toward Baihui (GV20); ② The needles are punctured from Baihui (GV20) toward Sishencong (Extra); and ③ The needles are all punctured toward the back on the point Sishencong (Extra). After removing the needles, apply scalp acupuncture with stimulation by frequent rotating of needles manually or with an electric machine, retaining the needle for 20 to 30 minutes.

[REMERKS]

1.   It takes a long time to treat this disease by acupuncture, so it is very necessary to continue the treatment to obtain the full effect.

2.   During the treatment, it is better to combine many kinds of therapies together, such as needling, massage, hydro-acupuncture, catgut-embedding method, and moxibustion.

3.   Speech and physical exercises should be taken at the same time to improve the restoration of brain intelligence.

4.   The prognosis of this problem in children is very bad. The importance is to prevent the occurrence of congenital diseases so as to protect fetus against them during pregnancy, and also try to avoid all kinds of injury.

CHAPTER FOUR
SURGERY

GOITER

[INTRODUCTION]

The disease is commonly located in the neck, manifested as diffuse swelling or masses, no skin discoloration, difficulty in removing masses and no diabrosis, corresponding to goiter, tumor of thyroid and hyperthyroidism in modern medicine. The disease is mostly caused by mutual stagnation of *qi,* phlegm and blood in the neck due to emotional depression, leading to *qi* and blood stagnation and retention of body fluid forming phlegm; or it is caused by invasion of six exogenous pathogenic factors and harmful *qi* from the mountain and river, or not being accustomed to the climate in a new place, resulting in stagnation of *qi* and blood blocking meridians and collaterals. The disease is treated by regulating *qi* circulation to resolve phlegm and removing stagnation to relieve swelling by the points on the Foot and Hand-Shaoyang and Yangming meridians, i.e., Tiantu (CV22), Tianding (LI17), Tianrong (SI17), Hegu (LI4), Shanzhong (CV17) and Zusanli (ST36), which are punctured by even-needling technique.

[CLINICAL EXPERIENCE]

1. CONVENTIONAL ACUPUNCTURE

(1) Interacting Puncturing of Upper and Lower Points

Points: Kunlun (BL60) and Renying (ST9)

Technique: The patient lies in a supine position with the legs extended. The operator stands opposite to the patient, and then punctures

Kunlun (BL60) bilaterally with rotating technique. When *qi* arrives, the needles are twisted with the thumb backward eight times. Reducing technique by rotating the needle is applied on Kunlun (BL60), while pricking is applied on Renying (ST9). The treatment is given once a day and five treatments make up one course. The therapy is given for hyperthyroidism.

(2) Puncturing Extra Point

Points: Pingyingxue (0.7 *cun* lateral to the interspace between C4 and C5), Shangtianzhu [0.5 *cun* above Tianzhu (BL10)], Fengchi (GB20), Jianshi (PC5) and Fuliu (KI7)

Technique: A perpendicular puncture is applied on Pingyingxue and Shangtianznu (Extra points), 0.5 *cun* deep, and a routine puncture on Fengchi (GB20), Jianshi (PC5) and Fuliu (KI7). All the points are punctured with even technique by the lifting, thrusting and rotating methods. The treatment is applied once a day, 10 treatments in a course. In 59 cases of hyperthyroidism that were treated by the therapy, the total effective rate was 92.6%.

(3) Surrounding Needling Method in the Local Area

Point: Tumor region

Technique: Puncture the center of the mass perpendicularly, 1 *cun* deep, penetrating two-thirds of the mass; then insert four to eight needles around the border of the mass according to its size; each needle is inserted transversely to half of the mass. The needles are withdrawn after being stimulated with even technique by the rotating method for 10 to 15 minutes. The treatment is given once every four days and 10 treatments form one course. The effective rate is 96.7%.

(4) Mother-Son Reinforcing and Reducing Method

Points: Jianshi (PC5), Neiguan (PC6), Shenmen (HT7), Sanyinjiao (SP6), Zhaohai (KI6), Taixi (KI6), Fuliu (KI7) and Qiyingxue [corresponding to Shuitu (ST10)].

Technique: Reducing technique, by lifting the needle forcefully and thrusting gently, is applied on Jianshi (PC5), Neiguan (PC6) and Shenmen (HT7); reinforcing technique, by thrusting the needle forcefully and lifting gently, is applied on Sanyinjiao (SP6), Taixi (KI3), Zhaohai (KI6) and Fuliu (KI7). For goiter, triple needling is adopted (one needle is inserted on the point and the other two on the lateral sides of the point). The needles are retained for 30 minutes. The treatment is applied once every other day for two to three months continuously. Clinically, the prescription is determined based on the concrete differentiation of symptoms and the points are combined and stimulated by reinforcing and reducing respectively according to the mother-son relationship of Zangfu organs relating to meridians and collaterals. Excellent therapeutic result is received by this method for hyperthyroidism.

2. CUTTING ROOT METHOD

Points: Feishu (BL13) and Xishu (BL15)

Technique: The epidermis of the point is cut 1 cm long after routine sterilization and local anesthesia, and then the subcutaneous fibrous tissue is pricked by a three-edged needle, 0.3 to 0.5 cm deep. After the point has been pricked for three to four seconds, iodine tincture is applied on the local area, and then the point is dressed by steriled gauze fixed by a plaster. The therapy is applied once every seven to 10 days, and two points are used alternatively in each treatment.

3. LASER THERAPY

Points: Main point: Futu (LI18). Supplementary point: Ermen (TE21) or Jingming (BL1)

Technique: The chief point is selected bilaterally, while the supplementary point is selected bilaterally and alternately in each treatment. The laser radiator 25 mW is applied on the chief point for five to seven minutes, and on the supplementary point for three to five minutes. The treatment is given once a day and 10 treatments form one course. Oryzanol is taken as an auxiliary treatment in some cases. The therapy is given for exophthalmic hyperthroidism.

[REMARKS]

1. For the treatment of simple goiter by acupuncture, iodine preparation is taken simultaneously to strengthen the therapeutic effect.

2.   Surgery should be applied in time for a large goiter associated with pressing sensation that is not suitable to be treated by acupuncture.

BREAST ABSCESS

[INTRODUCTION]

Breast abscess is acute suppurative mastitis in modern medicine. When it occurs in the pregnancy stage, it is called an internal breast abscess; and when it occurs in the lactation phase, it is known as external breast abscess. Most patients are breast-feeding phase women, especially primipara, suffering from the disease three to four weeks after delivery. Redness, swelling, feverish sensation and pain are the main manifestations. The disease is mainly caused by indulgence in greasy and sweet food leading to accumulation of heat in the stomach meridian; or worry, over thinking and anger leading to stagnation of the liver *qi*; or rupture of nipples leading to invasion of pathogenic toxic fire to the breasts blocking meridians and collaterals, resulting in retarded lactation, retention of toxic fire and milk until an abscess is finally forms. The treatment principle is to clear away heat and toxin, smooth liver and stomach *qi* to promote lactation and remove masses. The points are selected from Foot-Jueyin and Foot-Yangming meridians, i.e., Shaoze (SI1), Rugan (ST18), Shanzhong (CV17), Zhangmen (LR13), Qimen (LR14) and Xingjian (LR2), punctured by reducing technique, and needles retained for 20 minutes. The treatment is applied once or twice a day, 10 treatments forming one course.

[CLINICAL EXPERIENCE]

1.   CONVENTIONAL ACUPUNCTURE

(1) Puncturing Lou-Connecting Point
Point: Neiguan (PC6)
Technique: After routine sterilization on the point, insert a fili-

form needle swiftly and rotate, lift and thrust it repeatedly for one or two minutes after the arrival of *qi*. During the needling manipulation, the patient is asked to press the mass gently until the pain is relieved. The needle is manipulated three to five times during the 20-minute retention, and then the needle is removed with the point open. Strong stimulation is applied for severe general symptoms and short duration of illness, and moderate stimulation applied for mild general symptoms or long duration of illness. The treatment is given once or even two to three times a day for severe cases. Ten treatments form one course.

(2) PUNCTURING HE-SEA POINT

Point: Zusanli (ST36)

Technique: Insert a needle, 1.5 to 2 *cun* deep with the tip of the needle slightly to upward. Reducing needling technique with moderate stimulation is applied. During the 30-minute needle retention, it is manipulated once every five minutes. The treatment is given once a day and five times make a course. Xinshu (BL15), Daling (PC7) and Shaoze (SI1) are selected as supplementary points. The method is mostly effective for the early stage of acute breast abscess. But there is no effect for suppurative cases.

(3) *Puncturing Single Point*

Point: Jianjing (GB21)

Technique: Jianjing (GB21) on the contralateral side depending on the localization of the disease is punctured, 0.5 to 0.8 *cun* deep with the patient in a sitting position. Reducing technique with strong stimulation by swift rotation is applied for three to five minutes (10 minutes for severe cases). The treatment is given twice a day, avoiding lifting and thrusting the needle. The therapy is given for acute breast abscess.

(4) *Puncturing Double Points*

Points: Liangqu (ST34) and Taichong (LR3)

Technique: Reducing technique with strong stimulation is applied on both of the points, once a day, retaining the needles for 30 minutes. The therapy is given for acute breast abscess and two to three treatments are required generally.

2. MOXIBUSTION

(1) Indirect Moxibustion with Garlic
Point: The affected area

Technique: A 0.2 to 0.3 cm thick garlic slice (garlic cone is the best) is put on the swelling, and an ignited moxa cone of bean size is put on the garlic. The garlic slice is elevated or moved along the skin when the patient feels it becoming too hot to be tolerated, and then the slice is replaced on the same area after a while. A new garlic slice should be used when the previous one turns yellow. The moxa is given continuously until the local area turns red and lactation is excreted. The therapy was applied in ancient times for breast abscess.

(2) Indirect Moxibustion with Spring Onion
Point: The affected area

Technique: The clean white part of a spring onion in proper dosage is ground into paste that is put on the affected area, about 0.2 cm thick, and then mild moxibustion with a moxa stick is applied for 15 to 30 minutes each time. The treatment is given one to two times a day and three treatments make a course. The therapy is given for the early stage of non-suppurative mastitis with remarkable therapeutic effect.

(3) Steaming Moxibustion
Point: The affected area

Technique: The mixture of small pieces of the white part of a spring onion 500 g and the powder of Pugongying (Herba Taraxaci) 60 g and Yazao 15 g is decocted with a proper amount of water. The decoction is put in a big cup to steam and fumigate the affected area. The treatment is given one to two times a day, with a 30-minute steaming each time, for early stage non-suppurative mastitis.

3. AURICULAR THERAPY

Points: Tragus, Infra-tragic Apex, Ear-Shenmen, Mammary Gland, Liver, Stomach and Chest

Technique: All the points are used in turn in each treatment; two to four points are selected to be stimulated forcefully by reducing technique with short filiform needles. The needles are retained for 20 to 30 minutes and manipulated once every five minutes. The treatment is given one to three times a day and five treatments make up one course.

4. ELECTRIC ACUPUNCTURE

Points: Shanzhong (CV17), Quchi (LI11) or Hegu (LI4)

Technique: Reducing needling technique is applied on each point bilaterally until the patient feels soreness and distention. Then electric stimulation is added for 10 to 15 minutes.

5. BLEEDING METHOD

(1) Pricking According to the Types of Breast Abscess

Points: Upper breast type: Gaohuangshu (BL43), Pohu (BL42) and Fufen (BL41); Middle breast type: Gaohuangshu (BL43), Pohu (BL42) and Shentang (BL44); Lower breast type: Gaohuangshu (BL43), Shentang (BL44) and Yixi (BL45).

Technique: All points are pricked and cupped on the affected side after sterilization and three drops of blood are required on each point. The treatment is given once a day. Dazhui (GV14) and Taodao (GV13) are added for fever. After bleeding, the patient lies on one side with the upper arm flexed and the lower pressed under the body until the hand feels numb, while the local affected area is compressed by a hot towel for 30 minutes. Treatment is given three times a day.

(2) Pricking Affected Area

Points: Quze (PC3) and the affected area

Technique: An amount of 1-3 ml of blood is required on Quze (PC3) and pricking is applied on the local area with a three-edged needle after strict sterilization. The treatment is given once every other day and three treatments form one course. One to three drops of blood are required for patients with weak constitution.

6. WRIST-ANKLE ACUPUNCTURE

Point: No.2 area superior to the affected side (selecting two-finger breadth superior to the middle of the transverse crease of the wrist on the palm side of the left arm for left-side mastitis, or two-finger breadth superior to the middle of the transverse crease of the wrist on the palm side of the right arm for right-side mastitis).

Technique: An angle of 30° is formed between the needle body and skin surface during insertion, and then the needle is placed flat to be inserted 1.4 *cun* with the tip toward the elbow; and the handle of the needle is fixed by a plaster for one to three hours.

7. LASER THERAPY

Points: ① Shanzhong (CV17), Rugen (ST18), Jianjing (GB21), Shaoze (SI1), Ah-shi (the location of swelling and mass) and Zusanli (ST36). ② Shanzhong (CV17), Rugen (ST18), Liangqiu (ST34), Hegu (LI4), Ah-shi and Zusanli (ST36).

Technique: Two groups of points are used alternately in each treatment and each point is radiated for five minutes. The treatment is given twice a day and six treatments make up one course.

8. COMBINED TREATMENT

(1) Moxibustion and Pressing Method

Points: Shanzong (CV17) and Tianzong (SI11)

Technique: Indirect moxibustion with garlic is applied on Shanzhong (CV17), five to seven cones, until the local area turns slightly red. Then, the right thumb pushes while pressing on Tianzong (SI11) on the affected side forcefully for three to five minutes. The treatment is given twice a day.

(2) Puncturing and Massage

Points: Tianzong (SI11) and Ah-shi

Technique: Tianzong (SI11) on the affected side is massaged for two minutes at first; then, one to two Ah-shi points are detected around the inflammation area and the needles are inserted swiftly, then going deeply and slowly, finally being rotated for one to two minutes after the arrival of *qi*. The needles are retained for 10 minutes while gentle massage is given in the local area. After the needle is removed, forceful massage is applied to squeeze the breast along the mammary duct to the nipple to promote lactation. The treatment is applied once a day and three treatments form a course.

(3) Plum-Blossom Needle and Fumigation

Point: The affected area

Technique: After sterilization of the painful and swollen area of the breast, first take the cutaneous needle to tap the local area, and then tap the border of the mass before gradually moving to the center. Keep on tapping until there is slight bleeding. Afterward, fumigation is applied with the following prescription: Pugongying (Herba Taraxaci) 30 to 60 g is cooked with 1,000 to 3,000 ml water in an earthen pot for 10 to 15 minutes. Then the decoction is taken to fumigate and wash the affected area. The treatment is given once a day and three treatments make a course.

[REMARKS]

1. Acupuncture and moxibustion can achieve satisfactory therapeutic effects for acute breast abscess, especially for the early-stage non-suppurative case. Generally the disease is cured after one to three treatments by the methods introduced above. The in-time treatment is especially significant for the disease. For the suppurative case, acupuncture can promote diabrosis naturally, and the disease will be cured quickly after draining of pus.

2. Keep the nipples clean and keep lactation smooth and regular.

3. During weaning period, the feeding time is reduced gradually to prevent for the disease.

HEMORRHOIDS

[INTRODUCTION]

Hemorrhoids refer to small pieces of muscle exposed on the anus internally or externally. Where the growth is inside the anus, it is called internal hemorrhoids; a growth outside the anus is called external hemorrhoids. Where there is growth both inside and outside the anus, it is called mixed hemorrhoids. Clinically, internal hemorrhoids are very common. Piles may lead to swelling, pruritus, exudation and hemorrhage. The disease is commonly seen in adults, because of sitting for a long time, long distance walking while bearing a heavy burden, or improper diet, indulgence in alcohol and spicy food, or persistent diarrhea and delivery leading to sinking of the *qi* in the middle Energizer, or seven emotional stagnation leading to the *qi* failing to disperse. All the factors may cause irregular *qi* and blood circulation of the anus and intestines, stagnation in meridians and production of damp and heat. Finally, hemorrhoids result. The treatment principle is to clear away heat, eliminate damp, activate blood circulation to remove stasis and benefit *qi,* and to elevate the sunken *qi* by the main points from the urinary bladder meridian of foot-Taiyang, i.e., Changqiang (GV1), Huiyang (BL35), Erbai (Ex-UE2), Chengshan (BL57), Baihui (GV20) and Shenque (CV12), punctured by reducing technique.

[CLINICAL EXPERIENCE]

1. Conventional Acupuncture

(1) Puncturing Extra Point

Point: Erbai (Ex-UE2) [one of them is located between Jianshi (PC5) and Ximen (PC4) and the other one is between two tendons and one is on the radial side of the tendon.]

Technique: The point is punctured with reducing technique by lifting the needle three times and thrusting once. The needle is inserted 1 *cun* deep and retained for 20 minutes after the arrival of *qi,* with rotation once every five minutes. The treatment is given once a day and a two-week treatment makes up a course.

(2) Puncturing the Point in the Meridian

Point: Chengshan (BL57)

Technique: Take a 2-*cun* filiform needle (Size: No.26) to puncture the point swiftly about 1.5 *cun* deep, and then rotate the needle forcefully about 350 times to produce the radiation of soreness, distention and numbness to the popliteal fossa, leg and sole or cause local distending pain. The needle is retained for 30 minutes and manipulated once every five minutes.

(3) Combination of the Main and Supplementary Points

Points: Changqiang (GV1), Huiyang (BL35) and Chengshan (BL57)

Technique: All the points are punctured with reducing technique and retained for 15 to 20 minutes. The treatment is given once a day and 10 treatments make up a course. For hemorrhage, Erbai (Ex-UE2) and Sanyinjiao (SP6) are added; for fistula, Mingmen (GV4) and Shenshu (BL23) added; and for proctoptosis due to internal hemorrhoids, Shiqizhui (Ex-B9) and Baihui (GV20) added.

2. MOXIBUSTION

(1) Moxa on the Extra Point
Point: Anus

Technique: Vaseline is put on the anus, and then seven moxa cones in the size of a bean are added. Avoid burning the skin. The treatment is given once a day and the cones are replaced one after another until the burning sensation is present. This is for the early stage of hemorrhoids. It is said in *Classic of Fundamentals of Acupuncture and Moxibustion* that a remarkable effective is achieved by apply seven moxa cones on the anus for shallow piles.

(2) Moxibustion with Moxa Stick
Points: Taodao (GV13) and Yaoshu (GV2)

Technique: Apply 10 to 15 minutes of moxibustion with sticks on the two points until warming occurs, and then move the stick to descend along the Governor Vessel to the anus. A tense sensation in the anus indicates the best result. The treatment is given once a day and ten treatments make a course.

3. ELECTRIC ACUPUNCTURE

Points: Zhishu (Extra) [located 1 *cun* lateral to Mingmen (GV4)], Huiyang (BL35), Changqiang (GV1) and Chengshan (BL57). For hematochezia, Erbai (Ex-UE2) is added; and for prolapse of rectum, Qihai (CV6) and Shenshu (BL23) are added.

Technique: In each treatment, two to three points are selected with slightly forceful stimulation generally. For hematochezia, the stimulation is relatively mild on Erbai (Ex-UE2) or Chengshan (BL57). A certain intensity of electricity, determined by the patient's tolerance, is applied on each point for five minutes after the arrival of *qi*. The treatment is given once every two days and five treatments form one course.

4.   HOT-RED NEEDLING

Points: Changqiang (GV1) and Chengshan (BL57)

Technique: A prone position is adopted. Heat a 1.5-*cun* needle (Size: No.28) until the tip turns red, and then insert swiftly on Changqiang (GV1), 0.5 to 1 *cun* deep, rotating quickly for three to five seconds. Finally, remove the needle. The needle is inserted obliquely at an angle of 45° on Chengshan (BL57), 0.5 to 0.8 *cun* deep, with the tip upward, and is rotated continuously for three to five minutes. If the case is not cured by one treatment, another may be carried out three to five days later. The method is effective for internal and external hemorrhoids. Needling may remove swelling and pain quickly and the symptoms will be relieved after two days and disappear shortly afterward. Most cases are cured after no more than two treatments.

5.   PRICKING METHOD

(1) Pricking the Points on Meridians

Points: First select Xialiao (BL34), then Zhongliao (BL33)

Technique: After giving local anesthesia with 2% procaine 0.2 to 0.5 ml, take a three-edged needle to prick the subcutaneous fat on the point, 0.5 cm long, crossing the meridian to find a white, fiber-like object. Then sterilize the local area with 2% iodine tincture and compress. Simultaneously, a quick needling technique is applied on Changqiang (GV1) without needle retention. A second course of treatment follows seven days later.

(2) Pricking Reflecting Points

Points: The purplish or pink spots for T7 to the sacrum, those located on the lumbar-sacral region, close to Governor Vessel, may obtain better therapeutic effects.

Technique: Take a thick needle to prick the skin longitudinally, and then going deep to break the white fiber-like object. The treatment is given once a week and three or four treatments are required.

(3) Pricking Back-Shu Point

Point: Dachangshu (BL25)

Technique: Take a three-edged needle to prick Dachangshu (BL25) from the superficial to the deep to expose a white, fiber-like object; and dress the local area with a plaster. In each treatment, one point on one side is pricked, and the same is applied on the other side three to five days later. The method is effective for hematochezia due to internal hemorrhoids, since Dachangshu (BL25) is the Back-Shu point of the larger intestine, so that pricking on the point can promote the circulation of *qi* and blood there.

6. CUTTING METHOD ON ACU-POINT

Point: Yingjiao (CV7)

Technique: Turn the upper lip by the thumb and index finger of either hand to find folliculi and small white pimples in different shapes and sizes on the frenum. After sterilizing with merbromin, take small hemostatic forceps to fix the folliculi or small white pimples, then cut or remove them with a pair of small scissors or a small surgical knife to obtain a small amount of blood. The method once was applied to treat 100 cases of hemorrhoids, of which 64 cases were cured, 24 cases obtained remarkable effect, 10 cases were effective and there was no effect in only two cases.

7. MEDICINAL APPLICATION ON ACU-POINTS

Points: Baliao (BL3, one to three)

Technique: Firstly, tap the points with a seven-star needle to cause local congestion; then, put the powder of Dinggui on the points and cover them with plasters containing musk and tiger bone. After that, surrounding or sparrow-pecking moxibustion with a stick is applied above the plasters. The treatment is given once every other day and each treatment lasts 10 to 15 minutes.

[REMARKS]

1. Acupuncture and moxibustion help deal with inflammation, and stop the pain and bleeding, and is especially suitable for the inflammation period. Surgery is considered for the complete removal of hemorrhoids.

2. Pay attention to eating more fresh vegetables and fruits to keep a smooth bowel movement, do physical exercise and avoid anything irritable, like spicy foods, tobacco and alcohol.

3. Pay attention to anal hygiene. A hot water sitting bath is required every evening before retiring.

TETANUS

[INTRODUCTION]

The disease is characterized by opisthotonus and muscular spasm due to traumatic injury by pricking of a knife or bamboo leading to toxic pathogens attacking meridians and collaterals and further disturbing the whole body along the running courses of meridians and collaterals. Generally, the symptoms appear after a incubation period of two to 15 days after injury. At first, there is an aversion to cold, with fever and headache, gradually developing to lockjaw, inability to eat, forced smile, muscle stiffness of the nape and back, convulsion of the limbs; finally, there are general muscular spasms, opisthotonus, spasm attacking once every several minutes or several hours induced by outside irritants such as sound, light and vibration. The treatment principle is to clear away heat to eliminate toxin, deal with the spasms and expel wind, using the points on the Hand and Foot Taiyang, Yangming meridians and Governor Vessel, puncturing with reducing technique. Generally, the needles are retained for several hours, or even 24 to 48 hours depending on the condition of case. The points include Dazhui (GV14), Fengfu (GV16), Jinshuo (GV8), Yaoyangguan (GV3), Xiaguan (ST7), Jiache (ST6), Quchi (LI11), Kunlun (BL60), Taichong (LR3) and Shenmai (BL620).

[CLINICAL EXPERIENCE]

1. CONVENTIONAL ACUPUNCTURE

(1) Puncturing the Points Mainly on Governor Vessel

Points: Baihui (GV20), Fengfu (GV16), Dazhui (GV14), Shenzhu

(GV12), Zhiyang (GV9), Jinsuo (GV8), Yaoyangguan (GV3), Renzhong (GV26), Houxi (SI3), Weizhong (BL40), Fenglong (ST40), Sanjian (LI3) and Yanglingquan (GB34).

Technique: During spasms, all the points are stimulated forcefully without retaining the needles, twice a day or more depending on the condition. During the spasm relieving condition, the needles are retained for several hours, or 24 to 48 hours if it is necessary. After the needles removed, the subcutaneous needling method is applied on the key points, and retained for several hours or several days. For lockjaw, Jiache (ST6) and Hegu (LI4) are added; for convulsion of the four limbs, Shousanli (LI10) and Zusanli (ST36) are added; for dyspnoea, Chize (LU5), Tiantu (CV22), Sanzhong (CV17) and Neiguan (PC6) are added; and for retention of urine, Zhongji (CV3) and Ququan (LR8) are added. The therapy is applied for the early stage of tetanus.

(2) Puncturing the Points Mainly on Yangming and Shaoyang Meridians

Points: Dazhui (GV14), Shenzhu (GV12), Fengchi (GB20), Binao (LI14), Quchi (LI11), Hegu (LI4), Liangqu (ST34), Zusanli (ST36), Fenglong (ST40), Yanglingquan (GB34) and Taichong (LR3).

Technique: Even needling technique is applied after the arrival of *qi* and the needles are retained for 30 to 60 minutes. The treatment is given once a day and ten treatments make a course. The treatment is continuous after a three-day rest until the symptoms disappear. In each treatment, three to four points are selected for the sequelae of tetanus. For insufficiency of the anti-pathogenic *qi,* Guanyuan (CV4) and Qihai (CV6) are added.

(3) Puncturing Four-gate Points

Points: The four-gate points including Hegu (LI4) and Taichong (LR3) bilaterally, Baihui (GV20) and Yintang (Ex-HN3).

Technique: Reducing technique with forceful stimulation is applied on each point by rotating the needle for one to three minutes before removal. Clinically, the patients in the early stage of the disease suffer from constant spasm or sudden attack of spasms several days later. This technique may stop the spasms immediately or gradually.

2. MOXIBUSTION

Points: Rangu (KI2) and Shenque (CV8)

Technique: Mild moxibustion with stick is applied on each point for 10 minutes, once or twice a day, and is suitable for tetanus in a newborn baby (tetanus neonatorium).

3. MEDICINAL APPLICATION ON ACU-POINTS

Point: Shenque (CV8)

Technique: A fine powder mixed by Kufan (Alumen Exsiccatum) and Pengsha (Borax) 8 g for each, Zhusha (Cinnabaris) 2 g, Bingpian (Borneolum) 0.2 g and Yuancun 0.2 g is prepared. In each treatment, 2 g of the powder is put on the point and covered with gauze and fixed by plaster. The treatment is given once a day.

[REMARKS]

1. Since the disease is mainly manifested as the symptoms of Governor Vessel and three Yang meridians of Hand and Foot, the points are selected from the Governor Vessel and Yang meridians, i.e., Fengfu (GV16), Dazhui (GV14) and Houxi (SI3) for dispelling wind, calming down the mind and dealing with spasms; Baihui (GV20), Renzhong (GV26) and Neiguan (PC6) for regaining consciousness and relaxing the chest in an emergency; Hegu (LI4), Shousanli (LI10) and Zusanli (ST36) for clearing away heat from Yangming, Chengshan (BL57) and Rangu (KI2) for stopping spasms and convulsions; and Yanglingquan (GB34), the influence point of the tendons, for reducing wind and heat and strengthening tendons and bones.

2. More points are selected in the early stage by reducing technique and without retaining the needles during the spasms, and the needles are retained for 24 to 48 hours in the intermittent stage. In order to prevent re-occurrence of the spasms, the embedding needle method is applied on the key points.

3. For sequelae, less points are selected and stimulated with even technique. Patients should closely cooperate with doctors by keeping up the treatment.

TENNIS ELBOW

[INTRODUCTION]

Tennis elbow refers to aseptic inflammation of external humeral epicondyle, the head of radius and synovial bursa of humeroradial articulation. It is also called external humeral epicondylitis and humeroradial bursitis, but is known as "elbow pain" in TCM. The disease is caused by repeated twisting and traction movement of the forearms leading to the injury of *qi* and blood, lack of nourishment of the tendons and vessels. Because of persistent sickness and invasion of wind and cold, *qi* and blood in the elbow region becomes stagnated and blocks the circulation in the meridians. As a result, spasmodic pain in the elbow region occurs. The treatment principle is to disperse wind, warm *yang* and promote the circulation of *qi* and blood in the meridians and collaterals to stop pain by the points mainly on the Hand-Yangming meridian and Ah-shi points, i.e., Quchi (LI11), Shousanli (LI10), Hegu (LI4), Waiguan (TE5) and Ah-shi points. They are commonly punctured with even-needling technique associated with moxibustion.

[CLINICAL EXPERIENCE]

1. CONVENTIONAL ACUPUNCTURE

(1) Multi-direction Penetrating Puncturing
Points: Tender points
Technique: First, puncture the point perpendicularly to get the needling sensation, and then puncture to three directions (Hegu Needling, Chicken-claw Needling) by the reducing technique with strong stimulation. In each treatment, the needles are retained for 20 minutes. The treatment is given once a day, 10 treatments making up one course. Shousanli (LI10) and Hegu (LI4) are punctured in supplementation.

(2) Local Puncturing.
Points: The depression on the anterior border of the external hu-

meral epicondyle, and the depression on the posterior border of the external humeral epicondyle. For limited pronation of the forearm, Shousanli (LI10) is added; and for limited supination, Chize (LU5) is added.

Technique: Perpendicular (90°) and oblique (45°) puncturing is applied on the depressions of the anterior and posterior borders of the external humeral epicondyle respectively. Reducing technique with strong stimulation is applied for the patient with a strong constitution, and even-needling technique for those of a weak constitution. The needles are retained for 30 minutes and manipulated once every five minutes. The treatment is given once a day and 10 treatments form one course.

2. MOXIBUSTION

(1) Moxibustion with Sulfur
Points: Ah-shi points

Technique: A sitting position is selected, and crystal granules of sulfur in different sizes are put on the Ah-shi points depending on pain area, ignited and extinguished swiftly, avoiding burning that will cause blisters. The stimulation is determined by whether the patient feels any stabbing pain or not. Generally, the treatment is given once, but, if the case is not cured, another treatment is applied three days later. Avoid water in the local area on treatment day.

(2) Moxibustion with Herbal Paste
Points: Ah-shi points

Technique: Grind Baifuzi (Rhizoma Typhonii), Shenchuanwu (Radix Aconiti), Ruxiang (Resina Olibani), Xixin (Herba Asari) and Muoyao (Myrrha), 3 g each, into powder, mixing with yellow wine to create a herbal paste, 3 cm in diameter and 1 cm thick. Then, dozens of holes are pricked in the paste, which is put on the Ah-shi point and a moxa cone as big as a soybean is placed on top. Moxibustion lasts for 20 minutes. If the patient feels burning, a certain amount of medicinal cotton wool is put between the paste and the point to ensure the treatment can continue to the end. The treatment result is better if blisters are present in the point area. The blisters are pricked and sterilized with gentian violet, and a scab develops in four to five days.

3. AURICULAR THERAPY

Points: The corresponding sensitive points, Sub-cortex, Ear-Shenmen, Adrenal and Elbow

Technique: Reducing technique is applied with a filiform needle every day. The needles are retained for 30 minutes and manipulated several times intermittently. Ten treatments make up one course. Seed-pressing technique may also be given.

4. SUBCUTANEOUS NEEDLING TECHNIQUE

Points: Tender points

Technique: First, Hegu puncture is given with a filiform needle, the needle being removed after the arrival of *qi*. Secondly, a subcutaneous needle is embedded beneath the skin and the free movement of the joint is required. Generally, the subcutaneous needle is replaced once every three to five days.

5. HOT-RED NEEDLING

Points: The affected area

Technique: Insert a two-*cun* needle (Size: No.26) with a hot-red top swiftly right on the sterilized Ah-shi point and remove after the arrival of *qi*. Strict sterilization is applied in the local area after the treatment. Generally, the treatment is given once every other day or twice a week, and four treatments make one course.

6. ELECTRIC ACUPUNCTURE

Points: Ah-shi points, Quchi (LI11), Shousanli (LI10), Zhouliao (LI12), Tianjing (TE10) and Chize (LU5)

Technique: In each treatment, three to four points are selected and stimulated with electricity for 15 to 20 minutes after the arrival of *qi* by the filiform needles. The treatment is given once a day and 10 days make up a course.

7. CHINESE MASSAGE

Technique: The thumb of one hand is used to press the tender point on the lateral side of the elbow and the remaining fingers hold the medial side. The other hand holds the wrist. Elbow flexing and supination with traction are performed several times and during flexing, the tender area is pressed and kneaded repeatedly by the thumb and simultaneously the small head of the radial is pressed. The technique is called pressing-kneading with elbow flexing and taken as an auxiliary method after acupuncture.

8. LASER THERAPY

Points: Ah-shi points, Shousanli (LI10), Tianjing (TE10) and Chize (LU5)

Technique: Each point is radiated for 10 minutes with He-Ne laser, 25 mw. The treatment is given once a day, five treatments forming one course.

9. COMBINED TREATMENT

(1) Acupuncture and Moxibustion

Points: Quchi (LI11), Waiguan (TE5) and Ah-shi points

Technique: Reducing technique by the lifting, thrusting and rotating method is applied on Quchi (LI11)˙and Waiguan (TE5) and the needles are retained for 20 minutes after the arrival of *qi*. Moxibustion with a moxa cone as big as a half date stone is applied on the affected area (Ah-shi point) isolated with Vaseline or vegetable oil. Five to seven moxa cones are applied in each treatment until the skin turns to slightly red. The treatment is given once a day and seven treatments make up a course.

(2) Plum-blossom Needle and Moxibustion

Points: The affected area

Technique: Pressing and kneading by the thumb is applied on the affected area or the nearby points, i.e., Shousanli (LI10), Quchi (LI11), Chize (LU5) and Tianjing (TE10) to cause soreness and distention. After that, tapping with a plum-blossom needle is applied on the affected area to cause slight bleeding, and then surrounding moxibustion with moxa stick is given on the local area for 10 to 20 minutes after the blood has been wiped away. The treatment is given once a day.

[REMARKS]

1.   Certain therapeutic results can be obtained by acupuncture and moxibustion.

2.   During the treatment, it is required to rest the affected limb.

3.   Chinese massage or surgical treatment is applied if adhesion is present.

SCROFULA

[INTRODUCTION]

The disease is a chronic infectious disorder of the lymph node in the neck region and named because of beads of tuberculosis. The disease is commonly seen in children or young people, located in the neck or back of the ear and it happens slowly, with soybean-like tuberculosis, no discoloration and pain in the early stage. Gradually, it develops in a beading shape and the skin turns deep red after the formation of abscesses. Clear pus with a cotton-like substance is seen running after ulceration. The ulceration happens intermittently and a sinus is formed at the end, which is called cervical lymphoid tuberculosis in modern medicine. The disease is caused by stagnation of the liver *qi,* obstruction of *qi* activity, dysfunction of the spleen in transportation and transformation and combination of phlegm and *qi,* or caused by *yin* deficiency of the lung and kidney producing deficiency fire in the interior, phlegm-fire stagnated in the neck. The treatment principle is to smooth the liver *qi,* nourish blood, tonify the spleen to resolve phlegm and detoxification to drain the pus. The points are mainly selected from the liver and spleen meridians, i.e., Ganshu (BL18), Geshu (BL17), Pishu (BL20), Sanyinjiao (SP6), Xuehai (SP10) and Taichong (LR3). Even-needling technique and moxibustion are applied.

[CLINICAL EXPERIENCE]

1. CONVENTIONAL ACUPUNCTURE

(1) Penetrating Needling Technique

Points: Quchi (LI11) penetrating to Binao (LI14)

Technique: Before needling, rub the skin and muscle along the meridian from Quchi (LI11) to Binao (LI14), while holding the forearm. After routine sterilization, a six-*cun* filiform needle (Size: No.30) is inserted at an angle of 45° on Quchi (LI11), 0.5 to 1.0 cm deep. The needle is then moved slowly beneath the skin to penetrate to Binao (LI14) subcutaneously. During the 30-minute retention, the needle is rotated and the handle is scraped once respectively. Then the needle is withdrawn slowly. The treatment is given once a day and 12 treatments form one course. The therapy is given for lymphoid tuberculosis in the neck, axillary fossa, super-clavicular fossa, groin and mesentery. The effective rate is more than 96%.

(2) Coordination of Main and Supplementary Points

Points: Jianjing (GB21), Quchi (LI11), Tianjing (TE10), Sanyangluo (TE8) and Yinlingquan (GB34)

Technique: Even needling technique is applied on all the points and the needles are retained for 30 minutes. The treatment is given once a day and 10 treatments make a course.

2. MOXIBUSTION

(1) Scaring Moxibustion

Point: Scrofula points [taking the distance from the end of either right or left hand to the transverse cubital crease as the standard length to measure from Changqiang (GV1) upward along the center of the spine, then taking the terminal as the middle point to draw a transverse line as breadth as the width of the mouth. The two ends of the transverse line are taken as scrofula points].

Technique: Vaseline or tea oil is put on the points bilaterally, and then a moxa cone in the size of a soybean is applied on the point and is ignited until there is no smoke (local anesthesia by procaine of a certain dosage is given before moxibustion for children). After each moxibustion, boric acid is used to prevent infection. The second treatment is applied two months later. Generally, a moxa cone is put either on the inferior or the superior border of the point. In 139 cases of scrofula that once were treated by such method, 97 cases were cured, 28 cases improved and 14 cases saw no effect (no improvement after four treatments continuously).

(2) Non-Scaring Moxibustion

Points: Bailao, located 2 *cun* above Dazhui (GV14) and about 1 *cun* lateral, Tianjing (TE10), the end of the elbow and the local of scrofula

Technique: All the points are selected in turn and direct moxibustion with five to seven small cones is required on each point. Indirect moxibustion with garlic is applied on the affected area. For scrofula on the neck, Yifeng (TE17), Zulinqi (GB41), Binao (LI14) and Shousanli (LI10) are added and for scrofula on the axillary fossa, Jianjing (GB21) and Shaohai (HT3) are added. The treatment is given once a day and 10 treatments make up a course.

(3) Moxibustion with Moxa Stick

Point: Tianjing (TE10) or Zhoujian (Ex-UE1)

Technique: Keep on moxibustion on one point until a warm sensation is distributed from the end of the elbow, and from the upper arm to the shoulder and neck, everyday. Each treatment lasts about 10 to 15 minutes, and 10 treatments make up one course.

3. HOT-RED NEEDLING

Point: The local area of scrofula

Technique: After routine sterilization in the local area, the hard mass is fixed by the index finger and thumb of the left hand, then a hot-red needle is inserted on the center of the hard mass firstly and pricked three to four times around the mass, using two-thirds of the needle. For draining pus by the hot-red needle, gentle squeezing and pressing are applied after pricking. The wound is dressed with sterilized gauze afterwards. The method is suitable for illness of long duration, delayed removal of the tuberculosis or hard mass after treatment and an almost ulcerated abscess. Supplementary puncturing with the hot-red needle on Jianjing (GB21), Tianjing (TE10) and Shousanli (LI10) may also be carried out.

4. POINT CUTTING THERAPY

Points: Geshu (BL17), Ganshu (BL18), Feishu (BL13) and Jiuwei (CV15)

Technique: In each treatment, a pair of points are selected. After routine sterilization and local anesthesia, the skin and subcutaneous tissue are cut, one to two cm, to get few particles of fat until the patient feels soreness, numbness, distension and pain. No suture or dressing is applied after cutting. Generally, the treatment is given once every 15 days and two to six treatments make up one course.

[REMARKS]

1. In the early stage of acute scrofula, cold and heat are transmitted with each other, manifested as stiffness and pain of the neck, hard tuberculosis in the local area. For such cases, acupuncture and moxibustion are applied to cause dispersal. For cases of ulceration, Chinese herbs and Western drugs or surgical measures are used in combination. For suppurative scrofula, strict sterilization is required in the local area during acupuncture and moxibustion treatment to prevent super-infection.

2. Scrofula is a kind of chronic consumptive disease, so it is difficult to eliminate. Patience is required in keeping up the treatment. Generally, the effect is obtained after one to two courses of treatment. The curing of the disease depends on the severity of the case.

3. Light food is required for the patient during the treatment.

ACUTE INTESTINAL OBSTRUCTION

[INTRODUCTION]

Acute intestinal obstruction is manifested as distention, pain, vomiting and obstruction, mainly caused by obstruction of *qi* and blood, retention of cold and heat, accumulation of food and parasites, resulting in obstruction of transmission of stomach and separation of the upper from the lower. The treatment principle is to remove the retention, harmonize the stomach to stop vomiting and promote *qi* circulation in the intestines. The points are mainly selected from Foot-Yangming meridian, i.e., Shangjuxu (ST37), Xiajuxu (ST39), Guanyuan (CV4), Tianshu (ST25), Dachangshu (BL25), Neiguan (PC6) and Zusanli (ST36), stimulated by reducing needling technique.

[CLINICAL EXPERIENCE]

1. CONVENTIONAL ACUPUNCTURE

(1) Combination of Front-Mu and Back-Shu Points

Points: Main points: Tianshu (ST25), Dashangshu (BL25), Zusanli (ST36) and Ah-shi points. Supplementary points: Fujie (SP14), Guanyuan (CV4) and Daheng (SP15).

Technique: Strong stimulation is given until the presence of soreness and distention is felt after rotating the needle. During 30 to 60 minutes of retention, the needle is rotated once every five to 10 minutes depending on the case. By half-day observation after the pain has been relieved and there is no recurrence, anti-Ascaris of sufficient dosage is applied. The method is indicated in Ascaris intestinal obstruction. Fifteen cases were once treated by the method and pain in all the cases was removed and the remaining symptoms relieved. Among the 15 cases, one third were previously treated with acupuncture and moxibustion without effect. After being treated by the combination of Front-Mu and Back-Shu points, the pain stopped quickly and the symptoms were relieved. It is now thought that the combination of Front-Mu and Back-Shu points is effective for the treatment of the disease.

(2) Multiple-Needling Technique on Inferior He-Sea Points

Points: Shangjuxu (ST37), Xiajuxu (ST39) and Zusanli (ST36)

Technique: First, needle Zusanli (ST36) bilaterally, then needle Shangjuxu (ST37) and Xiajuxu (ST39) respectively. The needles are retained for an hour after the arrival of *qi*. Strong stimulation is applied by lifting, thrusting and rotating needles on the three points bilaterally in turn. Generally, pain and vomiting will stop after needling. Since Shangjuxu (ST37), Xiajuxu (ST39) and Zusanli (ST36) are located below the knee joint in a line, the technique is called the rowing-needling method. Stimulating several points on the same meridian can not only increase the treatment range in the local area, but also strengthen the regulating function of the internal organs and change the pathogenic reaction so as to remove intestinal obstruction by constant stimulation reaction and sensation transmission along the meridian.

(3) Single Needling Method

Point: Daheng (SP15)

Technique: Strong stimulation is applied on the point after the needle is inserted 4 *cun* deep without retention. Generally, the treatment is given twice a day. It is reported that this method can relieve acute intestinal obstruction in 24 to 48 hours after needling.

2.   INDIRECT MOXIBUSTION WITH GINGER

Point: Shenque (CV8)

Technique: A slice of ginger 0.1 cm thick is put on the point along with a moxa cone in the size of a Chinese date made of moxa wool mixed with Bingpian (Borneolum). In each treatment, three moxa cones (about 15 to 25 minutes) are required and moxibustion is applied three times a day.

3.   ELECTRIC ACUPUNCTURE

Combination of the Upper and Lower Points

Points: Tianshu (ST25) and Zusanli (ST36)

Technique: The method is suitable for adhesive ileus by applying Chinese herbs in combination. Generally, before the purgative is taken, Zusanli (ST36) is punctured and the needle retained for 10 minutes to prevent vomiting due to upward reverse of the stomach *qi*. One hour after taking the herbs, electric stimulation is applied on Tianshu (ST25) (negative electrode) and Zusanli (ST36) (positive electrode) with dense-sparse wave and the needles are retained for 30 minutes.

4. MEDICINAL APPLICATION ON ACU-POINTS

(1) Application with Spring Onion

Points: The local area

Technique: Small pieces of spring onions, 500 g, are stirred until they become hot, and then wrapped onto the abdomen, avoiding extreme heat. The spring onions are stirred once again when they get cold. The treatment continues until the symptoms are relieved.

(2) Application with Wuzhuyu (Fructus Euodiae)

Point: Shenque (CV8)

Technique: Coarse table salt 50 g and Wuzhuyu (Fructus Euodiae) 100 g are stirred together until they become hot. Then wrap the mixture onto Shenque (CV8) to allow the heat to penetrate the abdominal wall. The treatment is applied several times a day.

Note: The above-mentioned two methods are given for the early stage of abdominal distention, volvulus of the bowel with no signs of peritoneal irritation, intestinal adhesion and Ascaris intestinal obstruction.

5. AURICULAR THERAPY

Points: Ear-Shenmen, Large Intestine, Stomach, Small Intestine and Abdomen

Technique: When spasmodic abdominal pain occurs, the points are punctured with strong stimulation. During 30 to 60 minutes of retention, the needles are manipulated once every 10 minutes. The treatment is given once every four to six hours for pain and gastric-intestinal spasm relief.

[REMARKS]

1. Acupuncture and moxibustion can receive a certain effect for the disease. If there is no improvement within six to 24 hours of close observation, surgery should be considered.

2. Acupuncture and moxibustion can receive a better effect for stopping pain of dynamic obstruction and the effect lasts for a longer time. A certain therapeutic effect is also received for mechanical intestinal obstruction, but the effect can not be maintained for a longer time.

ACUTE APPENDICITIS

[INTRODUCTION]

Acute appendicitis is manifested as pain in Epigastrium or around the umbilicus in the early stage, then moving to the lower abdomen on the right side. The pain is characterized by being aggravated by pressure with a fixed location, a slight spasm in the abdomen, and difficulty in extending the right leg, fever and aversion to cold. The disease is mainly caused by irregular food intake, overeating and drinking, indulgence in greasy and cold food which injure the intestines and stomach, resulting in retention of damp and heat in the interior; or it is caused by violent movement after meal leading to dysfunction of the intestines in transportation and transmission and stagnation of *qi* and blood. Finally, an abscess is formed due to heat transmission in the intestines, stagnation and obstruction of *qi,* blood and phlegm. The treatment principle is to promote *qi* circulation of the Fu organ, and clear away stagnated heat. The points are mainly selected from Hand and Foot-Yangming meridians, i.e., Zusanli (ST36), Lanwei (Ex-LE7), Shangjuxu (ST37) and Quchi (LI11), stimulated with reducing technique. Generally, the treatment is given once or twice a day or once every four hours for severe case.

[CLINICAL EXPERIENCE]

1. CONVENTIONAL ACUPUNCTURE

(1) Needling Double Points

Points: Zusanli (ST36), Shangjuxu (ST37) or Lanwei (Ex-LE7)

Technique: Reducing technique with strong stimulation is applied on both points and the needles are retained for one hour. According to the severity of the case, the treatment is given one to three times a day until the complete disappearance of the pressing pain. For fever above 38°, Quchi (LI11) is added; and for abdominal distention, Dachangshu (BL25) and Ciliao (BL32) are added. A total of 590 cases of appendicitis were treated, among which, 356 cases were cured, 162 improved and 72 saw no effect. The total effective rate was 87.8%

(2) Puncturing Extra Points

Points: Xisi, bilaterally (located in 4 *cun* above the lateral border of the patella on the right side with the knee flexion in supine), Daheng (SP15), bilaterally.

Technique: To insert the needle perpendicularly on Xisi (Extra) swiftly and the depth of insertion is determined by *qi* arrival. The heavy reducing technique is applied to conduct the needle sensations to the leg, through groin, transmitting to the lower abdomen. Daheng (SP15) is punctured obliquely and bilaterally toward the groin to conduct the needling sensation to the groin. As a result, the needling sensations on the bilateral sides may connect with each other to obviously reduce or disappear abdominal tension. During 30-minute needle retaining after the arrival of *qi*, the needles are rotated once every 10 minutes.

(3) Puncturing the Reflection Area of the Small Intestine

Point: The reflection area of the small intestine (bilateral sides between ala nasi and zygoma) on the face. Before the treatment, the most sensitive point is detected by the meridian and collateral detector to determine the location of the reflection area of the small intestine.

Technique: 1. Oblique puncturing method: Insert the needle on the medial one third of the ala nasi groove and at an angle of 25° formed between the needle and the nasal longitudinal groove (GV 26), 0.2 to 0.3 cm deep. The arrival of *qi* is determined by local soreness, numbness and distention. Even-needling technique is applicable. 2. Perpendicular puncturing method: An angle of 90° is formed between the needle and nasal longitudinal axis when inserting the needle, about 0.1 cm deep. The same needling sensations are required. After the application of the needling technique, the needle is fixed with sterilized cotton and plaster and generally retained for 12 hours (12 to 24 hours in a few cases) and a good therapeutic result can be expected. The treatment is given once a day.

2. MOXIBUSTION

(1) Mild Moxibustion with Moxa Stick

Point: Qihai (CV6)

Technique: Mild moxibustion with the moxa stick is applied for 30 minutes once a day. Two or three daily treatments may be required in severe cases. A total of 40 cases of appendicitis were once treated by this method, with 38 cases cured and two showing no effect. Generally, the temperature is reduced in two to three treatments and the symptoms are reduced or disappear.

(2) Direct Moxibustion with Moxa Cone

Points: Dadun (LR1), bilaterally and the tender points on the right abdomen (McMurray point)

Technique: Direct moxibustion with moxa cones in the size of a piece of wheat is applied on Dadun (LR1) bilaterally. The cones are replaced one after another swiftly until a burning pain is felt and the treatment stops until the skin turns red. However, blistering should be avoided. Generally, five cones are required on each point. Mild surrounding moxibustion with the stick is applied around the tender point on the right abdomen (McMurray point), about 3 cm large, for about 20 to 30 minutes each time until the skin turns to red and strong heat sensation is felt while the heat is distributed to the muscle intermittently. Again, blistering should be avoided. In each treatment, moxibustion is given one to two times. In addition, a decoction of Juhua (Flos Chrysanthemi) or Jinyinhua (Flos Lonicerae) is applicable as tea in combination.

(3) Moxibustion on Zhoujian (Ex-UE1) Bilaterally

Points: Zhoujian (Ex-UE1) bilaterally

Technique: Surrounding moxibustion with moxa sticks is applied on Zhoujian (Ex-UE1) bilaterally for 30 to 60 minutes. This method is from *Moxibustion for Emergency*, which recorded that, "Sun Simiao said that intestinal abscesses were cured by swift moxibustion on Zhouliao (Ex-UE1) bilaterally with a hundred moxa cones in the size of a green bean, to cause defecation with blood and pus."

Note: Appendicitis is the interior heat syndromes of excess. Why is moxibustion effective? The writer views that since appendicitis is mainly caused by accumulation of stagnated blood, the treating principle is to dispel mass by the warming method and activate blood circulation to remove blood stasis. Moxibustion can produce warmth to remove stagnation, further regulate *qi* and blood circulation and strengthen anti-pathogenic *qi* to eliminate pathogenic factors.

3. PRICKING AND CUPPING

Points: ① Dazhui (GV14) and Pishu (BL20). ② Shenzhu (GV12) and Dachangshu (BL25). ③ Guanyuan (CV4), Qihai (CV6), Tianshu (ST25) and Ah-shi points.

Technique: In each treatment, one of the three groups' points is applied and the treatment is given one to three times daily. Firstly, prick the selected points, three seconds for each, with a three-edged needle, and then cup the points to cause bleeding. The cups are retained for 10 minutes.

4. AURICULAR THERAPY

Points: Tender point detected on either of Large or Small Intestines Area and Lanwei (Ex-LE7).

Technique: Strong stimulation is applied on both of the points and needles are retained for one to two hours. The treatment is given one to four times a day. Generally, after needling, pain in the lower abdomen on the right stops immediately or is reduced obviously. But it will take two to three days to relieve the pressing and rebounding pain gradually. A total of 25 cases were treated by this method, 21 being cured, with three more effective and one ineffective.

5. ELECTRIC ACUPUNCTURE

Points: Lanwei (Ex-LE7) bilaterally. Supplementary points: Tianshu (ST25) on the right side and Zusanli (ST36) on the right side.

Technique: Insert a needle on Lanwei (Ex-LE7), the main point, 1 *cun* deep. The sparrow-pecking needling technique is applied and the needle is retained for 30 minutes with endurable electric stimulation. The treatment is given three times a day. If the effect is not satisfactory, the supplementary points will be added.

6. LASER THERAPY

Points: Lanwei (Ex-LE7) bilaterally and McMurray Point.

Technique: He-Ne laser machine, output three to five mw, is applied to radiate the McMurray point for 10 minutes and Lanwei (Ex-LE7) for five minutes on each side, 30 to 60 cm away from the skin. The treatment is given twice a day for patients who are afraid of needling, children and ones with a weak constitution.

7. MEDICINAL APPLICATION ON ACU-POINTS

(1) Application with Jinhuangsan
Point: McMurray Point.

Technique: A paste of Jinhuangsan (Golden Medicinal Powder) and Yulusan (Jade Dew Medicinal Powder) mixed with water and honey is prepared and applied on a dressing on the McMurray point, twice a day.

(2) Application with Garlic Paste
Points: Ah-shi points on the lower abdomen of the right side

Technique: Garlic paste is made of garlic 60 g, Mangxiao (Natrii Sulphas) 30 g and Dahuang (Rhubarb) 30 g. First, garlic and Mangxiao (Natrii Sulphas) are ground together into a paste to dress the Ah-shi points. Two hours later, a paste prepared by the powder of Dahuang (Rhubarb) and vinegar is used as a dressing for six to eight hours. The therapy will be repeated several hours later if needed. A layer of Vaseline is used on the local area to prevent burning before the medicinal application.

[REMARKS]

1. Acupuncture and moxibustion are applicable for acute simple or mild suppurative appendicitis and are taken as the auxiliary therapy for the other types of appendicitis. If there is the tendency of appendicle perforation or necrosis, early surgery is recommended.

2. Acupuncture and moxibustion can improve the organic ability for anti-inflammation, strengthen phagocytosis of WBC, promote peristalsis of the appendix and benefit the secretion of the appendicle cavity and the improvement of blood circulation so as to promote anti-inflammation.

GALLSTONE AND CHOLECYSTITIS

[INTRODUCTION]

Gallstone and cholecystitis occur more in young and matured adults, more in females than in males. The two problems are closely related and can be induced by each other. Gallstones can induce both acute and chronic cholecystitis, while the inflammation of the gall-bladder is one of the major factors for the forming of gallstones. The two often exist together and the symptoms are similar, e.g., pain in the right upper quadrant or in the right rib arch radiating to the right scapular region. If it is the gallstone, there can be paroxysmal, colicky pain induced by excessive intake of a fatty diet. As far as the etiology and pathogenesis are concerned, it involves emotional depression, failure to adapt to weather changes, irregularity of food intake (excessive rich and greasy diet) or invasion of the exogenous pathogens. The accumulation of damp-heat and parasitosis leads to stagnant circulation of *qi* and blood especially in the liver and gallbladder so that the function of the liver and the purity and descending function of the gallbladder is disturbed. To treat the disease, the principle is to normalize the discharge of *qi* in the gallbladder, pacify the stomach and ease the middle-Jiao. Points are mainly selected from the foot Jueyin, Shaoyang and Yangming meridians, such as Riyue (GB24), Qimen (LR14), Yanglingquan (GB34), Taichong (LR3) and Zusanli (ST36). Reinforcing needling technique is performed for the syndrome of excess, and reducing technique for deficiency.

[CLINICAL EXPERIENCE]

1. CONVENTIONAL ACUPUNCTURE

(1) Puncturing Front-Mu Points

Points: Riyue (GB24), Zhongwan (CV12), and Tianshu (ST25). Supplementary points: Qimen (LR14) and Yanglingquan (GB34). All the points are selected from the right side except Zhongwan (CV12).

Technique: The points are the Front-Mu points of liver, gallbladder, stomach and large intestine; the Lower He-Sea point of gallbladder is combined. The reducing technique is applied and the needle-rotating method is used for insertion at a fairly large angle and with rapid frequency. Stimulation should be strong. The needles are retained for 10 minutes after the arrival of *qi* and then removed, with the needle holes opened.

(2) Puncturing Extra Points

Points: Xisixue (4 *cun* above the lateral border of the knee with the joint flexed), Yanglingquan (GB34) and Qimen (LR14).

Technique: The patient lies supine, and the point on the right leg is selected. A perpendicularly thrust for rapid insertion is made at Xisixue, stopping with the arrival of *qi*. The needle is then rotated counterclockwise. Yanglingquan (GB34) is also punctured perpendicularly and performed with counterclockwise rotation. If the technique is properly made, there should be a needling sensation running upward along the thigh. Qimen (LR14) is thrust obliquely. After the arrival of *qi*, the needle is rotated clockwise and a sensation of soreness and numbness. Distention should be conducted down so the abdominal distention is markedly relieved. The needles are retained for 30 minutes and are rotated once every 10 minutes.

(3) Penetrating Puncture

Point: Penetrating from Qimen (LR14) to Zhangmen (LR13) with strict caution to prevent the penetration of the thoracic cavity; from Juque (CV14) to Shangwan (CV13); from the 9th thoracic vertebra to the 10th (i.e., right-side Jiaji); and from Ganshu (BL18) to Danshu (BL19).

Technique: Take two-*cun* or three-*cun* stainless needle (Size: No.28) according to the distance of the penetration, and insert perpendicularly for 0.3 cun; then, penetrate to the other point. When there is a needling sensation, the proper reinforcing-reducing technique is performed in light of syndrome differentiation. Then the needles are fixed with plasters and embedded for two to three days. During the embedding, if there appears to be a sharp pain in the loci of the embedding, the needles should be removed. This method was used to treat five cases of cholecystitis, all of which were basically cured. Auricular therapy can be combined with needles embedded in Ear-Shenmen, Gallbladder, Stomach, etc.

(4) Puncturing Reacting Tender Points

Point: The primary point is the tender spot on the scapular region. Dazhui (GV14) and Quchi (LI11) are combined when there is running of fever; Yanglingquan (SP9) is supplemented for the costal pain; and Zhongwan (CV12) and Zusanli (ST36) are added for vomiting and epigastric distention.

Technique: Taking a sitting position, the patient crosses the arms to embrace the shoulders, so as to project the scapular region. The physician is searching for the tender spot between the right side of the spine and the scapula by palpation with the face of the right thumb. The tender spot is mostly located in the middle or lower portion of the right scapular region. A 1.5-*cun* or two-*cun* needle is thrust obliquely at an angle of 30° into the tender spot and the needling manipulation of lifting-thrusting and rotation is performed for five to 10 minutes. Cupping is combined after the removal of the needle for 10 to 15 minutes. The other points are punctured with needles retained for 15 to 30 minutes during which manipulation is given once every five minutes. However, in case of high fever of the acute cholecystitis, the needles can be retained for one hour with manipulation once every 10 to 20 minutes. Five to seven days are taken as one course of treatment, and there is a one- or two-day break after every course. This method was once used to treat 21 cases of cholecystitis, and the condition improved after a couple of sessions, with remarkable improvement, or even disappearance of the symptoms, after five to seven sessions. To treat acute cholecystitis, 30 to 60 minutes after the needling the abdominal pain was alleviated and the fever was reduced; and with three to five sessions, the symptoms disappeared. Since chronic cholecystitis is susceptible the recurrence, the treatment can be resumed with positive effect.

(5) Contralateral Puncture

Point: Penetrating from Qiuxu (GB40) to Zhaohai (KI6).

Technique: Needle the points on the right side when the pain appears on the left, and vice versa. The physician holds a two-*cun* filiform needle with the right hand and grips the shaft of the needle just above the tip with the left thumb and index finger to insert by rotation toward the point Zhaohai (KI6), which is located 1 *cun* below the medial malleolus. When the needling sensation appears, or there is a kind of radiating sensation in the point, the treatment is starting to take effect. The method is indicated for pain in the chest or lateral chest.

2. ELECTRIC ACUPUNCTURE

Points: Auricular points (right side): Ear-Shenmen, Sympathetic, Pancreas, Gallbladder, and Dannangxia (about 0.2 cm below Pancreas/Gallbladder). Auricular points (left side): penetrating from Pancreas/Gallbladder to Duodenum. Body points: Yanglingquan (GB34) and Dannangxue (EX-LE6). To those with physical asthenia, Zusanli (ST36) and Dannangxue (EX-LE6) are selected or a tender point should be found on the running course of the Gallbladder Meridian. Neiguan (PC6) is combined for nausea and vomiting.

Technique: When the points are selected, the Acupuncture-Anesthesia Apparatus is connected with either auricular points or body points for 20 to 45 minutes until the abdominal pain is relieved and the abdominal wall is relaxed. The needling is given once daily, three to five sessions making up one course of treatment. While using the electric acupuncture, oral medication of 10 ml of 33% magnesium sulfate is taken three times daily.

3. ORBITAL ACUPUNCTURE

Point: Bilateral gallbladder zone and right Middle-Jiao.

Technique: Use 0.5-*cun* stainless filiform needles (Size: Nos.30 to 32) and gently thrust them perpendicularly to reach the periosteum, as deep as 0.2 to 0.3 *cun*. No manipulation is normally performed. In case there is no arrival of *qi,* lift the needle and thrust again. The needles are retained for five to 10 minutes. After the removal of needles, the pain should be alleviated immediately. This can be taken as the supplementary method for treating an attack of biliary colic.

4. AURICULAR ACUPUNCTURE

(1) Embedding of Ear Seed

Point: For the cholecystolithiasis, such points as Pancreas/Gallbladder, Liver, Stomach, Middle of Cymba Concha, Brain and Lower Intertragic Space are prescribed as the primary ones while Intertragic Space, Occiput, Sanjiao, and Duodenum as the secondary ones; for choledocholithiasis, Pancreas/Gallbladder, Liver, Brain, Subcortex, and Lower End of Crus are as the primary points and Kidney, Lower Intertragic Space, and Duodenum as the secondary. If the manifestations of dull pain, distending pain, radiating pain on the back, or appearance of pain after consuming a fatty diet, Ear-Shenmen, Diaphragm, Lung and other points are added.

Technique: Before the treatment, the auricle is observed to see if there are any positive reaction points (roughness of skin as orange peel, or redness, rashes, pimples, etc.) of the liver/gallbladder diseases around the point Pancreas/Gallbladder; if there are no such positive reaction, detection should be done to find the tender spots on which the Semen Vaccaria are stuck. The two ears are alternated, once every other day. Ten sessions are taken as one course of treatment. To treat the onset of acute cholecystitis, bilateral Ear-Shenmen, Lower End of Crus, Posterior Vagus Nerve, and Duodenum can be pressed for analgesia. This method was used to treat 500 cases of gallstone, of which 46 cases (9.2%) were cured, 293 (59%) markedly improved; 145 (29%) improved; and 14 (2.8%) unchanged. The total effective rate was 97.2%.

5. LASER THERAPY

Points: Riyue (GB24) and Qimen (LR14).

Technique: The 7 ma He-Ne Laser Apparatus is used to irradiate through optical fiber the points Riyue (GB24) and Qimen (LR14), 10 minutes for each, once daily. Ten sessions make one course of treatment.

6. COMBINED TREATMENT

Points: Primary points (auricular): Liver, Gallbladder, Spleen,

Stomach, Duodenum and Ear-Shenmen. Secondary points (auricular): Lower portion of rectum, Sub-cortex, Endocrine, Sympathetic Nerve, Large Intestine and Small Intestine.

Technique: In each treatment, altogether eight to 10 points are selected from the primary and secondary groups. Semen Vaccaria are stuck on the points with adhesive plaster, once every other day. The seeds are pressed for 30 minutes every time some 20 minutes after meals. Alternatively, the seeds can be pressed whenever the pain starts. Simultaneously, herbal medication of the Formula 1 Lidanpaishi (Promoting the Gallbladder Function and Evacuating the Stones) was taken which includes Jinqiancao (loose strife) 30-100 g, Yujin (turmeric root) 30 g, fried Zhiqiao (bitter orange) 30 g, Jineijin (chicken's gizzard-skin) 5-10 g; or, the Formula 2 Lidanpaishi, including Formula 1 plus Yinchen (oriental wormwood) 30 g, Pugongying (dandelion) 30 g, Huangqin (skullcap root) 10 g, and Muxiang (costus root) 5 g (boiled for a shorter time). The prescription can be modified according to the symptoms. An appropriate amount of fatty food can be consumed, e.g., pig's feet at breakfast.

[REMARKS]

Acupuncture has a fairly satisfactory effect in evacuating stones, but it takes one to four courses for complete relief. When the diameter of the stones is smaller than 8 mm, the effect of evacuation is more satisfactory, while those with the diameter over 12 mm can hardly be discharged. Among the evacuated stones, those with a mixture of bile pigment calculus and bile pigment cholesterol are up to 2/3. Therefore, patients treated with acupuncture are required to wash the stones out of the stools so as to observe the therapeutic effect.

BILIARY ASCARIASIS

[INTRODUCTION]

The disease is characterized chiefly by paroxysmal, excruciating "drilling" and "tearing" pain, or colicky pain in the sub-xiphoid region, usually accompanied by nausea and vomiting. When the roundworm moves out of the biliary tract, sudden remission from pain is achieved, but a relapse can occur at any moment. The disease is mostly due to improper food intake and emotional upset, leading to coldness in the Zang-organs and heat in the stomach; hence, the roundworms may move up in a reverse way to obstruct the flow of *qi,* and the biliary tract then becomes blocked. The points of the gallbladder and liver meridians are mainly prescribed in the treatment, and Yanglingquan (GB34), Riyue (GB24), Taichong (LR3), Zhongwan (CV12), Danshu (BL19), and Dannangxue (EX-LE6) are taken in the primary prescription. The prescription serves to regain the normal flow of *qi* in liver and gallbladder so as to release the spasm for analgesia. When the pain is alleviated, the spleen should be regulated, its *qi* harmonized and the roundworms are eliminated to prevent the recurrence.

[CLINICAL EXPERIENCE]

1. CONVENTIONAL ACUPUNCTURE

(1) Penetrating Puncture (1)

Points: From Yingxiang (LI20) to Sibai (ST2).

Technique: Use a filiform needle to thrust bilateral Yingxiang (LI20) perpendicularly 0.5 cm and then puncture obliquely upward to Sibai (ST2) after the arrival of *qi.* When the needle reaches Sibai (ST2), the patient will feel a sensation of numbness and distention, sometimes even down to the upper lip. If it is not possible to make sure whether the needle tip reaches Sibai (ST2), the physician should press with the other index finger the orbital ridge lateral to Chengqi (ST1) and feel the needle tip. Then the needle should be withdrawn a bit and needle tip fixed at Sibai (ST2). Thereafter, the handle of the needle is fixed with adhesive plaster at the place just above the upper lip. Intense stimulation is performed and the needles are retained for 12 to 24 hours. The method was used to treat 22 cases of biliary ascriasis, and the pain was usually relieved half an hour after the acupuncture treatment and disappeared after about two hours.

(2) Penetrating Puncture (2)

Point: From Gaohuang (BL43) to Geshu (BL17) on the right side.

Technique: Use a filiform needle (Size: No.32) and thrust it horizontally in the subcutaneous layer from Gaohuang (BL43) to Geshu (BL17). The needle is then twirled for three minutes and retained for one hour. The liver and gallbladder are located in the right upper quadrant of abdomen, so the "back points are utilized to treat the front disease," usually with satisfactory results.

(3) Puncturing Front-Mu Points

Points: Juque (CV14) and Tianshu (ST25) on the right side

Technique: Routine needling technique. The needle is retained for 60 minutes and is rotated once every five minutes.

(4) Corresponding Points

Point: Bilateral Jiaji at the level of the 7th thoracic vertebra or Zhiyang (GV9) as the primary points and Danshu (BL19), Pishu (BL20), and Weicang (BL50) mainly on the right side as the secondary points.

Technique: The Jiaji points are needled perpendicularly to the subcutaneous layer and then thrust obliquely at an angle of 65° for about 1 *cun* toward the thoracic spine until the needle tip reaches the periosteum of the spine. The reducing method by small amplitude of needle rotation is performed so as to enable the patient to have a relaxing feeling in the chest and abdomen. The needle is retained for 20 to 30 minutes. The secondary points are needled with routine technique.

(5) Puncturing Huijuexue (Point for Syncope due to Ascriasis)

Point: Huijuexue (in the depression below the 8th thoracic spinous process).

Technique: The patient lies prone, and a 2.5-*cun* disinfected stainless steel needle is obliquely thrust for 1.5 to 2 *cun* slightly upward along the inter-spinous space. The needle is manipulated once every five minutes and retained for 15 to 30 minutes.

(6) Reacting Point of Biliary Ascriasis

Point: Tender spot of biliary ascriasis, it may be found below Zusanli (ST36).

Technique: Thrust a 3.5-*cun* or 4-*cun* needle (Size: Nos.28-30) into the point. When *qi* arrives, the needle is further thrust for about 3 *cun* and there will be the arrival of *qi* once more. It is the most optimal to produce the centripetal propagation of *qi*. The same needling is performed on the other side, and then the reducing technique is manipulated simultaneously with both hands by means of lifting-thrusting and rotating the needles until the pain is relieved or even disappears. The needles are retained for 30 minutes during which manipulation is given a couple of times.

(7) Long-needle Puncture

Point: Jiuwei (CV 15)

Technique: Thrust a 5-*cun* to 7-*cun* needle (Size: No.28) slowly from Jiuwei (CV 15) toward Shenque (CV8). When moving down to Shuifen (CV9), manipulate the needle with lifting-thrusting and rotating technique until the pain is alleviated. The needle is then retained for 10 to 20 minutes. Usually one session can relieve the pain.

2. INDIRECT MOXIBUSTION WITH SALT

Point: Shenque (CV8).

Technique: Place stir-fried salt powder into the point (umbilicus), and conduct heavy moxibustion with 10 to 100 moxa cones. The moxibustion should exert certain effect since the roundworms tend to "move up on cold and move down on warmth." This type of moxibustion is applicable to the "ascriasis syncope." When the pain is alleviated, mild moxibustion with moxa stick is given over Danshu (BL19), Riyue (GB24), Qimen (LR14), and Yanglingquan (GB34), all on the right side, 10 to 20 minutes for each point, once daily.

3. Electrical Acupuncture

Points: Shangwan (CV13) and Danshu (BL19) on the right side

Technique: The patient should be in a lying position. When the arrival of *qi* is achieved in the points, the electro-acupuncture apparatus is connected with the needles to produce a tolerable intensity of stimulation to the patient. The current is given for five to 20 seconds each time, and there is an interval of several minutes after each episode of stimulation. After the first episode of stimulation, the pain is usually greatly relieved, and the stimulation should be repeated for several times until the symptoms totally disappear.

4. Auricular Acupuncture

Point: ① Large Intestine, Gallbladder, Duodenum, Liver, Pancreas and Sympathetic Nerve. ② Root of Vagus Nerve.

Technique: Puncture the first group of points and retain the needles for 30 to 60 minutes. Puncture the second group with a silver needle thrusting toward the external acoustic foramen for about 0.5 *cun*. There will be a feeling of heat and a distending sensation in the ear with the arrival of *qi*. The needle is retained for five to 10 minutes. To start with, one ear is needled and, if the pain is not alleviated in five minutes, the other ear is needled alike. The needle is retained for 10 to 15 minutes, so the analgesic effect is noticeable in the majority of cases.

5. Thick-needle Puncture

Points: From Jinsuo (GV8) to Jizhong (GV6), Shendao (GV11) to Bazhuixia (EX); and Yanglingquan (GB34).

Technique: The first two groups are performed with the penetrating method by means of a one-mm thick needle, which is retained for four hours. Yanglingquan is stimulated intensely. This method was used to treat 95 cases of biliary ascriasis in young children and the effective rate was up to 92.6%.

[REMARKS]

1. In treating biliary ascariasis, acupuncture is positively effective in relieving pain and easing vomiting. However, in order to consolidate the therapeutic effect, a sufficient dosage of herbal anti-parasitic e.g., Jiaweiwumeiwan (Modified Black Plum Pill) and Huachongwan (Anthelmintic Pill) should be administered.

2. Treatment beforehand of intestinal ascariasis may easily prevent the occurrence of biliary ascariasis.

HERNIA

[INTRODUCTION]

There are descriptions of this disease recorded in TCM involving a variety of disorders. All those that feature a contracting pain of the testis and lower abdomen, swelling and dragging sensation of the scrotum, or lumps and masses as a cup or a plate, can be called hernia. The commonly seen types of hernia in TCM include "cold hernia," "damp-heat hernia," and "foxy hernia." Cold hernia results from the excess of endogenous *yin*-cold due to constitutional weakness plus the invasion of exogenous cold that leads to stagnation of *qi* and blood in the Ren and liver meridians. Damp-heat hernia is caused by the downward flow of damp-heat to the Ren and liver meridians. Foxy hernia is due to the sinking of *qi* resulting from physical over-exertion e.g., carrying extra heavy loads. Cold hernia should be treated by the principle of warming the meridians and dissipating the cold with such points from the Ren and liver meridians as Guanyuan (CV4), Sanyinjiao (SP6), Dadun (LR1), etc. To treat damp-heat hernia, the principle is to clear the damp-heat with reducing needling technique in the points from Ren, spleen, and liver meridians. On the treatment of foxy hernia, the primordial *qi* is cultivated by means of reinforcing needling technique and moxibustion at such points from Ren and kidney meridians as Guanyuan (CV4), Taixi (KI3), and Ququan (LR8). The disorders in modern medicine such as oblique hernia, femoral hernia, direct hernia, umbilical hernia, incarcerated hernia, scrotal hydrocele, hydrocele of tunica vaginalis, varicocele, orchitis, and epididymitis can be treated by referring to the above-mentioned.

[CLINICAL EXPERIENCE]

1. CONVENTIONAL ACUPUNCTURE

(1) Groups of Points
   Points: Taichong (LR3) and Zhongji (CV3), and Guanyuan (CV4)

and Sanyinjiao (SP6).

Technique: The two groups are alternately punctured with reducing technique. The needle is withdrawn after the arrival of *qi*. Treatment is given once a day. This method is applicable to hydrocele of tunica vaginalis.

(2) Puncturing the Luo-Connecting Point of Liver

Point: Ligou (LR5).

Technique: The needle is inserted at an angle of 15° between the needle tip and the skin for 0.5 to 0.8 *cun* along the running course of the meridian and is manipulated with neutral technique. The treatment is given once daily. Other points, such as Qihai (CV8), Sanyinjiao (SP6), Taixi (KI3), and Dadun (LR1), can also be combined.

(3) Puncturing Point Zhishanxue

Point: Zhishanxue, anterior and inferior to the medial malleolus, 0.5 *cun* anterior to Zhaohai (KI6).

Technique: Make a contralateral puncture; the needle is thrust obliquely for 0.3 to 0.5 *cun* and is retained for five minutes, once a day. This method is indicated for hernia in young children with marked therapeutic effect.

(4) Combining the Upper Points with the Lower Points

Points: The primary points include Chongmen (SP12) located at the painful swelling in the inguinal region, and Sanyinjiao (SP6). Quchi (LI11) and Zusanli (ST36) are combined in case of running fever.

Technique: The point at the painful swelling in the inguinal region is punctured with a one-*cun* or 1.5-*cun* needle obliquely at an angle of 30° toward the perineum (avoid the artery), and the needling manipulation of lifting, thrusting and scraping the needle-handle is performed. The other points are punctured with routine technique. The needles are retained for 30 to 60 minutes, during which they are manipulated every 15 to 20 minutes. The treatment is given once daily. This method is mainly for acute epididymitis.

2.   MOXIBUSTION

(1) Triangular Moxibustion

Point: Point Sanjiao (triangle).

Technique: Measure the distance between the corners of the patient's mouth which is taken as one unit, and divide a piece of clean grass (cogongrass or wheat straw is best) into three units the same as above, to make a triangle. One angle is set at the navel while the other two are set below, which are taken as the points. Contralateral moxibustion is performed or bilateral moxibustion instead in case of affection on both sides. With a garlic slice on the point, the moxa cone as big as a pea is put on the garlic, and moxibustion is performed until the slice becomes yellow. This is the remarkable therapy for long-term hernia.

(2) Moxibustion at Dadun (LR1)

Point: Dadun (LR1).

Technique: Contralateral indirect moxibustion is given with ginger or garlic; three to five moxa cones as big as a jujube pit are used until the onset of an intolerable burning pain. This method is efficacious to all the types of hernia. The treatment is given once a day and 10 sessions make up one course.

(3) Direct moxibustion with moxa cones

Point: Yangchi (TE4).

Technique: A small amount of Vaseline is applied on the point and a moxa cone as big as a mung bean is placed on top. Three cones are used in each session. Treatment is given once daily and consecutively for seven days. This method was used to treat acute orchitis with marked effect. The longest course was seven days, and the shortest 10 hours.

3. BLEEDING METHOD

Point: Xinjian (LR2)

Technique: Use a three-edged needle to prick Xingjian (LR2) on the affected side to cause slight bleeding. Teatment is performed once every three to seven days.

4. HERBAL APPLICATION ON ACUPOINTS

Point: Yongquan (KI1).

Technique: Mix seven pieces of pure castor bean with an appropriate amount of wheat flour and make it into a paste that is applied on the point contralaterally. Then cover it by gauze and fix it with adhesive plaster. It is changed twice a day.

[REMARKS]

1.   Dr. Zhang Zihe (1156-1228) said: "All the types of hernia are attributable to liver meridian." Since "liver meridian runs on the medial aspect of the thigh, enters the pubic hair, curves over the genitalia, and reaches up to the lower abdomen," it is the meridian most closely related with the focus of hernia. Therefore in terms of the principle that "a meridian is indicated for the disorders near its running course," it is an approach to deal with the liver when treating hernia in spite of the modification of various therapeutic methods, e.g., taking heart meridian, spleen meridian, stomach meridian, kidney meridian, etc.

2.   Acupuncture claims satisfactory effect in treating cold and damp-heat hernia.

3.   Foxy hernia, also known as "*qi* of the small intestine" by laymen, can be treated when it is mild at the beginning; but as it gets worse in the advanced stage, radical treatment with surgery is advisable.

UROLITH DISEASE

[INTRODUCTION]

Urolith disease is referred to as stones of the kidney, urinary bladder and urethra, which cause local injury, infarction, and complicated infection in the urinary system. This disease is mostly caused by an excessive intake of spicy, hot and greasy food, or an over-indulgence in alcohol, leading to damp-heat flowing downward to the urinary bladder; or when the genital region fails to be kept clean, the pathogens of dirt and turbidity invade the urinary bladder, generating damp-heat. The protracted accumulation of damp-heat turns into sand and stone, which might block the urinary bladder, disturb the discharge of urine, and obstruct the flow of *qi*. The disease is characterized by the chief complaints of sudden lancing pain in the lumbar region or in the lower abdomen and hematuria. The pain is a kind of paroxysm lasting for several or scores of minutes, and even several hours, radiating from the kidney region to the urethra, external genitalia, and the medial side of the thigh. Nausea and vomiting or even syncope are associated with it. The principle of treatment is to eliminate damp-heat, ease pain, and restore normal urination. Points are mainly selected from the bladder, kidney, and spleen meridians, such as Shenshu (BL23), Zhishi (BL52), Yinlingquan (SP9), Sanyinjiao (SP6), Taixi (KI3) and Pangguangshu (BL28). The reducing technique is applied and intermittent needling manipulation should be performed during the retention of needles.

[CLINICAL EXPERIENCE]

1. CONVENTIONAL ACUPUNCTURE

(1) Puncture According to the Located Parts of the Stone

Points: The primary points are Ah-shi points. Shenshu (BL23) and Jingmen (GB25) are combined for the stones in the kidney and upper part of the urethra; Yanglingquan (GB34) for the stones in the middle and lower parts of the urethra; and the penetrating method from Guanyuan (CV4) to Zhongji (CV3) is used for stones in the bladder.

The Ah-shi points include those as: 1) Tender points: These will be found by palpation at the innervations from the 10th thoracic vertebra to the 1st lumbar vertebra when the stones are in the kidney and the upper part of the urethra, while in the lower part of the lower abdomen when the stones are in the bladder. 2) Radiating tenderness: When the colic occurs, most of tender points caused by the radiating pain from the lumbar and abdominal region, e.g., from the kidney and urethra stones, are located in the kidney region, lower abdomen, and the medial aspect of the thigh, and the pain resulting from stones in the bladder may radiate to the perineum. 3) The projected points of the focus of the stones found by X-ray plain film on the body surface.

Technique: Those above the 2nd lumbar vertebra are punctured obliquely toward the spine for 1 *cun* to 1.2 *cun* with the rotating technique; and those below the 2nd lumbar vertebra are needled perpendicularly for 1 *cun* to 2 *cun* with lifting-thrusting and handle-scraping techniques. The Ah-shi points in the abdomen should be thrust deep down to the peritoneum with slow lifting-thrusting or handle-scraping technique. To perform the penetrating method from Guanyuan (CV4) to Zhongji (CV3), a three-*cun* needle is used to thrust perpendicularly at Guanyuan (CV4), 1.5 *cun* to 2 *cun* deep. After a feeling of emptiness appears under the needle, make a slow lifting-thrusting a couple of times, producing a sensation of soreness and distention radiating down to the external genitalia or the perineum. The needle is then lifted to the subcutaneous layer and thrust again deep down to Zhongji (CV3). On the arrival of the point, lifting-thrusting is performed a couple of times. Yanglingquan (GB34) and Jingmen (GB25) are punctured with routine technique. During the colic attack, all the points mentioned above must be performed with needling manipulation until the pain is relieved and disappears. The needles are retained for an hour or two, once a day. When there is no attack, the needles are retained for 30 to 60 minutes during which the needling manipulation is performed every 10 to 20 minutes. The treatment is also given once daily, and seven sessions make up one course. Attention should be paid to the fact that, sometimes, when the needles are retained for the period of 10 to 30 minutes, the patients complain of aggravated colic, but this is a sign of the effectiveness of the acupuncture treatment.

(2) Puncturing Xi-Cleft Points

Points: Main points: Shuiquan (KI5), Jiaoxin (KI8), and Yangjiao (GB35). Supplementary points: Shenshu (BL23), Kunlun (BL60), Fujie (SP14), Guanyuan (CV4) and Ah-shi.

Technique: All the primary points are the Xi-Cleft points. Shuiquan (KI5) is the Xi-Cleft point for the kidney, Jiaoxin (KI8) for the Yinqiao meridian, and Yangjiao (GB35) for the Yangwei meridian. All of them are punctured with intense stimulation. When needling Jiaoxin (KI8), sometimes there is an electric-shock sensation moving to the kidney region, or just a warm sensation extending to the lumbar region and to the anterior and inferior side, with slight paroxysmal pain in the lower abdomen and increased frequency of urination. To needle the other points, to those who are physically weak, moderate stimulation is given; for those with a strong constitution, strong stimulation is given. The needles are retained for 15 to 30 minutes during which stimulation is performed from time to time. The treatment may be performed several times a day.

(3) Puncturing Yuan-Source Points

Point: Taixi (KI3)

Technique: Puncture bilateral Taixi (KI3) with moderate stimulation until the patient has a numb and distending sensation radiating to the feet. The needles are retained for 30 to 90 minutes. Intermittent needling manipulation can be given during the retention of needles to intensify the needling sensation. If there are remarkable symptoms of nausea and vomiting, bilateral Neiguan (PC6) are punctured. This method was used to treat 23 cases of urolith colic. After one to three sessions of acupuncture treatment, the pain basically disappeared in 18 cases and was markedly alleviated in the remaining five.

2. MOXIBUSTION

Points: Guanyuan (CV4) and Dadun (LR1)

Technique: Moxibustion is performed with either moxa cones or moxa sticks at the points to reopen the meridians and ease the pain. Moxibustion is given when the pain strikes, and may be given several times a day. There is marked effect of this method. As it is said in the book *Classic of Fundamentals of Acupuncture and Moxibustion*: "Stone-Lin syndrome (urolith) is treated by moxibustion at Guanyuan (CV4) or Qimen (EX) or Dadun (LR1) for 30 moxa cones."

3. ELECTRIC ACUPUNCTURE

Points: Select the points from the bladder meridian near the kidney and urethra. For intra-renal calculus, Ah-shi points (where the stones are located) and Shenshu (BL23) are selected; for stones in the upper urethra, Shenshu (BL23) and Pangguangshu (BL28) or Guanyuan (CV4) instead of Pangguangshu (BL28) are selected; for stones in the middle urethra, Shenshu (BL23) and Guanyuan (CV4) or Ah-shi point (1 cm above the location of the stone) instead of Shenshu

(BL23) are selected; and for stones in the lower urethra, Ah-shi point and Guanyuan (CV4) or Sanyinjiao (SP6) instead of the Ah-shi point are selected.

Technique: Thirty minutes before the treatment, the patient is required to drink 1,000 ml of water, or at least as much of that amount as possible, and then lie supine or prone. The needles are inserted in the points and are connected with an electro-acupuncture apparatus (with fairly strong current). The negative pole is connected with points near the kidney and the positive pole with the points near the bladder. The insertion is as deep as the strongest needling sensation can be made and the intensity of the electric current is up to the patient's tolerance. The dense-disperse wave is used for 30 minutes. The treatment is given once daily, 10 sessions making up one course. During the treatment, the patient should feel a pushing-down sensation from the upper to the lower urethra. There should be no other kind of discomfort. Most patients urinate right after the treatment and feel comfortable, while the stones may also be discharged.

4.   AURICULAR ACUPRESSURE

Points: Kidney, Urinary Bladder, Urethra, Sanjiao, Ear-Shenmen, External Genitalia, etc.

Technique: Semen Vaccaria are fixed with plasters on the points for three days, 10 sessions making up one course of treatment. The patients are required to press the seeds several times daily and drink 250 ml to 500 ml of liquid every time before the ear pressure. Appropriate exercise should be done to promote the discharge of the stones. In 41 cases of stones treated with this method, 21 saw the stones discharged (11 cases were cured and 10 were markedly effective), eight cases were effective (the stones moved down 2-5 cm), and 12 cases were unchanged.

5.   BLEEDING THERAPY

Points: Primary points: Shenshu (BL23) and Yaoyangguan (GV3). Supplementary points: Yinlingquan (SP9) and Yangjiao (G35)

Technique: A three-edged needle is used to cause a small amount of bleeding and the pain should disappear. This is because bleeding can promote the circulation of blood and resolve the inflammation of the urinary tract, so the spasm of the urethra is relieved and the excruciating pain in the lumbar region alleviated.

6. COMBINED TREATMENT

(1) The Combination of Conventional Acupuncture, Cupping and Cutaneous Needing

Points: Shenshu (BL23) and Jingmen (GB25), all on the affected side.

Technique: The patient lies in a recumbent position with the affected side on top. Shenshu (BL23) and Jingmen (GB25) are punctured with reducing technique and are connected with an electro-acupuncture apparatus after the appearance of the needling sensation of soreness, numbness, distention and heaviness. Continuous wave is given with frequency of 200 beats per minute. The needles are retained for 15 minutes and then plum-blossom needling is performed around the points in combination with cupping for a short period. After the cupping, plum-blossom needling is gently resumed for a further minute. The treatment is given once a day and 10 sessions form one course. Usually, small stones can be discharged after one course.

(2) The Combination of Acupuncture and Chinese Herbs

Points: Taixi (KI3), Feiyang (BL58), Jingmen (GB25) and Sanyinjiao (SP6).

Technique: Reinforcing-reducing technique upon the running orientation of meridians is applied with Taixi (KI3) reinforced, Feiyang (BL58) reduced, Jingmen (GB25) punctured neutrally and Sanyinjiao (SP6) reduced. During the attack of kidney colic, Yongquan (KI1) is reduced heavily. The needles are retained for 30 to 60 minutes and are manipulated every six minutes. The treatment is given once daily, 10 sessions in one course, with a four-day interval between two courses. The Chinese herbs are administered one dose a day, primarily including Dongkuizi (cluster mallow fruit seeds), Shiwei (pyrosia leaf), talcum, Xueduan, Baizhu (bighead atractylodes rhizome), Biejia (tortoise carapace and plastron), Wangbuliuxing (cow soapwort seed),

Chuanniuxi (cyathula root), Puhuang (cat-tail pollen), walnut kernel, amber powder, and Cheqiancao (plantain). The prescription can be modified according to the manifestations.

(3) The Strategic Offensive with Both Acupuncture and Chinese Herbs

Points: Shenshu (BL23), Pangguangshu (BL28), Ah-shi point, and Sanyinjiao (SP6) for the upper and middle urinary stones; and Shenshu (BL23), Shuidao (ST28), Ah-shi point and Sanyinjiao (SP6) for the lower urinary stones.

Technique: At 6:00, 7:00, 8:00 a.m. the patient drinks respectively 500 ml of water. At 9:00 in the morning, the stone-discharging herbal decoction is administered, including Jinqiancao (loosestrife), Haijinsha (climbing-fern spores), Niuxi (cyathula root), Zexie (water-plantain tuber), Cheqiancao, Dongkuizi (plantain), talcum, and licorice root, 200 ml for one dose. At 10:20 a.m., 0.5 mg of Atropine is injected intramuscularly or in the acupoints. At 10:30 a.m., routine technique is performed on all the points mentioned above and the needles are connected with G6805 Electro-Acupuncture Apparatus with the positive pole at Shenshu (BL23), Pangguangshu (BL28) and Shuidao (ST28) and the negative pole at Ah-shi point, and Sanyinjiao (SP6). The needles are retained for 20 to 30 minutes and the treatment is finished at 11:00 a.m., so the patient is required to exercise a bit. This method is applicable to patients with normal kidney function and smaller stones of diameter less than 1 cm. In case of complicated infection, anti-infection therapy should be given first and the Strategic Offensive is given later after the infection is under control.

[REMARKS]

1. Acupuncture claims certain analgesic effect, but if the pain is so excruciating that it cannot be controlled, combined treatment of Western and traditional Chinese medicine should be taken into consideration.

2. It is easier to discharge the stones for those who are younger with short duration of disease and at the onset of the acute stage, preferably drinking more water and exercising vigorously.

3. At ordinary times, in order to prevent the occurrence of this disease, sufficient water should be drunk and the intake of food with an excess of calcium should be avoided.

4. To treat the pyelolithasis, when the stone is in the lower part, the patient should adopt Trendelenburg's position in the treatment; and when the stones are in the lateral side, the lateral recumbent position should be adopted with the healthy side on the bottom and the kidney region should also be patted during the treatment.

TENOSYNOVITIS AND THECAL CYST

[INTRODUCTION]

Tenosynovitis and thecal cyst mainly occur on the dorsal aspect of the wrist when the tendon sheath is inflamed and cyst-genetic (the cysts are round-shaped and enveloped with connective tissue capsule and contain colloidal mucus), and the cysts are hard. It occurs chiefly among the young and matured adults. It is understood in traditional Chinese medicine that the disease is caused by overstrain which harms the tendon-muscle meridians so the circulation of *qi* and blood is disturbed. The treating principle is to ease the tendons, dredging the collaterals, promoting blood circulation and dispersing the stagnation. Such points as Ah-shi point, Yangxi (LI5), Lieque (LU7), and Hegu (LI4) are selected for acupuncture, moxibustion, or the combined treatment.

[CLINICAL EXPERIENCE]

1. CONVENTIONAL ACUPUNCTURE

(1) Needling in a Plum-blossom Way

Point: Ah-shi point.

Technique: At the midpoint of the cyst, a needle is thrust perpendicularly deep down to penetrate the base of the cyst and four more needles are thrust symmetrically from four directions horizontally toward the base, forming a plum-blossom shape. The reducing method is performed, but the needles are not retained. The treatment is given once daily and 10 sessions constitute one course.

(2) Cross-like Puncture

Points: The affected area.

Technique: Puncture perpendicularly the midpoint of the cyst to penetrate its base; then lift the needle slowly to the inside of the cyst, and thrust horizontally into the cyst wall in all the directions in a cross-like way. Reducing technique is used and the needle is not retained. After the removal of the needle, squeeze out the liquid from the needle hole. The treatment is given once every other day, and the cyst usually disappears after five or six sessions.

(3) Three-edged Needle Puncture

Point: The affected area.

Technique: The physician fixes the cyst with the left hand and grips a three-edged needle with the right hand. If it is a single cyst, the needle is thrust into its topmost point; if there are multiple cysts, every nodule-like topmost point is penetrated. After the insertion of the needle, the tip punctures circularly deep inside the cyst, but not too fiercely. On the removal of the needle, squeeze the cyst toward the needle hole, trying to squeeze up all the intracystal contents. Afterward, the needle hole is sterilized with 75% alcohol and covered by a dried, sterilized cotton ball with a coin on it. The cotton and the coin are finally fixed by circular-compression with an adhesive plaster three to five cm in breadth. After three to five days, the coin is removed. If no cure is achieved, the same therapy is resumed. The majority of patients are usually cured after two or three treatments.

2.   RED-HOT NEEDLING

Points: The affected area.

Technique: Pushing the intracystal contents aside and using a needle (Size: Nos.22-24) to thrust deep into the cyst. Be sure to avoid the blood vessels. The needle is withdrawn rapidly and the intracystal liquid is squeezed out right away. The needle hole is sterilized with alcohol and bandaged with compression. The therapy can be resumed on recurrence of the problem.

3. PRICKING METHOD

Point: Ah-shi point.

Technique: Use a fine needle to prick the fibers in the Ah-shi point, swaying up and down a bit each time, with moderate stimulation. The needle is then retained for 30 minutes. If the focus is small, the pricking can be done every three to five days, but if it is fairly large, the pricking is given once a day for the first three sessions. Usually, two to five sessions are taken as one course.

4. WARMING-NEEDLE METHOD

Point: The affected area.

Technique: A mild case needs only a thrust in the middle of the cyst, deep down to its base, and then the warming-needle method is combined for 30 minutes. For protracted and intractable cases, triple needling (one thrust in the middle and one from both the left and right sides) must be combined to enhance the efficacy of needling. Moreover, moxibustion should also be added. If cupping with a small cup is given after the removal of the needle to suck out some sticky liquid, it will be even more effective.

5. HYDRO-ACUPUNCTURE

Point: The tenderest spot of the swelling sheath.

Technique: After sterilization, 2 ml of Antongting injection, or 4 ml of 0.25% procaine hydrochloride, or 2 ml of 5% to 10% glucose injection, is injected slowly into the point. If it is not cured with one session, one more treatment can be given on the third day.

6. SEVEN-STAR NEEDLING (A KIND OF CUTANEOUS NEEDLING)

Points: The affected area.

Technique: After the sterile technique in the local region, a seven-star needle is used to tap the cyst surface circularly from the middle to the border. The tapping should be fairly strong so as to cause flushing of the skin in the local region, or even slight leopard-like bleeding. One session or two sessions should be enough for a cure.

7. COMBINED TREATMENT

Points: Primary points: Ah-shi point around the cyst. Secondary points: adjacent points from the involved meridians.

Technique: Usually, the primary points are effective enough to cure acute and small-sized cysts, while in treating middle or large sized ones, the intracystal mucous fluid should be drawn out. Then, four one-*cun* needles (Size: No.28) are used to thrust symmetrically from outside the cyst to its center; the secondary points are combined as well. The needles are connected with direct current to create stimulation for 10 minutes. After the removal of the needles, mild moxibustion is given with moxa stick over the cyst for 10 minutes. Finally, fixation is made with an aseptic dressing and adhesive plaster. The treatment is given once daily and 10 sessions form one course of treatment.

[REMARKS]

1. After the acupuncture treatment, a pressure bandage should be applied on the cyst for three to five days.

2. Acupuncture claims fairly satisfactory effect in treating the disease in spite of a susceptibility of recurrence. Hence, the above-mentioned methods can be resumed to achieve a complete cure after recurrence.

PROSTATIC HYPERPLASIA AND CHRONIC PROSTATITIS

[INTRODUCTION]

Prostatic hyperplasia is characterized chiefly by increased nocturnal urination, delayed urination, a weak stream, and even acute retention of urine; chronic prostatitis is featured by dysuria, discomfort or burning sensation during urination, the dropping of white secretes at the end of urination or during bowel movement, pain in the genital region sometimes including the penis and testis, and sexual disorders, e.g., hyposexuality, prospermia, impotence, seminal emission, etc. It is held in traditional Chinese medicine that this disease is due to constitutional deficiency with weakness of kidney *qi,* or immoderate consumption of rich food and alcohol leading to stagnation of *qi* and blood and endogenous accumulation of damp-heat; or over-indulgence in sexual activities giving rise to deficiency of kidney *yin,* which subsequently leads to the undermining of kidney *yang* as well, hence the disorder of *yin* and *yang* in the kidney. Accordingly, the principle of treatment is, on the one hand, to nourish *yin* and replenish the kidney, and, on the other hand, to eliminate damp-heat. The points are mainly selected from the kidney, bladder, and liver meridians, including Taixi (KI3), Ququan (LR8), Taichong (LR3), Yinlingquan (SP9) and Sanyinjiao (SP6). Even needling technique is performed, and moxibustion is combined according to the individual conditions.

[CLINICAL EXPERIENCE]

1. CONVENTIONAL ACUPUNCTURE

(1) Penetrating Puncture

Points: Primary points: From Qihai (CV6) to Guanyuan (CV4) or from Guanyuan (CV4) to Zhongji (CV3), and Shenshu (BL23). Secondary points: Shuidao (ST28) and Sanyinjiao (SP6).

Technique: The penetrated primary points are punctured horizontally downward, and the needle is retained and manipulated with reducing needling technique after the arrival of *qi.* Meanwhile, Shenshu (BL23) is needled perpendicularly for 0.3 to 0.5 *cun* or with the reinforcing method. Bilateral Shuidao (ST28) are punctured obliquely to the medial side down to the wall of the bladder, while Sanyinjiao (SP6) is penetrated horizontally down to Taixi (KI3), or needled perpendicularly for 1 to 1.5 *cun,* usually with moderate stimulation.

(2) Puncturing Huiyinpangxue ("Point Lateral to Huiyin CV1")
Points: Huiyinpangxue (Located 1 *cun* lateral to Huiyin CV1).

Technique: Before the puncture, the left index finger covered with a rubber glove or finger-guard is inserted into the anus to feel the prostate gland for guiding the needling orientation, while the right hand grips the needle to thrust "Huiyinpangxue," and as deep as 2 to 2.5 *cun*. The needle is then inserted in the prostate gland. The continuous lifting-thrusting technique is performed and the needle is retained for 30 minutes. During the treatment, the retained urethral catheter should be kept through. This method can obtain satisfactory short-term effect in treating prostatic hyperplasia.

(3) Strong Needling-Stimulation Method
Points: Primary points: Shenshu (BL23), Guanyuan (CV4), and Sanyinjiao (SP6). Secondary points: Zusanli (ST36) and Hegu (LI4).

Technique: Two to four points are selected each session. After routine sterilization, 1.5-*cun* filiform needles (Size: Nos.26-28) are used to thrust rapidly into the points and then retained for 30 minutes after the arrival of *qi*. The treatment is given once a day and 15 sessions form one course of treatment.

2. MOXIBUSTION WITH MOXA STICK

Points: Mingmen (GV4) and Guanyuan (CV4).

Technique: The moxa stick is ignited to perform sparrow-pecking moxibustion, five to 10 minutes for each point, twice a day. This is applicable to treat protatitis or retention of urine due to the prostatic hyperplasia.

3. ELECTRIC ACUPUNCTURE

Points: Around the anus (at loci of 10 and 3 points).

Technique: Under the guidance of anal digital examination, needles are thrust from the two points to the prostate gland and then are connected with an electro-acupuncture apparatus for 30 to 40 minutes. Ten days make up one course of treatment. Five cases of prostatic hyperplasia were treated with this method with satisfactory results, including shrinking of the hyperplastic gland, and there were no more complaints of clinical symptoms.

4. AURICULAR THERAPY

Points: Prostate Gland, Urinary Bladder, Endocrine, Adrenal Gland and Pelvis. Subcortex and External Genitalia are combined in case of the complication of epididymitis.

Technique: Strong stimulation is given, with needles retained for five to 15 minutes; or ear seeds can also be embedded. The treatment is given once a day and 10 sessions make up one course of treatment.

5. CUTANEOUS PUNCTURE

Points: Both sides of the spine from the 1st lumbar to the 5th sacral vertebrae, inguinal region, and perineum.

Technique: Tap once a day in order to cause skin flushing.

6. PRICKING METHOD

Points: To find the reacting points around Dachangshu (BL25) and Pangguangshu (BL28).

Technique: Two reacting points are selected in each session. If there is no reacting point, just prick Dachangshu (BL25) and Pangguangshu (BL28) to cause bleeding with a three-edged needle. The pricking is given once every seven to 10 days and five sessions form one course.

7. BLEEDING METHOD

(1) Bleeding Jing-Well Points

Points: Zhiyin (BL67) and Inner Zhiyin, which is located at the place 0.1 *cun* lateral to the medial corner of the nail of the little toe, also understood as the extension of Yongquan (KI1), hence a Jing-Well point.

Technique: Use a three-edged needle to bleed each point, drawing about 20 drops of blood; the points of the two feet are alternated day by day. The method helps regulate and open the Lower-Jiao and eliminate damp-heat, implying that "the disorders of Zang-organs are treated by Jing-Well points."

(2) Bleeding Two Points

Points: Yaoshu (GV2) and Yinlingquan (SP9).

Technique: The points are bled each time, three to five drops, to relieve the congestion of the prostate gland. Usually, the method has immediate effect. Xialiao (BL34) and Sanyinjiao (SP6) can be combined in the bleeding to consolidate the effect.

8. ACUPOINT HERBAL APPLICATION

Points: Zhongji (CV3).

Technique: Nine grams of ground Gansui powder are mixed with an appropriate amount of borneol and flour, and made into the paste with lukewarm water. The paste is applied on the point to a diameter of 9 *cun*, and is covered with plastic film and fixed with adhesive plaster. The treatment is given once or twice a day and the herbal paste is taken off after urination. When it is ineffective, a heat compress can be combined. The method has fairly good effect to treat acute retention of urine resulting from prostatic hyperplasia or prostatitis.

9. COMBINED TREATMENT: ACUPUNCTURE, MOXIBUS-TION, AND MASSAGE

Points: Guanyuan (CV4), Zhongji (CV3), Taixi (KI3), Taichong (LR3) and Huiyin (CV1).

Technique: All the points are punctured with even technique and the needles are retained after the arrival of *qi*. The needling sensation at Zhongji (CV3) should be conducted downward. Moxibustion with three moxa cones is performed on Guanyuan (CV4) and Taixi (KI3), while acupressure massage and moxa-stick moxibustion are applied on Huiyin (CV1) alternately for 15 to 30 minutes. The treatment is given once every other day. The method was used to treat 44 cases of chronic prostatitis, and 37 were cured, with the remaining seven unchanged.

[REMARKS]

Acupuncture claims a certain effect in treating this disease. When there are manifestations of chills and fever, the combination of Western and traditional Chinese medicine should be taken into consideration.

THROMBOANGITIS OBLITERANS

[INTRODUCTION]

Thromboangitis obliterans, a chronic peripheral vascular disease, is the periodic segmental inflammatory disorder of arteries and veins. It is characterized by ischemic symptoms, such as excruciating pain, coldness of the affected limbs, feeble pulse, intermittent claudication, and even acromelic gangrene. It is understood in traditional Chinese medicine that the disease is mainly due to the invasion of meridians and collaterals by exogenous pathogenic cold or dampness resulting in the stagnation of *qi* and blood; or it is caused by immoderate smoking and alcohol consumption leading to the endogenous generation of toxic fire, which disturbs the emotions, hence the stagnation of *qi* and blood. In addition, traumatic injuries can also give rise to stagnation of *qi* and blood. The treating principle is to activate the circulation of blood, reopen the meridians and collaterals, warm *yang* by dissipating the cold, and eliminate the heat and toxic matters. The prescription includes Quchi (LI11), Neiguan (PC6), Hegu (LI4), Xuehai (SP10), Yanglingquan (GB34), Zusanli (ST36), Taichong (LR3), Kunlun (BL60), Taixi (KI3), and Ah-shi points. To start with, there is the congealment of cold and dampness, so acupuncture is performed with the combination of reducing technique and moxibustion. When the pathogens are transformed into heat, the reducing technique should be performed likewise, but moxibustion is no longer used. In the remission stage, the reinforcing technique of acupuncture is given and moxibustion is resumed.

[CLINICAL EXPERIENCE]

1. CONVENTIONAL ACUPUNCTURE

(1) Penetrating Puncture

Points: Upper limb: from Quchi (LI11) to Shaohai (HT3), and from Waiguan (TE5) to Neiguan (PC6). Lower limb: from Yanglingquan (GB34) to Yinlingquan (SP9) and from Xuanzhong (GB39) to

Sanyinjiao (SP6).

Technique: All the points are punctured with strong stimulation and the needles are manipulated for two to three minutes. When the pain of fingers and toes is severe, Baxie (EX-UE9) and Bafeng (EX-LE10) are combined.

(2) Selection of Points According to Syndrome Differentiation

Points: Upper limb: Primary points: Quchi (LI11), Ximen (PC4), and Qingling (HT2); Secondary points: Shousanli (LI10) for the thumb and index finger, Neiguan (PC6) for the middle finger, Tongli (HT5) for little finger, Waiguan (TE5) for the ring finger, and Daling (PC7) for the palm and forearm. Lower limb: primary points: Xuehai (SP10) and Yinbao (LR9); secondary points: Yinlingquan (SP9) and Diji (SP8) for the 1st toe, Zusanli (ST36) and Fenglong (ST40) for the 2nd and 3rd toes, Yanglingquan (GB34) and Xuanzhong (GB39) for the 4th toe and the lateral aspect of the calf, Chengshan (BL57) and Kunlun (BL60) for the 5th toe and the posterior aspect of the calf, and Taixi (KI3) for the sole of planter.

Technique: Select the sensitively-reacting acupoints in the involved meridians from the affected limbs as the primary points and combine the ones selected according to the differentiation of symptoms and the affected areas. After the arrival of *qi,* the needle is scraped outward 10 times for excess-heat syndrome, or gently inward three to five times for cold-deficiency syndrome; for a mixture of both, the needle is scraped with even technique up and down repeatedly. One to five points can be selected each session and the treatment is given once every day or every other day. Fifteen sessions form one course of treatment, and there is a break of three to five days after each course. Antibiotics should be combined for infection during ulceration and the surface of eruption can be applied with "Hong Yi Xiao Gao (Red Powerful Effect Cream)."

2. MOXIBUSTION

(1) Mild Moxibustion with Moxa Stick

    A. Point: The affected area.

Technique: Moxibustion over the affected area for five to 10 minutes, once daily. Ten sessions make up one course.

B. Points: Select points around the ankle of the affect limb e.g., Fuliu (KI7), Taixi (KI3), Zhongfeng (LR4), Shangqiu (SP5), Kunlun (BL60), Guangming (GB37), Qiuxu (GB40), Zhaohai (KI6) and Shenmai (BL62); and Xuehai (SP10), Shenshu (BL23), Weizhong (BL40) and Chengjin (BL56).

Technique: Apply moxibustion with a moxa-stick to make the patient feel comfortable, two to four times a day. Patients may treat themselves. The method was used to treat 30 cases of this disease and 21 cases showed marked analgesic effect.

(2) Moxibustion with Moxa Cones

Points: Qihai (CV6), Zhongwan (CV12), Danzhong (CV17), Yangchi (TE4), Zusanli (ST36), Chongyang (ST42), Taixi (KI3), Feishu (BL13), Xinshu (BL15), Ganshu (BL18), Pishu (BL20), Shenshu (BL23), Pohu (BL42), Shentang (BL44), Geshu (BL17), Geguan (BL46), and Zhubin (KI9).

Technique: Three or four points are selected each session so that all the points are alternated for the puncture. Every time there must be a Back-Shu point in the prescription. Indirect moxibustion with a ginger slice is performed on the points, three cones for each point, once a day and five sessions in a course. The method is applicable to the early and convalescence stage of this disease.

3. AURICULAR THERAPY

Points: Heat Point (a bit inferior to the junction of the upper and lower crura of the antihelix) and the corresponding parts of the affected limbs. The secondary points: Sympathetic Nerve, Kidney, Subcortex, Heart, Lung, Liver, Spleen, Clavicle when the upper limb is affected and Hip Joint when the lower limb is affected.

Technique: Two or three pairs of points are selected each time and strong stimulation is given with needles rotated continuously for half to one minute, and then the needles are retained for one to two hours during which needling manipulation is carried out every 30 minutes. The treatment is given once daily, 10 to 12 days making up a course of treatment. The method has fair analgesic effect, but decreases with repeated use.

4. BLEEDING METHOD

(1) Intravenous Bleeding

Points: Yaoshu (GV2), Weizhong (BL40), Zulinqi (GB41), Taichong (LR3), and Jiexi (ST41).

Technique: Two points are selected each time and bled with a three-edged needle to draw out 3 ml of blood. The bleeding is given once every 12 days, six sessions making up one course of treatment. Consistent treatment with this method will surely obtain good effect. This disease has obstruction as its root cause and the manifestations of coldness, pain, claudication and ulceration as secondary superficiality. So the treatment principle aims at activating the circulation of blood and reopening the meridians and collaterals, which is why bleeding therapy is helpful.

(2) Leopard-spotted Puncture

Points: Primary points: affected area. Secondary points: 1) Zusanli (ST36) and Xuanzhong (GB39); 2) Yanglingquan (GB34) and Chengshan (BL57); 3) Xuehai (SP10) and Ququan (LR8); and 4) Yinlingquan (SP9) and Fuliu (KI7).

Technique: The affected area is given a leopard-spotted puncture to thrust the capillaries so that the stagnated blood is eliminated and the circulation of *qi* and blood is promoted. Then the secondary points are selected according to the affected areas: If the lateral aspect of the calf is affected, either A and or B group is recommended so the two can be alternated; if the medial aspect is affected, either C or D group can be prescribed. Conventional acupuncture is performed at the points, once daily, and one week is taken as a treatment course.

5. CATGUT-EMBEDDING METHOD

Points: Xuehai (SP10), Zusanli (ST36), Siqiang, Chengshan (BL57), and Fenglong (ST40).

Technique: No.2 or No.3 chromic catgut is used to penetrate the point for a transverse sewing. The distance between the two ends is 3 cm and is deep inside the muscles. The catgut is then pulled back from the same needle hole subcutaneously; no incision is made and neither is there ligation. The catgut is cut, patting the cut end under the skin. This treatment is given once every 10 to 15 days, with two or three points selected each session. Four to five sessions are taken as one course of treatment. There can be a two- or even three-month break between treatment courses.

6. OMBINED TREATMENT

Early stage (cold-damp syndrome): Neiguan (PC6), Taiyuan (LU9), Zusanli (ST36), Yanglingquan (GB34), Sanyinjiao (SP6) and Taixi (KI3). The first two are used for the affected upper limbs and the last two are for the lower limbs. All the points are performed with "Setting Mountain on Fire" needling technique and warming-needle moxibustion. Middle stage (heat syndrome): Besides the above points, Shenmen (HT7) is added and the "Through the Sky Cool" technique is used instead of the above. Weizhong (BL40) and Pangguangshu (BL28) are bled with a three-edged needle for a small amount of blood and cupping is added thereafter. Advanced stage (heat-toxin syndrome): The above treatment for the middle stage is combined with indirect moxibustion taking garlic as the media on Chongyang (ST42) and Taixi (KI3) and the area around the ulceration. In addition, a decoction made of Tougucao, Zhuidifeng, Dongguapi, Aiye and Chishao is administered, once in the morning and once in the evening. The residue is decocted with more water to fumigate and wash the affected area. "Yu Hong Gao (Jade Red Cream)" is used to dress the affected area once every other day.

[REMARKS]

1. Patients are required to stop smoking and prevent the invasion of the limbs by coldness and dampness. No tight and hard socks and shoes should be worn so as to avoid long-lasting compression to the blood vessels of the limbs. Vasoconstrictors are prohibited.

2. The affected limbs should be kept warm and the exercise of the affected limbs should be encouraged for elevating-dropping movement (lying supine and lifting the affected limbs to 45° and

keeping them there for two to three minutes, and then dropping the limb down below the bed for three to five minutes; finally, positioning the limb flat on the bed for two to three minutes) so that the formation of collateral circulation can be promoted.

3. To treat the disease with acupuncture, it should start as early as possible since acupuncture has satisfactory analgesia effect. In the later stage, surgical remedies should be combined for ulceration.

PANCREATITIS

[INTRODUCTION]

Pancreatitis is divided into two types, acute and chronic. Acute pancreatitis, occurring mainly among the young and matured adults, is characterized by such acute abdomen symptoms as sudden onset of upper abdominal pain associated with fever, nausea and vomiting, and its incidence is higher in females than in males. Chronic pancreatitis, which is featured by abdominal distention, diarrhea, etc., occurs more in males than in females. This disease is mainly caused by such factors as irregularity of food intake, an excessive greasy diet, and long-term immoderation in alcohol consumption, which would contribute to the accumulation of damp-heat and retention of food in the Middle-Jiao leading to the drastic harm to the spleen and stomach and dysfunction of liver and gallbladder in maintaining the flow of qi. Alternatively, it can be due to the liver being harmed by emotional disorders, e.g., depression and anger. Hence liver qi attacks the spleen transversely and results in disharmony between the liver and stomach. It can also be induced by roundworms, which may disturb the liver and gallbladder. The treatment is based on the principle of returning liver and gallbladder functions to normal, while the pancreas is cleared and the pain alleviated. Points of stomach and liver meridians are mainly selected, e.g., Ganshu (BL18), Danshu (BL19), Zhongwan (CV12), Liangmen (ST21), Neiguan (PC6), Yanglingquan (GB34), and Zusanli (ST36). All the points are punctured with reducing needling technique for acute pancreatitis and an attack of chronic pancreatitis, the needles being retained for 15 to 60 minutes several times daily. For chronic pancreatitis without attack, two or three points are punctured with reinforcing needling technique each time.

[CLINICAL EXPERIENCE]

1. CONVENTIONAL ACUPUNCTURE

(1) Hegu-Puncturing Method

Points: Zusanli (ST36) and Yanglingquan (GB34).

Technique: Both points are performed with reducing technique, and needles are retained for one hour, two or three times a day. In order to enhance the therapeutic effect, other points should be added according to syndrome differentiation, i.e., Taichong (LR3) for liver *qi* stagnation; Zhongwan (CV12), Quchi (LI11), and Xiangu (ST43) for excessive heat of spleen and stomach; Yinlingquan (SP9) for damp-heat in spleen and stomach; Neiguan (PC6) and Zhongwan (CV12) for nausea and vomiting; and Zhongwan (CV12) for severe abdominal pain.

(2) Puncturing Xi-Cleft Points

Points: Liangqiu (ST34), Neiguan (PC6), Gongsun (SP4), Taichong (LR3), and Ah-shi point.

Technique: The bilateral Xi-Cleft points of the stomach meridian are needled first with reducing technique and the needles are rotated for five minutes. Usually, the pain can be slightly eased after needling. Then the Ah-shi point should be found about 1 *cun* below Zusanli (ST36) and punctured with reducing technique. All the needles are retained for 30 to 60 minutes. Puncturing should be applied several times daily according to the individual condition.

(3) Penetrating Method for Four Points

Points: From Shangwan (CV13) to Zhongwan (CV12), Jianli (CV11), and Xiawan (CV10).

Technique: The patient lies supine and both legs are bent upward slightly. The physician, stretching the skin of Shangwan (CV13) with the left hand and holding a three-*cun* filiform needle with the right, inserts it from Shangwan (CV13) after sterilization, and thrusts it horizontally down to penetrate the other three points, Zhongwan (CV12), Jianli (CV11) and Xiawan (CV10). Then the needle is rotated continuously and retained for 10 to 30 minutes after the arrival of *qi*. Needling manipulation is given intermittently until the pain is relieved or disappears. Then large amplitude of rotation of needle is made three to five times and the needle is withdrawn slowly. Usually, the abdominal pain can be alleviated in 30 minutes.

2. INDIRECT MOXIBUSTION WITH SALT ON SHENQUE (CV8)

Points: Shenque (CV8).

Technique: Stir-fried salt powder is spread on the point up to the level of the abdomen surface, and three to five moxa cones are laid on top in succession. The method is used for severe abdominal pain due to the acute pancreatitis.

3. ELECTRIC ACUPUNCTURE

(1) Puncturing the Reacting Points in the Lower Limb

Points: Ah-shi point.

Technique: Tender spots can be found around Xiajuxu (ST39) or Diji (SP8), or on the medial aspect of the knee and 3 *cun* above. A two-*cun* needle is used to puncture perpendicularly these Ah-shi points to a depth of 1 or 1.5 *cun* with strong stimulation. The needles are then connected with an electro-acupuncture apparatus, the intensity of stimulation being based on the patient's tolerance. Needles are retained for 30 to 60 minutes. Three or four daily treatments are permissible during the acute stage.

(2) Puncturing Ah-shi Points at the Pancreas

Points: Abdominal Ah-shi point in combination of the points in lower limbs.

Technique: After ensuring the absence of remarkable peritonitis, the tender spot is found at the pancreas and the needle is thrust perpendicularly there. The needling depth depends on the patient's body build, but is usually between 3 to 7 *cun*. Strong stimulation is given and the needles are retained for 15 minutes. Then Yanglingquan (GB34) or Zusanli (ST36) can be punctured bilaterally with an electro-acupuncture apparatus for one hour. The treatment is given once or twice a day.

4. AURICULAR THERAPY

Points: Gallbladder, Pancreas, Sympathetic Nerve and Ear-Shenmen.

Technique: Usually, when there is attack of pancreatitis, the above points will be tender. Strong stimulation is given, and the needles retained for 60 minutes, several times a day. Alternatively, the subcutaneous needle-embedding method can be used.

5. HYDRO ACUPUNCTURE

Points: Zusanli (ST36) or Xiajuxu (ST39).

Technique: Five to 10 ml of 10% glucose injection is injected into each point, or a small dosage of compound wintermin is injected to stop vomiting. Or 0.25 mg of Atropine is injected in each point for analgesia. For chronic pancreatitis without an attack, 2 ml of Astragalus Injection and 2 ml of Angelica Injection are injected into the above points.

6. LASER THERAPY

Points: Ganshu (BL18), Pishu (BL20), Zhongwan (CV12), Zhangmen (LR13), Neiguan (PC6) and Zusanli (ST36).

Technique: The 3 to 25 mw He-Ne laser needle is used to irradiate the points for five minutes each time. This method is applicable to chronic pancreatitis and mild cases of acute pancreatitis.

7. ACUPOINT MASSAGE

Points: Liangmen (ST21), Zhangmen (LR13), Zusanli (ST36) and some Back-Shu points.

Technique: The abdominal points are taken as the primary points, i.e., Liangmen (ST21) and Zhangmen (LR13); while the points at the medial as well as the lateral aspects of the lower leg (from the ankle to the knee) are also performed with massage, and Zusanli (ST36) is pressed heavily; then the Back-Shu points from Shenshu (BL23) up to Xinshu (BL15) are selected for massage. During the attack, one session is given once every two to four hours, five to 15 minutes each time. When the condition is not so drastic, it can be done once or twice a day.

[REMARKS]

1.   For mild pancreatitis, acupuncture can be used alone since it is multiply effective for anti-inflammation, analgesia, regulating gastrointestinal functions, anti-infection, decreasing pancreatic secretion, and for anti-spasmodic and anti-emetic purpose. However, the medication should be combined in severe cases so as to have better therapeutic effect.

2.   Approximately half of the cases of acute pancreatitis are complicated by biliary disorders, so biliary diseases should be actively treated and prevented.

CHAPTER FIVE
OPHTHALMOLOGY AND OTORHINOLARYNGOLOGY

CONJUNCTIVITIS

[INTRODUCTION]

Conjunctivitis is caused by the infection of the conjunctiva by bacteria and viruses, and it is epidemic chiefly in summer and autumn. Clinically, this disease is divided into acute and chronic types. The acute type is characterized by congested conjunctiva, increased secretion from the eyes, burning sensation in the eyes, photophobia, acute onset and susceptibility to the epidemic. The chronic is featured by the thickness of the conjunctiva with a velvet surface, itching, burning, dryness and fatigue of the eyes. It is understood in traditional Chinese medicine that the acute form is due to the epidemic of pestilential factors, with the invasion by exogenous toxins, and the pathogenic heat is mixed with the wind, attacking the eyes. Meanwhile, the chronic form results from endogenous heat caused by *yin*-deficiency, or by the excessive intake of rich and spicy food giving rise to the fumigating of damp-heat to the eyes, or by the stimulus from dust and smoke. To treat the acute form, the principle is to expel the wind and heat, disperse the pestilential factors, and regain the normal functions of the liver and gallbladder; to treat the chronic form, the principle is to soothe the liver and subdue the endogenous wind, nourish *yin* and clear away the heat. Points are mainly selected from the gallbladder and bladder meridians, such as Jingming (BL1), Fengchi (GB20), Taiyang (EX-HN5), Hegu (LI4), Shangxing (GV23), Ganshu (BL18) and Zusanli (ST36). The reducing technique is used for acute cases and the even technique for chronic cases. The treatment is given once daily and the needles are retained for 10 to 20 minutes each time.

[CLINICAL EXPERIENCE]

1. CONVENTIONAL ACUPUNCTURE

(1) Puncturing Binao (LI14) as the Primary Point

Points: Main points: Binao (LI14). Supplementary points: Taiyang (EX-HN5), Jingming (BL1), Daling (PC7), Yangbai (GB14), Guangming (GB37) and Ganshu (BL18).

Technique: Needle Binao (LI14), the needle inserted along the running course of the large intestine meridian at an angle of 30°, and is then rotated rapidly for one to two minutes to produce the reducing technique. The needle is retained for 15 to 20 minutes. One to three secondary points can be selected each time.

(2) Selection of Points on the Syndrome Differentiation

Points: Jingming (BL1), Taiyang (EX-HN5), Chengqi (ST1), Zanzhu (BL2), Sizhukong (TE23), Fengchi (GB20) and Hegu (LI4). Shaoshang (HT3) and Shangxing (GV23) are combined for the syndrome of wind-heat; Taichong (LR3) and Yuyao (EX-HN4) are for the headache and eye pain; Daling (PC7) for the severe congestion of eyes; Yemen (TE2) for the congestion and dryness of the eyes; Shangxing (GV23) and Ganshu (BL18) for the pain in the inner canthus; Xiaxi (GB43) for the pain in the outer canthus, Ganshu (BL18), Erjian (LI2) and Zusanli (ST36) for the blurred vision; and Guangming (GB37), Sanyinjiao (SP6), Zusanli (ST36), Ganshu (BL18), Taichong (LR3) and Shuaigu (GB8) for the chronic type.

Technique: To treat acute cases, the penetrating method is carried out from Taiyang (EX-HN5) to Shuaigu (GB8), or just bleeding Taiyang (EX-HN5), or the bleeding is combined with cupping; Jingming (BL1) and Hegu (LI4) are treated with mild stimulation; Fengchi (GB20) is given mild sparrow-pecking to conduct the needling sensation to the eyes. The needles are retained for 10 to 20 minutes, once daily. The effect is fairly satisfactory.

2. MOXIBUSTION

(1) Mild Moxibustion with Moxa Stick

Points: Liangyanxue (Point for Measuring the Eyes).

Technique: The point is selected first in the following way: The patient takes a sitting position, and the ipsilateral elbow of the affected eye is flexed 170° to 180°. Then the arm is lifted upward and backward with the elbow put on the ipsilateral side of the head, and the elbow joint superior to the shoulder. At this time the forearm is over the shoulder and extended down to the ipsilateral side of the back. The middle finger is put two-finger breadth lateral to the spine, which is the location of the point [roughly the equivalent to the point Xinshu (BL15) or Dushu (BL 16)]. If both eyes are affected, both arms are used to find the point. Every time, mild moxibustion is given with moxa stick for five to 10 minutes until the skin becomes moderately flushed in the local region. The treatment is made once daily.

(2) Moxibustion for Extra Points

Points: Taiyang (EX-HN5), Dagukong (EX-UE5) and Xiaogukong (EX-UE6).

Technique: Taiyang (EX-HN5) is bled with a thick needle to let out one to three drops of blood, and then Dagukong (EX-UE5) and Xiaogukong (EX-UE6) are treated with non-scarring moxibustion with small moxa cones as big as the core of a jujube. Three cones are given each time. Alternatively, sparrow-pecking moxibustion with moxa stick can be given for three to five minutes.

3. AURICULAR THERAPY

(1) Auricular Needling

Points: Eye, Ear Apex, Lung and Liver.

Technique: All the points are needled with reducing needling technique, once daily or twice for acute and severe cases.

(2) Burning-Rush Moxibustion

Points: The upper part and the conjunction of capillary on the ipsilateral posterior auricular triangular fossa.

Technique: A piece of rush is taken and soaked with vegetable oil at the tip. After igniting, it is used to burn rapidly the above points and the skin burning sound must be heard clearly. If it is ineffective, the method is repeated the next day.

(3) Bleeding Method

Points: Primary points: Ear Apex, Eye, or the tender point on the auricle. Secondary points: Hypertensive Groove.

Technique: If there is tender point found on the auricle (looks like a millet-sized nodule), it is chosen first, otherwise the other points are selected. A three-edged needle is used to prick to a depth of 0.1 to 0.2 cm, and about three drops of blood are squeezed out. When the inflammation is remarkable, several spots of the Hypertensive Groove are punctured. The method was used to treat 30 cases of this disease and the patients were treated twice on average. The total effective rate was 96.7%.

4. PRICKING METHOD

Points: 1 *cun* lateral to Dazhui (GV14) up and down on both sides.

Technique: Strict sterilization is carried out on the above points, and they are then pricked with a three-edged needle to cut the subcutaneous fibers. Usually, one session can achieve a complete cure. In order to enhance the therapeutic effect, cupping should be combined for 10 minutes after the pricking.

5. SCALP ACUPUNCTURE

Points: Bilateral Vision Zone.

Technique: The 2.5-*cun* needles (Size: No.28) are used to puncture the points obliquely and the needles are connected with G6805 Electro-acupuncture Apparatus after being rotated for one minute. The dense-disperse wave is employed with a frequency of 200 beats per second. The needles are retained for 30 minutes. This method was used to treat 13 cases and all were cured.

6. INTRO-DERMAL NEEDLING

Points: ① Taiyang (EX-HN5) and Ganshu (BL18). ② Auricular points: Eye and Liver.

Technique: The wheat-grain-like intro-dermal needles are embedded each time in two points, e.g., left Taiyang (EX-HN5) with right Ganshu (BL18), and vice versa. The embedding normally is changed every second or third day, but is changed every day in summer.

7. LASER THERAPY

Points: ① Ipsilateral Jingming (BL1), Waiming (EX), Qiuhou (EX-HN7), Ah-shi point (the affected part of the bulbar conjunctiva), and Fengchi (GB20). ② Ipsilateral Jingming (BL1), Taiyang (EX-HN5), Ah-shi point and bilateral Fengchi (GB20) and Hegu (LI4).

Technique: The He-Ne laser, with a wavelength of 6328 A and output power of 5 mw in the needle, is used to treat conjunctivitis catarrhalis aestiva with the first group of points and sore conjunctivitis with the second group.

8. MEDICINAL APPLICATION ON ACUPOINTS

Points: Shaoshang (LU1).

Technique: An appropriate amount of fresh buttercup is mixed with a little salt and mashed into a paste. A soybean-sized paste is applied on the point contralaterally if only one eye is affected and bilaterally when both eyes are affected. When a blister appears, the paste is removed and the blister is just covered with a dressing so that it will be cured spontaneously.

[REMARKS]

1. Conjunctivitis is a common ophthalmic problem which responds well to acupuncture, especially the acute type. After the acupuncture treatment, there is a feeling of comfort and brightness in the eyes since the acupuncture is effective in analgesia and promoting the circulation of blood. If eye douche is combined during the treatment, the effect can be enhanced.

2. It is very important to prevent infectious conjunctivitis, so materials, such as towels and basin, should be disinfected by boiling and exposure to the sun. Attention should be paid to the isolation of the patients.

3. Spicy and hot food is prohibited in the duration of the disease.

STY

[INTRODUCTION]

Sty is an acute purulent inflammation at the margin of the eyelid or inside it, and is usually divided into external sty (occurs at the outer surface of the eyelid skin and the purulence moves out on the skin surface after diabrosis) and internal sty (occurs at the inner surface of the eyelid skin and the purulence moves out on the surface of the palpebral conjunctiva after diabrosis). This disease is often multiple or recurrent, and usually occurs fairly abrupt, mostly in one eye, but possibly in both eyes in some cases. It is maintained in traditional Chinese medicine that the disease is mainly caused by the exogenous wind-heat pathogen invading the eyelid, or by the excessive intake of fried, roasted, and spicy food, which leads to damp-heat in the spleen and stomach. When the damp-heat runs up and the heat toxin accumulates in the skin and meridians of the eyelid, there occurs the disease. The recurrence is due to the lingering toxin or the susceptibility to the invasion of the wind-toxin because of the insufficiency of the *qi* and blood. Clinically, it is manifested as the congestion of the eyelid, edema, tenderness, and hard nodules. The principle of treatment is to dissipate the wind, clear away the heat, and disperse the stagnation. To the chronic cases, the spleen should be built up and the *qi* is replenished. Points of the stomach and bladder meridians are selected mainly, e.g., Jingming (BL1), Zanzhu (BL2), Chengqi (ST1), Hegu (LI4), Xingjian (LR2), etc. Reducing needling technique is performed.

[CLINICAL EXPERIENCE]

1. CONVENTIONAL ACUPUNCTURE

(1) Puncturing Yangming Points Alone
Points: Hegu (LI4) and Quchi (LI11).

Technique: The ipsilateral Hegu (LI4) and Quchi (LI11) (or bilateral when both eyes are affected) are punctured for 0.5 to 1 *cun*, the rotation technique is employed to carry the needling sensation upward, and the needles are retained for 10 minutes.

(2) Single-Point Puncture

Points: Sanyinjiao (SP6).

Technique: The point is selected ipsilaterally or the bilaterally when both eyes are affected; the puncture goes for 1.5 to 2 *cun* with strong stimulation. The needle is not retained. Hairy needling is combined all around the orbital ridge repeatedly for two or three times. The treatment is given once a day, consecutively for three to four days.

(3) Extra-Point Puncture

Points: Ah-shi point.

Technique: If the sty is on the upper eyelid, a filiform needle is inserted horizontally at the level of the upper border of the lump from the lateral-superior or from the medial-superior side; the tip of the needle should reach the lump. If the lump is fairly big, the needle tip reaches its upper border; and if the lump is big and in the middle of the lower lid, the needle tip should reach the lower border of the lump. The needle is retained for five minutes. If the sty is close to the inner canthus, the needle is inserted through the medial aspect; and if the sty is close to the outer canthus, the needle is inserted from the lateral aspect.

2. MOXIBUSTION

(1) Moxibustion at Meridian Points

Points: Houxi (SI3).

Technique: The contralateral selection of point is mainly adopted; the disease in the right eye is treated by the point on the left, and vice versa. Two millet-sized moxa cones are positioned directly on the skin of the point successively. When the second cone is finished, the ash is pressed slightly on the point rapidly with the hand. Usually, the problem should be cured in two to four days. It is more effective for early cases without purulence.

(2) Burning-Rush Moxibustion

Points: The local part of the disease and the reacting spots on both sides of the thoracic spine and the scapular region.

Technique: First, find the reacting spots in the scapular region (the red-colored or black- or brown-colored millet-sized spots). A piece of rush soaked with vegetable oil is ignited and moxibustion carried out on three to five spots. The lump should disappear the next day. But it is not so effective for purulent sties.

3.   BLEEDING METHOD

(1) *Bleeding He-Sea Points*
Points: Quchi (LI11).

Technique: The contralateral Quchi (LI11) is pricked with a three-edged needle and a small drop of blood squeezed out, once a day.

(2) *Bleeding Back-Shu Points*
Points: Ganshu (BL18).

Technique: The ipsilateral Ganshu (BL18) is bled, or the bilateral ones are bled if both eyes are affected, with a needle (Size: No.26 or No.28). The needle is thrust obliquely for 0.4 to 0.6 *cun*. After the arrival of *qi,* reducing technique with strong stimulation is performed and after rotating the needle several times, it is taken out slowly with the swaying method to enlarge the needle hole. When the needle is removed, the needle hole is not pressed, but is squeezed to let out a small drop of blood.

(3) *Bleeding Extra Points*
Points: The tips of the middle toes.

Technique: The tips of middle toes are pricked to let out three to five drops of blood. Routine sterilization is carried out before and after the bleeding to prevent infection.

(4) *Bleeding the Reacting Points*
Points: Sty point on the back.

Technique: Find the sty points (look like pimples) on the back, usually in the area between the 1st to the 7th thoracic vertebrae and 3 *cun* lateral. The ones in the area between the 4th and the 7th thoracic vertebrae are the most effective. If there are no such sty points, Gao-huang (BL43) or Jiaji (EX-B2) between the 3rd and the 9th thoracic vertebrae can be prescribed. After local sterilization, a three-edged needle, or an injection needle, is used to prick the points for 1 mm. The skin is pricked and the cutaneous fibers are cut. Then a small amount of blood is squeezed out and cupping is combined over the points for five to 10 minutes.

3. WRIST-ANKLE ACUPUNCTURE

Points: Zone 1 and Zone 2 above the wrist.

Technique: When the sty is at the inner canthus, Zone 1 above the wrist [equivalent to the place 0.5 *cun* above the point Lingdao (HT4)] is selected; if the sty is at the outer canthus, Zone 2 above the wrist [equivalent to the point Neiguan (PC6)] is used; and if the sty is located in between, a needle is added lateral to Zone 2. For severe cases, auricular acupressure with embedding of Semen Vaccaria can be combined on the points Eye, Ear-Shenmen, and Liver. Usually 1.5-*cun* needles (Size: No.30) are used to make a horizontal puncture for 1.2 *cun*, and the patient can experience the sensation of soreness, numbness, distension and pain. The needles are fixed with adhesive plaster and retained for half a day.

4. AURICULAR THERAPY

(1) Moxibustion

Point: Eye.

Technique: A moxa stick is used for moxibustion over the point Eye (located at the ear lobe) for five minutes, once in both morning and afternoon. The effect is fairly satisfactory.

(2) Bleeding Method

Points: Ear Apex or the vein in the back of the auricle.

Technique: After sterilization, a three-edged needle is used to prick the point and three drops of blood are squeezed out from the needle hole. Then the needle hole is pressed close with a dry cotton ball. The method has an effective rate of 90%.

(3) Needle-Embedding Method

Points: Eye, Eye 1, Eye 2, Liver, Ear-Shenmen, and Subcortex.

Technique: After sterilization, two or three points are selected each time. The thumb-tag needles are thrust in the points and are fixed with adhesive plaster. The patient is required to press the needles three to five times a day, one to three minutes each time. Re-examination is carried out three days after. If it is found to be ineffective, the treatment is repeated. The cure time on average is 1.5 days. This method is inapplicable during pregnancy and for inflammatory disorders of the auricle.

5. CUTANEOUS PUNCTURE

Points: Around the affected part, Yintang (EX-HN3) and Taiyang (EX-HN5).

Technique: If the sty is on the upper eyelid, the skin between the upper lid and the eyebrow is tapped; and the skin between the lower lid and the point Chengqi (ST1) is tapped if the sty is on the lower eyelid. The tapping is performed to create a burning sensation in the local region or to make the skin flushed. The treatment is given three times a day, three to five days forming one course of treatment. To treat phlyctenular conjunctivitis, the peri-orbital skin is tapped as well as Yintang (EX-HN3) and Taiyang (EX-HN5) on the affected side until there is slight bleeding.

6. CUTTING THERAPY

Points: Near the scapula.

Technique: The cutting is done contralaterally, i.e., cutting the right scapular region when the left eye is affected, and vice versa. The local area is first sterilized, and then 0.2 ml of 2% procaine is injected. A small vessel forceps is used to clamp the point and a small operating knife is used to make the circular cut of the skin. The fibrous tissues must be severed and anti-inflammatory cream applied. Finally, it is covered with the small gauze.

7. INTRAVENOUS BLEEDING PLUS CUPPING

Points: Dazhui (GV14).

Technique: After the point is sterilized, a three-edged needle is used to bleed it and cupping is then combined thereafter for about 10 minutes.

[REMARKS]

1. To treat the disease in the early stage of inflammation, acupuncture can promote the absorption and repercussion and is also effective for analgesia. When there is suppuration, acupuncture can be helpful to further phylogenic maturation. When the suppuration is erupted, acupuncture can decrease the discharge of pus. Clinically speaking, the effect of acupuncture in the treatment of this disease is the most optimal in non-suppurative cases. In early non-suppurative cases, the pricking therapy is also satisfactorily effective.

2. It is not permitted to press or squeeze the affected area so as to avoid spreading the inflammation to prevent the occurrence of palpebral or orbital cell ulitis or even the cavernous sinus emboli or hematocepsis.

DACRYORRHEA

[INTRODUCTION]

This disease is divided into "cold tear" and "heat tear" in traditional Chinese medicine. The "heat tear" is mainly due to "fire" while "cold tear" is chiefly due to "coldness." If the heat tear is characterized by the running of hot tears when exposed to the wind, it is caused by accumulated heat in the liver meridian plus the invasion of exogenous pathogenic wind; the flaming up of fire resulting from *yin* deficiency in the liver and kidney means it is unable to balance *yang*. The cold tear can also takes place in exposure of wind and it is attributable to insufficiency of liver blood plus the invasion by exogenous pathogenic wind cold; and the cold tear, appearing at any time despite the absence of exposure to wind, is brought on by a coexistent deficiency of liver and kidney and the consumption of *yin* and blood leading to the harming of *yang*. Thus the tears cannot be controlled. In the cases of cold tear, there can be such manifestations as normal appearance of the eyes, lacrimation only in exposure of wind or at any time without the wind, clearness and thinness of the tears without hot feeling, or just moisture in the inner canthus in a mild case, but the running of tears out of the eyelids and even down to the cheek in severe cases. In the case of heat tear, there can be manifestations as reddened and swollen eyes, burning pain, photophobia, running of turbid tears aggravated when exposed to wind, and hot feeling from the tears. To treat heat tears, the principle is to expel the wind and clear away the heat, dispersing the stagnation of liver *qi* to brighten the eyes; for cold tear, the treatment serves to reinforce the liver and kidney, disperse the wind and stop the abnormal running of tears. Such points as Jingming (BL1), Zanzhu (BL2), Fengchi (GB20), Hegu (LI4), Taichong (LR3), Ganshu (BL18), Danshu (BL19) and Shenshu (BL23) are prescribed in the treatment and the reinforcing and reducing needling techniques are combined.

[CLINICAL EXPERIENCE]

1. CONVENTIONAL ACUPUNCTURE

(1) Midnight-Noon Ebb-Flow Acupuncture

Points: ① Ququan (LR8) and Fuliu (KI7). ② Chize (LU5) and Shugu (BL65).

Technique: For cold tear, reinforcing Ququan (LR8) at 3:00 to 5:00 a.m. and Fuliu (KI7) at 7:00 to 9:00 p.m.; and for heat tear, reducing Chize (LU5) at 3:00 to 5:00 a.m. and Shugu (BL65) at 3:00 to 5:00 p.m.

(2) Selection of Points According to Differentiation

Points: Jingming (BL1), Yingxiang (LI20), Sibai (ST2), Fengchi (GB20) and Hegu (LI4).

Technique: For cold tear, the reinforcing technique is performed with filiform needles, and for heat tear, the reducing technique is given. The needles are retained for 30 minutes.

(3) Grouping of Points

Points: Main points: Jingming (BL1). Supplementary points: Zanzhu (BL2), Touwei (ST8), Juliao (ST3) and Fengchi (GB20).

Technique: In the first day of treatment, Jingming (BL1) is selected; on the second day, Jingming (BL1) is combined with Zanzhu

(BL2); on the third day, Jingming (BL1) with Touwei (ST8); on the fourth day, Jingming (BL1) with Juliao (ST3); and on the fifth day, Jingming (BL1) with Fengchi (GB20). The needle-rotating technique is combined with sparrow-pecking technique and mild stimulation is given on all the points except Jingming (BL1), which is performed only with perpendicular thrust and free from any other techniques in order to prevent bleeding. The needles are not retained. Five days form one course of treatment, and there should be a two-day break between two courses. According to observation, this method is helpful to open the lachrymal passage.

(4) Treatment Based on Classical Literature

Point: Tianzhu (BL10).

Technique: The point is thrust perpendicularly and is performed with rotating and lifting-thrusting techniques for reinforcement. This method is selected from *Inquiry. Miraculous Pivot* in which it says: "Tianzhu (BL10) is reinforced for the cases of deficiency with uncontrolled running of tears, for the meridian is traveling along the nape of the neck." Later Dr. Yang Yongxuan, a famous acupuncture physician, also used this method to treat uncontrollable running of tears due to the emotional depression and pathogenic factors attacking upward into the eyes, and obtained immediate effect.

2. MOXIBUSTION

Points: Ganshu (BL18), Baihui (GV20), Fengchi (GB20), Houxi (SI3), Dagukong (EX-UE5), Xiaogukong (EX-UE6) and Touwei (ST8).

Technique: All the points are performed with non-scarring moxibustion by means of moxa cones, seven cones for Ganshu (BL18), three cones for Baihui (GV20), five to seven cones for Fengchi (GB20), five to seven cones for Dagukong (EX-UE5) and Xiaogukong (EX-UE6) each, five cones for Houxi (SI3), and three cones for Touwei (ST8).

3. AURICULAR THERAPY

Points: Eye, Liver, Eye and Kidney.

Technique: All the points are punctured or given acupressure with

Semen Vaccaria. The puncture is made with even technique and the needles are retained for 30 minutes. The needling is given once daily, while acupressure is used once every three days in summer and once every five days in winter.

4. Intravenous Bleeding Plus Cupping

Points: Taiyang (EX-HN5).

Technique: A needle (Size: No.28) is used to thrust perpendicularly the ipsilateral Taiyang (EX-HN5), and after the arrival of *qi,* the needle is retained for 20 to 30 minutes with manipulation every 10 minutes. After the removal of the needle, cupping is made on the point for 10 minutes and a herbal plaster is applied on the point when the cupping is finished.

5. Pricking Method

Points: The tender spots in the scapular region.

Technique: One tender spot or two should be selected and pricked with a three-edged needle. The muscle fibers should be cut off and cupping is combined after pricking for 10 minutes. The method is given once every six days. It is fairly effective for heat tear.

[REMARKS]

1.   Acupuncture is satisfactorily effective in the treatment of heat tear, but the effectiveness is not so satisfactory for cold tear.

2.   Attention should be paid to maintaining good eye hygiene.

MYOPIA

[INTRODUCTION]

Myopia is one of the ametropic disorders. In terms of traditional Chinese medicine, it is due to innate insufficiency or inheritance; or due to working and studying under dim light, or in an improper position, so that there is over-exertion of the heart and mind, the heart

Yang is lessened, the eye collaterals stagnate so that the vital light in the eye becomes unable to reach very far. Alternatively it can be caused by chronic illness, postpartum exhaustion, over-indulgence in sexual activities giving rise to the deficiency of the liver and kidney and insufficiency of essence and blood. Thus the eyes are not well nourished and the vital light declines, limiting vision. To treat this disorder, the principle is to activate the circulation of *qi* and blood and to refresh the tendons and collaterals to brighten the eyes. Such points as Zanzhu (BL2), Chengqi (ST1), Taiyang (EX-HN5), Fengchi (GB20), Hegu (LI4), Guangming (GB37) and Taichong (LR3) are selected. Other points can be combined including Ganshu (BL18), Shenshu (BL23) and Taixi (KI3) for deficiency of the liver and kidney; Neiguan (PC6), Shenmen (HT7) and Xinshu (BL15) for weakness of the heart and mind. Attention should be paid to an appropriate combination of local and distant points. The primary points are performed with even needling technique, but with reinforcing technique by rotating the needles for the secondary points.

[CLINICAL EXPERIENCE]

1. CONVENTIONAL ACUPUNCTURE

(1) Taking Chengqi (ST1) as the Primary Point

Points: Main points: Chengqi (ST1). Supplementary points: Yiming (EX-HN14) and Fengchi (GB20).

Technique: A 1.5-*cun* needle (Size: No.30) is thrust at Chengqi (ST1) obliquely toward Jingming (BL1) at an angle of 30° for about 1 *cun* deep. The needle is retained for five minutes after the appearance of a sensation such as soreness and distention in the orbital region and running tears. After withdrawal, the needle hole should be pressed with a dry cotton ball for couple of minutes to avoid bleeding. Both Yiming (EX-HN14) and Fengchi (GB20) are punctured for 0.8 *cun* and the needles are retained for 10 minutes after the arrival of *qi*. The treatment is given once a day and 10 sessions are taken as one course of treatment with the three-day interval after each course. A total of 1,894 eyes were treated with this method, among which 360 (19.5%)

were cured in the short-term, 555 (29.2%) were showed marked improvement, 773 (40.8%) were improved, and 198 (10.5%) were unchanged.

(2) Inducing the Extension of Needling Sensation

Points: Guangming (GB37) in combination of Waiguan (TE5); and Taichong (LR3) in combination with Hegu (LI4).

Technique: The two groups of points are alternated for the needling. After the arrival of *qi* the needles are rotated in small amplitude to maintain the extension of the needling sensation so as to conduct it up to the face. Or if the needling sensation fails to move up to the face, but it is extended halfway along the running course of the meridian, it is also considered as a success. The treatment is given once daily and 15 days make up one course of treatment. There is a seven-day break after each course. A total of 182 eyes were treated with this method, and 157 (86.3%) were improved to varying degrees, among which 42 (23.1%) were restored to normal vision (above 1.0).

(3) Puncturing Extra Points

Points: Huiguang (located at the crossing point between the longitudinal line from the mastoid process and the parallel line drawn backward from the cricoid cartilage when the patient lies supine with the head turning to one side), Mingchaxue (at the anterior border of the fibula and 8 *cun* above the external malleolus), and Xiaoyixue (0.2 *cun* below the midpoint of the lateral orbital margin).

Technique: Huiguang is punctured perpendicularly for 0.3 *cun* and the needling sensation should reach the ipsilateral temporal region and the orbital margin. Mingchaxue is needled perpendicularly for 1 *cun* to 1.5 *cun* to conduct the needling sensation down to the lateral aspect of the lower limb, and the needle is retained for 10 minutes. Xiaoyixue is thrust when the patient is lying supine; the needle is inserted perpendicular from below the lateral orbital margin between the margin and the eyeball with the tip of needle backward, inward and slightly upward, so the needle body is very close to the eyeball and the depth of puncture is 1 *cun* to 1.5 *cun*. However, for those under 14 years of age, the depth should only be less than 0.8 *cun*. The needle is retained for 10 to 15 minutes and manipulation is given once every five minutes so as to send the needling sensation to the entire orbital region. The treatment is given once for every other day and 10 sessions make up one course. Acupressure on the eyes should be combined. The cure/marked-effect rate for true myopia is up to 68%. The therapeutic actions of these three points were compared with some conventional meridian points, i.e., needling Tongziliao (GB1), Sibai (ST2) and Guangming (GB37), of which the cure/marked-effect rate is only 25% for true myopia.

2. ELECTRO-IMPULSE THERAPY

Points: ① bilateral Jingming (BL1). ② bilateral Taiyang (EX-HN5). ③ bilateral Sibai (ST2).

Technique: The electric poles are placed on the points of both sides, and each group is stimulated for five minutes with the frequency of 80 to 100 beats/minute. The intensity should be strong enough to produce the feeling of vibration but not beyond the patient's tolerance. The treatment is given once daily and 10 sessions form one course. Acupressure is combined on the points, such as Jingming (BL1), Yuyao (EX-HN4), Xuanli (GB6) or just the infraorbitale margin, twice a day.

3. PLUM-BLOSSOM ACUPUNCTURE

Points: ① Both sides of the cervical spine, from the external occipital protuberance to Dazhui (GV14). ② The orbital region.

Technique: Tapping is made for five to 10 times from the top to the bottom on both sides of the cervical spine with heavier stimulation to make small bleeding spots after the treatment. The orbital region is tapped from the medial to the lateral three to five times with mild stimulation to make the skin flush and produce a burning sensation. The treatment is given once daily, 10 sessions in one course, and there is a three to five-day break after each course.

4. ELECTRIC PLUM-BLOSSOM ACUPUNCTURE

(1) Method 1
Points: ① Jingming (BL1) and Chengqi (ST1). ② Sizhukong (TE23)

and Qiuhou (EX-HN7).

Technique: In the treatment, two electric plum-blossom needles are positioned perpendicularly on the above points with the current strong enough to give a mild tingling sensation in the local region. Continuous wave is applied, about two to three Hz/second. The treatment is performed once daily for five to 10 minutes each time, and 10 sessions form one course. After a seven-day break, a re-examination is carried out, and if the treatment appears effective, a further course will be implemented. In the first two courses, Jingming (BL1) and Chengqi (ST1) are used, and in the third and fourth courses, Sizhukong (TE23) and Qiuhou (EX-HN7) are selected.

(2) Method 2

Points: ① Primary points: $Zhengguang_1$ [the midpoint between Yuyao (EX-HN 4) and Zanzhu (BL2), at the junction of the 3/4 of the medial side of the supraorbitale margin] and $Zhengguang_2$ [the midpoint between Sizhukong (TE23) and Yuyao (EX-HN 4)]. Secondary points: Fengchi (GB20), Neiguan (PC6) and Dazhui (GV14). ② The points are selected in terms of areas, i.e., nape, orbital region and temporal region.

Technique: The two groups of points are alternated. Altogether, 1,158 cases involving 2,284 eyes were treated with this method. Of these, 494 eyes (21.6%) were cured, 1,307 (57.4%) were markedly improved, 461 (20.2%) were improved, and 22 (1%) were unchanged. From the view of clinical effect, the smaller the diopter, the better the therapeutic effect; it is more effective to stimulate the points than to do the areas; and electric plum-blossom needling is more effective than ordinary plum-blossom needling. Plum-blossom needle tapping, or just massage at Zhengguang can all increase visual acuity.

5. AURICULAR THERAPY

(1) Needle-Embedding in Auricular Points

Points: Liver, Kidney, Heart, Eye_1, Eye_2 and Eye.

Technique: The contralateral points are selected; or if both eyes are affected, in the first session the left eye and the right liver and kidney are used; in the second session, the left liver and kidney and the right eye are used; and in the third session, the left eye_2 and the right heart are selected. Eye_2 is combined all the time for those with astigmia. All the points are sterilized and then sterilized forceps are used to grip the disinfected thumb-tag auricular needles for insertion, after which these are fixed with plaster. Usually, the needles are changed every five days but this should be reduced to every four days in summer. Altogether, 207 cases of myopia are treated, among which 21 (10.1%) were basically cured, 41 (19.8%) were markedly effective, 128 (61.8%) were improved, and 17 (8.2%) were unchanged.

(2) Ear-Seed Method

Points: Main points: The junction between the endocrine and subcortex, liver and kidney. Supplementary points: Eye, Eye_1 and Eye_2.

Technique: Three to four points are selected each time from the primary and secondary points. Both ears are treated simultaneously. Semen Vaccaria are pressed on the points with adhesive plaster. The seeds should be pressed three to four times a day, one or two minutes each time. One session is given every five to seven days in winter, and every two to three days in summer. There is a break of a couple of days after each session and four sessions form one course. A total of 517 cases were treated with the method and the total effective rate was 75%.

6. WRIST-ANKLE ACUPUNCTURE

Points: $Upper_1$ point (in the depression anterior to the ulnar border on the side of the 5th finger, the thumb is used to press the point).

Technique: Bilateral points are used if both eyes are affected and the ipsilateral point is selected when only one eye is affected. There should be no pain when the needle is inserted. The needle is retained for one hour, during which the patient must stare into the distance. Needling is given once a day and 10 sessions form one course. There is a five-day break after each course. Usually two or three courses are needed. The total effective rate is 84.9%.

7. LASER THERAPY

Points: Jingming (BL1), Chengqi (ST1) and Guangming (GB37).

Technique: The 3 to 7 mw He-Ne laser therapeutic apparatus is used to perform acupoint irradiation, five minutes each time, once a day. Ten sessions form one course of treatment.

[REMARKS]

1. Myopia is a common juvenile disease. Acupuncture can obtain certain effect in treating simple myopia, especially the satisfactory short-term effect; but it is not indicated for the underdevelopment or mal-development of the orbital tissues due to congenital factors.

2. During the treatment, or for a period after the treatment, good habits of protecting the eyes should be established, e.g., try to avoid watching TV, don't read under a dim light or read for a long time (a rest for five or 10 minutes is necessary after study or reading for one hour) in order to avoid exertion of the orbital muscles that will lessen the effect of the acupuncture treatment. Regular self-massage protection on the peri-orbital acupoints is quite significant to consolidating the therapeutic effect.

STRABISMUS

[INTRODUCTION]

Strabismus is referred to as a disorder whereby both eyes are unable to focus together straight ahead. Clinically, the disease is divided according to the symptoms into esotropia (paralysis of the bulbar abductor muscle) and exotropia (paralysis of the bulbar adductor muscle). The chief complaints include the deviation of the cornea and iris to the inner or outer canthus, impaired bulbar motion, and double vision. The pathogenesis of the disease is related to the invasion of the meridians and collaterals by exogenous pathogenic wind, giving rise to contraction and cramp of the tendons and vessels; or to weakness of the spleen and stomach leading to inadequate transportation and transformation of dietary nutrients, resulting in the tendons and vessels being malnourished and the ocular system becoming flaccid; or deficiency of the kidney and liver in their essence and blood, leading to failure of the eyeball to be well maintained; or traumatic injury on the head and eyes damaging the tendons and vessels bringing on stagnation of *qi* and blood and malnourishment of the optic system. To treat the disease, the principle is to expel the wind and reopen the meridians and collaterals, reinforce *qi* in the middle-Jiao, tonify the kidney and liver, and regulate the flow of *qi* and blood to disperse the stagnation. Hand and foot Taiyang, Shaoyang and Yangming meridians are mainly prescribed, such as: Fengchi (GB20), Chengqi (ST1), Yangbai (GB14), Jingming (BL1), Hegu (LI4), Zusanli (ST36), Taichong (LR3) and Zulinqi (GB41). All the points are performed with moderate stimulation, except those in the ocular region, which are stimulated mildly. The needles are retained for 10 to 20 minutes. Ten sessions make up one course of treatment.

[CLINICAL EXPERIENCE]

1. CONVENTIONAL ACUPUNCTURE

Points: Esotropia: ① Tongziliao (GB1), Fengchi (GB20), Sibai (ST2) and Taichong (LR3). ② Qiuhou (EX-HN7), Taiyang (EX-HN5), Muchuang (GB16) and Waiguan (TE5). ③ Sizhukong (TE23), Yuyao (EX-HN4), Touwei (ST8) and Guangming (GB37). Exotropia: ① Jingming (BL1), Meichong (BL3), Yuyao (EX-HN4) and Hegu (LI4). ② Zanzhu (BL2), Sibai (ST2), Fengchi (GB20) and Taichong (LR3).

Technique: The groups of points are used alternately, and the treatment is given once daily. There are 12 sessions in one course, with a five to seven-day break between two courses. Points are needled bilaterally if both eyes are affected and ipsilaterally when only one eye is affected. For children under five, the rotating needling technique is adopted for the in-and-out needling, with no retention. Juveniles who can cooperate with the treatment receive even needling technique but the lifting-thrusting needling technique is avoided for the points in the ocular region. Needles are retained for 30 minutes, during which manipulation is given twice. This method can play a role of dredging the meridians, promoting the local nerves by changing from paralysis to excitation, and the muscles from asthenia or paralysis to normal function.

2. ELECTRIC PLUM-BLOSSOM NEEDLING

Points: Zhengguang$_1$ [the midpoint between Yuyao (EX-HN 4) and Zanzhu (BL2), inferior to the supraorbitale margin], Zhengguang$_2$ [the midpoint between Sizhukong (TE23) and Yuyao (EX-HN 4), inferior to the supraorbitale margin], Fengchi (GB20), Neiguan (PC6), Dazhui (GV14), Baihui (GV20), Ganshu (BL18), Danshu (BL19), Pishu (BL20), Shenshu (BL23), Zhongwan (CV12), and both sides from the 8th to the 12th thoracic vertebrae and the lumbar region.

Technique: The disease is treated stage by stage. In the first stage, Zhengguang$_1$, Zhengguang$_2$, Fengchi (GB20), Neiguan (PC6), Dazhui (GV14), Baihui (GV20), Ganshu (BL18) and Danshu (BL19) are selected. After the attainment of the effect, both sides from the 8th to the 12th thoracic vertebrae and the lumbar region, Pishu (BL20), Shenshu (BL23) and Zhongwan (CV12) are added to the above points. The plum-blossom needle is connected with electricity through the transistor therapeutic apparatus; the electric voltage is 9 v and the current is less than 5 ma. The intensity of the current is based on patient tolerance. Tapping is carried out 20 to 50 times on each point in the area of 0.5 to 1 cm in diameter. On both sides of the thoracic and lumbar spine, the tapping is performed from the top to the bottom in three lines (the first is 1 cm lateral to the spine, the second 2 cm and the third 3 or 4 cm). The treatment is given once every other day and 15 sessions form a course. A half-month break is given before the next course. The tapping force should be moderate. Patients are required to do self-massage on the Zhengguang point bilaterally, 50 to 100 times of manipulation each time, three sessions a day. The wearing of spectacles should be avoid during the treatment. The method was used to treat 103 cases of concomitant strabismus; after 15 to 105 sessions (36.5 sessions on average), the total effective rate was up to 98.3%. The less severe cases obtained more satisfactory therapeutic effect, while for the more severe cases, the effectiveness was less satisfactory.

3. LASER THERAPY

Points: Qiuhou (EX-HN7), Jingming (BL1), Tongziliao (GB1), Hegu (LI4) and Taichong (LR3).

Technique: The 3 to 7 mw He-Ne laser needle is used to irradiate the above points, five minutes for each, once a day.

4. AURICULAR THERAPY

Points: Eye, Liver, Kidney, Eye_1, Eye_2, Sympathetic Nerve, and Ear-Shenmen.

Technique: Short filiform needles are used to give moderate stimulation and the needles are retained for 30 minutes, during which manipulation is given intermittently. After the removal of the needles, Semen Vaccaria are stuck on the points for one or two days in summer and three to five days in winter.

5. MAGNET-ELECTRIC THERAPY

Points: Sibai (ST2), Yangbai (GB14), Taiyang (EX-HN5), Zanzhu (BL2), Pishu (BL20), Weishu (BL21), Guangming (GB37) and Fengchi (GB20).

Technique: Two or three points are selected each time and all the points are alternated in the treatment. The therapy is given once a day, 30 minutes each time with intermittent wave. Twenty sessions form one course of treatment and there is a three to five-day break after each course.

[REMARKS]

1. Acupuncture has fairly good therapeutic effect in treating this disease.

2. If it is paralytic strabismus (mostly in children), further examination should be made and etiological treatment given thereafter. If it is concomitant strabismus, eyeglasses can be worn to improve vision.

3. After obtaining the effect, further treatment should be done for consolidation and to prevent recurrence.

RETINOPATHY

[INTRODUCTION]

Retinopathy includes central retinitis, central retinochorioiditis, retinal vein obstruction, obstruction of the retinal artery, retinal hemorrhage, and arteriosclerosis of the retina. This disease occurs more in male adults. The chief complaints are diminution of vision in varying degrees, and sudden loss of partial or entire vision, central darkness, metamorphopsia, micropsia and deviated vision in those with obstruction of the retinal artery. Lateral headache is often present in the early stage. In terms of traditional Chinese medicine, the pathogenesis of this disease involves mental fatigue and over-exertion of the eyes, or insufficiency of the liver and kidney in their blood and essence being unable to nourish the eyes; or *yin*-deficiency leading to the flaring-up of fire which disturbs upward the ocular orifice; or emotional abnormality giving rise to the stagnation of liver *qi,* leading to stagnant flow of *qi* and blood obstructing the meridians and collaterals; or weakness of the spleen and stomach resulting in the failure of clear-*yang* ascending and turbid-*yin* descending, thus blocking the ocular collaterals. The treatment serves to tonify the liver and kidney, regulate the flow of *qi* and blood, build up the spleen to resolve the phlegm, and disperse the obstruction in the meridians and collaterals. The local points in the ocular region and the Back-Shu points are mainly selected, such as Jingming (BL1), Taiyang (EX-HN5), Yangbai (GB14), Qiuhou (EX-HN7), Hegu (LI4), Guangming (GB37), Taichong (LR3), Ganshu (BL18), Pishu (BL20) and Shenshu (BL23), all of which are performed with even needling technique.

[CLINICAL EXPERIENCE]

1. CONVENTIONAL ACUPUNCTURE

(1) Combining the Primary and Secondary Points

Points: Group 1: Main points: Qiuhou (EX-HN7), Jingming (BL1), Jianming (EX) and Chengqi (ST1); Supplementary points:

Sibai (ST2), Yiming (EX-HN14), Fengchi (GB20), Quchi (LI11) and Hegu (LI4). Group 2: Main points: the same as those in Group 1; Supplementary points: Quchi (LI11), Yifeng (TE17), Tianzhu (BL10), Guangming (GB37), Waiguan (TE5), Dazhui (GV14), Fengchi (GB20), Mingmen (GV4), Shenshu (BL23) and Taichong (LR3).

Technique: Treatment is given once daily, one primary point and two secondary points being used each time. All the points are needled alternately with even needling technique. Ten sessions make one course. If the points of Group 1 are getting less effective after repeated needling, those of Group 2 can be used instead.

(2) Puncturing Extra Points

Points: Xinming$_1$ (new brightness) and Xinming$_2$.

Technique: The location of points and the needling technique are described in the chapter "Disorders of the Optic Nerve." The method was used to treat pigmentary degeneration of retina and retinal periphlebitis, and the total effective rate was 82.4% for the former and 76.2% for the latter.

(3) Puncturing Meridian Points

Points: Jingming (BL1) and Hegu (LI4).

Technique: Bilateral Jingming (BL1) is needled slowly for 1 *cun* and the handle-scraping technique is also performed so that the needling sensation of soreness, numbness and distention can radiate to the fundus and outer canthus, and tears flow. Then Hegu (LI4) is needled with rotating technique. All the needles are retained for 15 to 20 minutes and manipulation is given every five or 10 minutes. The treatment is made once daily. This method is indicated for obstruction of retinal artery.

(4) Puncturing Point Xiangyang

Points: Xiangyang$_1$ (the crossing point between the extending horizontal line from both sides of the hyoid bone and the medial border of sternocleidomastoid muscle), and Xiangyang$_2$ (the crossing point between the extending line from both sides of the superior thyroid notch and the medial border of sternocleidomastoid muscle).

Technique: The patient lies supine with the neck fully exposed. After ensuring the location of the carotid artery, the needle is inserted between the medial border of the sternocleidomastoid muscle and the artery backward and upward for 1.5 to 2 *cun* at an angle of 45°. After the arrival of *qi* (i.e., the sensation of soreness and distention to the ocular region), the needle is rotated and then is retained for 10 minutes. Either of the points can be selected and the needling is given once daily. If both eyes are affected, any can be needled bilaterally. Ten sessions make a course of treatment and there is a break of three to five days after each course. This method was used to treat central retinitis and the total effective rate was 92.85%.

2. AURICULAR THERAPY

(1) Auricular Hydro-Acupuncture

Points: ① Kidney and Eye. ② Liver and Eye_1.

Technique: 200% of "Qianliguang Injection (Ragwort Injection)" is used to inject the above auricular points. The two groups are alternated. 0.1 ml is injected into the liver and kidney and 0.4 ml is for Eye and Eye_1. The treatment is given once a day and 10 sessions make up one course with a two to three-day break between courses. This method was used to treat central retinochorioiditis, and the total effective rate was 90.3%.

(2) Auricular Seed-Embedding

Points: Liver, Kidney, Heart, Eye, Eye_1, Eye_2 and Sympathetic Nerve.

Technique: Semen Vaccaria are used to press the points. The seeds are retained for one or two days in summer, and three to five days in winter, 10 sessions forming one course of treatment.

3. HYDRO-ACUPUNCTURE

Points: Zanzhu (BL1), Qiuhou (EX-HN7), Fengchi (GB20), Ganshu (BL18), Shenshu (BL23), Xuanzhong (GB39), and the round or flat nodules on the side of the 4th, 5th, and 6th cervical vertebrae.

Technique: Angelica Injection, Vitamin B_{12}, or Placenta Tissue Injection can be used to inject one point on the head and one distant point each time; 1 ml of medicine is injected into each point. To inject Qiuhou (EX-HN7), a dental syringe needle (Size: No.5) is needed.

After sterilization, the physician gently pushes the eyeball upward with the left thumb and thrusts the needle slowly for 1 *cun*; when no return blood is found on the initial extraction, the medicine is injected slowly. The point must be pressed with a dry cotton ball for a moment after the injection is completed in order to prevent bleeding. The injection is given twice a week.

4. ELECTRIC ACUPUNCTURE

Points: Penetrating from Yifeng (TE17) to Qubin (GB7), then to Sizhukong (TE23).

Technique: All the points are needled with even needling technique and the needling sensation should be conducted to the ocular region. The needles are connected with the electro-acupuncture apparatus for 20 to 30 minutes. If only one eye is affected, the ipsilateral points are selected; otherwise bilateral points are needled. The penetration can be alternated between Qubin (GB7) and Sizhukong (TE23). The treatment is given three times a week, 10 sessions making up one course, with a three-day break between each course. A total of 90 eyes were treated with the method, of which 42 (46.67%) were cured; 16 (17.78%) markedly improved; 24 (26.67%) improved; and 8 (8.89%) unchanged.

5. COMBINED TREATMENT (Auricular Therapy and Herbal Medication)

Points: Eye_1, Eye_2, Liver and Sub-cortex.

Technique: The points are needled once every four days on alternate ears. The needles are retained for 30 to 60 minutes. The Chinese herbal medication "Yan Guang Ming He Ji (Mixture for Brightness of Eyes)" is given, one dose a day. The formula consists of Qianliguang 15 g; Yemingsha, Muzeicao (scouring rush), Baijili, Heshouwu (the tuber of multiflower knodweed) and Gujingcao (pipewort flower), 9 g for each; and Chantui 3 g.

6. MAGNETIC THERAPY

Points: The periocular points or auricular points.

Technique: ① Magnet-Rotating Method: The output pole is sterilized and then disposed on two periocular points each time [such as Jingming (BL1), Zanzhu (BL2), Tongziliao (GB1), Taiyang (EX-HN5), Yangbai (GB14) and Sibai (ST2)], 20 minutes for each point. ② Auricular Magnet Method: Auricular points Eye, Liver, Eye₁, Eye₂ and Sub-cortex are selected and stuck with a small magnetic bead changed once a week.

7. SCALP ACUPUNCTURE

Point: Vision Zone.

Technique: A 1.5-*cun* or 2-*cun* filiform needle is thrust into the bilateral point, and rapid rotating needling technique is performed 150 times per minute. Thereafter the needles are connected with the electro-acupuncture apparatus for 15 to 20 minutes. The treatment is given once every other day and 10 sessions make a course.

[REMARKS]

1. Retinopathy, the multiple disorders of ocular fundus, is common but intractable in the ophthalmologic clinic. Acupuncture can obtain certain effect in the treatment of the disease, but there is a difficulty with objective indices and the lack of the control observation and long-term follow-up.

2. Since the treatment of the disease with acupuncture requires fairly long treatment, patience is vital.

3. It has been observed that acupuncture at Binao (LI14) can improve visual acuity, so it can be combined with all the above methods. The needling is performed as: a 1.5-*cun* needle (Size: No.28) is slowly thrust upward obliquely at an angle of 45° [to the point Jianyu (LI15)]; with rotating technique the arrival of *qi* can be obtained and then the needle is withdrawn one-third; the rotation is repeated for further arrival of *qi,* and the needle is lifted a further one-third and rotation resumed; then the needle is slowly thrust again in the original direction with the same technique as before. This procedure is repeated three times and the needle is retained for 30 minutes. Before the treatment, the patient is required to close the eyes for rest and after the treatment the eyes are open. Vision should be improved.

OPTIC NERVOUS LESION

[INTRODUCTION]

Optic nervous lesion includes optic neuritis and optic atrophy. In traditional Chinese medicine, the former is known as "Sudden Blindness" and the latter as "Green Blindness." "Sudden blindness" is due to furiousness leading to the rise of hyperactive liver *yang* which makes the eyes lose their function; or due to the stagnation of *qi* and blood resulting in their failure to circulate to the eyes; or due to immoderate alcohol and spicy-food intake giving rise to an accumulation of heat. The disease is characterized by abrupt onset, sudden loss or drastic decrease of vision. When it is the syndrome of liver-*yang* hyperactivity, headache, vertigo, blurred vision, irritability, and hot temper are associated. When it is stagnation of *qi* and blood, there will be a purple or purple-spotted tongue and hesitant pulse. Accumulation of heat in the stomach is revealed by irritability, thirst, constipation, concentrated urine, and rapid and forceful pulse. "Green blindness" is mainly attributable to *yin*-deficiency of the liver and kidney and the depletion of essence and blood so the essence and *qi* are unable to nourish the eyes; or to an insufficiency of heart *yin* and weakness of vitality leading to the decline of the vital brightness, leading to gradual decrease of vision. There will be nothing abnormal about the appearance of the eyes, but the patient feels a progressive decrease of visual acuity and gradually the inability to distinguish people and objects, even darkness and brightness, and eventually total loss of vision. Dizziness, blurred vision, palpitation, soreness in the lumbar region, tinnitus, insomnia, pale tongue and a thready and weak pulse can be present. The principle of treatment is to activate the circulation of blood, nourish the blood, clear the heat in the liver, tonify the kidney, and brighten the eyes. Points from Foot-Taiyang, Foot-Yamgming and Hand-Yangming meridians are mainly selected, including Jingming (BL1), Chengqi (ST1), Fengchi (GB20), Hegu (LI4), Taichong (LR3), Guangming (GB37), Ganshu (BL18), Xinshu (BL15) and Shenshu (BL23). The periocular points are given mild stimulation while the distant ones are performed with moderate stimulation.

[CLINICAL EXPERIENCE]

1. CONVENTIONAL ACUPUNCTURE

(1) Needling New Points

Points: Xinming$_1$ and Xinming$_2$.

Technique: When needling Xinming$_1$, the needle is rapidly inserted upward and forward with the shaft at an angle of 60° with the skin, and when the needle tip reaches the posterior side of the Intertragic notch, the ear lobe is pulled slightly to the anteriolateral side and the needle is thrust slowly further at an angle of 45°. When the needle shaft reaches the sallow side of the sub-mandibular styloid process for 1 *cun* to 1.5 *cun*, the needling sensation will appear. If the sensation is not remarkable, the needle can be thrust a further 0.5 *cun*. If the needling sensation is even now not remarkable, the direction of the needle tip can be changed slightly to find the satisfactory sensation. To those being sensitive to the needling sensation, the rotating technique is combined with small amplitude of lifting-thrusting technique; to those being less sensitive to the needling sensation, the needle-twisting technique should be performed to conduct the needling sensation to the ocular region. In needling Xinming$_2$, the needle tip is thrust toward the forehead at the horizontal level slowly for 0.5 to 0.8 *cun* and after the appearance of needling sensation manipulation is employed to produce a strong needling sensation in the eyeball. The needling manipulation is done for one or two minutes for each point. The needles are then retained for 30 minutes. The treatment is given once a day, 10 sessions forming one course, with a three-day break after each course. This method is applicable for optic neuritis and optic atrophy; it is satisfactorily effective to treat acute optic neuritis, but much less effective for optic atrophy.

(2) Needling Extra Points

Point: Qiuhou (EX-HN7). Secondary point: Yiming (EX-HN14).

Technique: A two-*cun* needle (Size: Nos.30-32) is used. The patient is required to look straight ahead and the needle is inserted for 0.5 or 0.6 *cun* at the junction of the lateral 1/4 and medial 3/4 of the infra-orbital margin with the needle tip thrust slightly upward and medially along the margin for 1.5 *cun*. After the needling sensation is obtained with gentle rotating technique, the needle is removed and the needle hole is pressed with a cotton ball for a while. If there is resistance during the insertion of needle, it should be withdrawn slowly and changed slightly to another direction in order to avoid injury to the eyeball or bleeding. To needle Yiming (EX-HN14), an upright sitting position is required for the patient, and a 1.5 *cun* needle is inserted perpendicularly for about 1 *cun* and is removed after the appearance of the needling sensation. The treatment is given once every other day, 10 sessions forming one course of treatment, with a break for three to five days after each course. A total of 34 cases of optic atrophy were treated with this method and the total effective rate reached 68.3%.

(3) Multiple Groups of Points

Points: There are altogether 7 groups of points: ① Fengfu (GV16), Fengchi (GB20), and Taiyang (EX-HN5). ② Shangxing (GV23), Muchuang (GB16) and Yingxiang (LI20). ③ Binao (LI14), Hegu (LI4) and Guangming (GB37). ④ Zhaohai (KI6), Hegu (LI4), and Zanzhu (BL2). ⑤ Yuyao (EX-HN4), Sibai (ST2) and Shenmai (BL62). ⑥ Jingming (BL1), Tongziliao (GB1) and Toulinqi (GB15). ⑦ Mingmen (GV4) and Ganshu (BL18).

Technique: The seven groups of points are used in alternation, one a day, with one course of treatment lasting seven days. Ganshu (BL18) and Mingmen (GV4) are treated with the rotating or handle-scraping method in a rapid and short way. Fengfu (GV16) is punctured perpendicularly for 0.3 to 0.5 *cun* with the needle inserted slowly; deep insertion is forbidden in order to avoid injury to the medullar bulb. The handle-scraping method is also given. Muchuang (GB16) is thrust horizontally forward for 0.3 to 0.5 *cun* with rotating or handle-scraping method. Binao (LI14) is thrust upward for 0.8 to 1 *cun* at an angle of 45°. Zhaohai (KI6) is punctured perpendicularly for 0.3 to 0.5 *cun* with the rotating method. Zanzhu (BL2) is needled with penetrating method toward Yuyao (EX-HN4); Shenmai (BL62) is punctured perpendicularly for 0.3 to 0.5 *cun*; Toulinqi (GB15) is thrust horizontally forward for 0.3 to 0.5 *cun*, and all three are performed with rotating technique. The other points are needled with routine technique.

2. MOXIBUSTION

(1) Moxibustion with Moxa Cones (Non-scarring Moxibustion)

Points: Juliao (ST3), Ganshu (BL18), Shangyang (LI1) and Mingmen (GV4).

Technique: Three cones are given on Juliao (ST3), seven on Ganshu (BL18), and three on Mingmen (GV4). Shangyang (LI1) is treated with bleeding technique. This method is applicable to "green blindness."

(2) Indirect Moxibustion with Ginger

Points: Dagukong (EX-UE5) and Xiaogukong (EX-UE6).

Technique: Ginger slices are normally used, with three to five moxa cones on each point, once a day.

3. BLEEDING METHOD

(1) Puncturing Meridian Points

Points: Zanzhu (BL2), Shenting (GV24) and Shangxing (GV23).

Technique: All the three points are bled with a three-edged needle to obtain one to three drops of blood. This method is indicated for optic neuritis.

(2) Acupuncture Plus Bleeding

Points: Zanzhu (BL2), Shenting (GV24), Shangxing (GV23), Xinhui (GV22), Qianding (GV21), Baihui (GV20) and Weizhong (BL40).

Technique: Zanzhu (BL2) and the other five points on the vertex are punctured with reducing needling technique and the needles are retained for 10 minutes. Weizhong (BL40) is bled for three to five drops of blood. The needling is given once a day. It is satisfactorily effective for " sudden blindness" due to the acute optic neuritis.

4. ELECTRIC ACUPUNCTURE

Points: Primary points: Upper Jingming (BL$_1$) and Qiuhou (EX-

HN4). Secondary points: Taiyang (EX-HN5), Fengchi (GB20), Hegu (LI4) and Guangming (GB37).

Technique: In every session, one primary and two secondary points are selected. After the arrival of *qi,* the needles are connected with the electro-acupuncture apparatus for 15 minutes. The treatment is given once every other day, seven sessions forming one course.

5. SCALP ACUPUNCTURE

Points: Bilateral Vision Zone.

Technique: The tip of needle points downward and is thrust horizontally for 1.5 to 2 *cun.* Then the rapid needle-rotating technique is performed for one minute to produce the needling sensation of pain, distention, numbness and heat. The needles are retained for 20 minutes. The treatment is given once a day, and 10 sessions comprise one course of treatment. Conventional acupuncture should be combined. In ordinary cases, the marked effect can be obtained after three or four courses.

6. AURICULAR THERAPY

Points: Eye$_1$, Eye$_2$, Eye, Liver, Kidney, Sub-cortex, Apex of Tragus, and the tender spots in the area of occiput.

Technique: In each session, three to four points (bilateral) are punctured with filiform needles by means of rapid needle-rotating technique for one minute. Then the needles are removed and the intradermal needles or the Semen Vaccaria are fixed on the points for one or two days. The treatment is given once daily. It is also believed that this method is useful as an auxiliary therapy or is chosen when other measures prove ineffective.

7. HYDRO-ACUPUNCTURE

Points: Primary points: Qiuhou (EX-HN7) and Chengqi (ST1). Secondary points: Zusanli (ST36), Guangming (GB37), Taichong (LR3), Ganshu (BL18) and Shenshu (BL23).

Technique: One primary point and one secondary point are selected in each session. The compound Red-Sage (or Angelica) Injection, or a mixture of vitamin B_1 and B_2, or 0.5% procaine is taken for the acupoint injection; 1 ml of Chinese herbal injection or 0.5 to 1 ml of Western injection is administered in each point. The injection is given once every other day, and 10 sessions comprise a course of treatment. The method should be suspended if there is no effect after three sessions.

8. LASER THERAPY

Points: Jingming (BL1), Zanzhu (BL2), Shangxing (GV23), Chengqi (ST1), Qiuhou (EX-HN7), Hegu (LI4), Fengchi (GB20), Taichong (LR3), Guangming (GB37), Ganshu (BL18), Pishu (BL20) and Shenshu (BL23).

Technique: Two local and two distant points are selected each session. A 3 to 7 mw He-Ne laser is used to irradiate the points, five minutes for each, once a day. Ten sessions form one course of treatment, and there is a three-day break after each course.

[REMARKS]

1.   There is not yet an ideal therapeutic method to treat this disease. In recent years, fairly satisfactory effect has been achieved with acupuncture treatment, however.

2.   The patients are required to take care of the eyes by closing them for rest. Meanwhile, vitamin B_1 and B_{12} are combined for administration. Breast-feeding patients should stop lactation.

CATARACT

[INTRODUCTION]

The disease is divided into congenital and acquired types. The latter is subdivided into the senile, traumatic, and complicated ones. Senile cataract is the one most commonly seen in clinical studies, mainly affecting those over 50, and is characterized by chronic progressive disorder in both eyes. In terms of traditional Chinese medicine, this disease is attributable to deficiency of both the liver and kidney because of the high age, thus the eyes are unable to be nourished; or to weakness of the spleen and stomach leading to failure to generate the essence and blood to prevent eye malnourishment; or to an innate insufficiency of essence and blood to nourish the eyes; or to wind-heat in the liver meridian depleting *yin* and blood, leading to malnourishment of the eyes; or to traumatic injury which causes turbidity and cloudiness of the pupil. The chief complaints are blurred vision or the visual disturbance of a dark shadow in front of the eyes, or dark objects following the movement of the eyeball, double vision in one eye, and gradual decrease of visual acuity. Finally, the pupil becomes totally silver-white, so that vision is so poor that it is unable to distinguish people's features, but just able to see the movement of the hands. The affected eyes look normal with the congestion, the pain, and the lacrimation denied. The pupil also remains intact, the light reflex is sensitive, and the movement is normal. The treatment serves to nourish *yin* and replenish the blood. Such points are selected as Tongziliao (GB1), Yifeng (TE17), Fengchi (GB20), Guangming (GB37), Zusanli (ST36), Ganshu (BL18) and Shenshu (BL23). The reinforcing needling technique is performed.

[CLINICAL EXPERIENCE]

1. CONVENTIONAL ACUPUNCTURE

(1) Multiple Groups of Points

Points: ① Jingming (BL1), Yangbai (GB14), Fengchi (GB20) and Hegu (LI4). ② Qiuhou (EX-HN7), Taiyang (EX-HN5), Yiming (EX-HN14) and Binao (LI14).

Technique: The two groups are used in alternation, one group for seven days (a course of treatment), and the needling is given once a day. A break for two or three days is essential after each course.

(2) Single-Point Puncture

Point: Bilateral Binao (LI14).

Technique: After insertion, the needle is thrust obliquely upward with strong stimulation until an intense sensation of soreness and distention is felt. The needles are not retained.

2. HYDRO-ACUPUNCTURE

Points: Guangming (GB37), Zusanli (ST36), Sanyinjiao (SP6), Yanglao (SI6), Quchi (LI11) and Hegu (LI4). Shenshu (BL23) and Ganshu (BL18) or Xuehai (SP10) are combined to those with constitutional weakness and *qi* deficiency.

Technique: All the points are selected bilaterally and every point (a pair) is taken as one group. In the first and third courses, 20 ml of Angelica Injection and 500 mg of vitamin C are injected; in the second course, 50 mg of vitamin B_1, 100 mg of vitamin B_2 and 1 ml of Angelica Injection are mixed and 1.5 ml of the mixture is injected into each point. Seven days are taken as a course of treatment. A break of five to seven days is given after each course.

3. PRICKING METHOD

(1) Puncturing Extra Points

Points: The spinous processes of the 6th and 7th cervical vertebrae and the 1st thoracic vertebra.

Technique: Each of the above points is taken as a center and six spots are selected around the center in a diameter of 0.6 cm, so there are altogether seven points in each place, and 21 points can be pricked one after another. After sterilization, a three-edged needle is used to prick the skin deep enough to cut several white fibers from the point. After pricking, cupping takes place until there is a small amount of bleeding. The above-mentioned pricking is given consecutively for four days, seven points each time. From the fifth time, the pricking is made once a week on the two points symmetrically on both sides of the above spinous processes. Twelve sessions make up a course of treatment and a one-month break is taken after each course.

(2) Pricking the Scapular Region

Points: Ah-shi points in the scapular region.

Technique: If the right eye is affected, the patient is required to move the left palm back to the right shoulder and place closely on the skin of the scapular region; in the area three finger-breadth below the tip of the middle finger, one to three red pimples can be found and they are pricked out. The opposite is done when the left eye is affected.

4. AURICULAR THERAPY

(1) Needling a Single Point
Point: Eye area.

Technique: The needle is thrust and retained for 15 to 30 minutes, once a day or every other day. Twenty sessions form one course.

(2) Embedding of Needles or Seeds
Points: Eye, Liver, Kidney, Adrenal Gland, Heart, and Sympathetic Nerve.

Technique: The tender spots are found in the above points and the thumb-tag needles or the ear seeds are embedded on them. Two or three spots are used each time and the change is given for every three to five days. The two ears are alternated.

[REMARKS]

1. Acupuncture does have certain effect in treating the early stage of senile cataract, and it is especially significant to those unwilling or unable to have the operative treatment, since acupuncture can control or delay the progress of the disease.

2. If the disease is incurable with acupuncture and medication, it is only when the cataract nebula becomes ripe in pure white color that cataractopiesis can be performed with a gold needle.

GLAUCOMA

[INTRODUCTION]

There are different types of glaucoma, i.e., primary, secondary and congenital. The primary type is subdivided into non-congestive glaucoma (chronic simple glaucoma) and congestive glaucoma (acute or chronic congestive glaucoma) and it is suitable for treatment by acupuncture. As far as secondary glaucoma is concerned, the treatment should aim to deal with the primary diseases, while the congenital type is indicated for a surgical operation. To understand the etiology and the pathogenesis, this disease is caused by an emotional stir which leads to the transformation of fire in the liver and gallbladder flaring up to the eyes so that the ocular fluid cannot be properly discharged; or by depression of liver *qi* and weakness of the spleen, which results in the dysfunction of transportation and transformation and the disharmony of *qi* and blood; or the retention of harmful fluid in the body running to block the eyes; or by depletion of the primordial *yin* so that imbalanced and preponderant *yang* turns to fire and induces the wind, which boils the ocular fluid. In the initial stage, there are manifestations of headache, slight distention of the eyes, decrease in visual acuity. Gradually, the headache becomes severe and is associated with nausea, vomiting, congested conjunctiva, cloudiness of the cornea, and eventually a drastic increase in intra-ocular pressure, optic atrophy in the fundus and blindness. To treat this disease, the principle is to expel the wind, brighten the eyes, nourish *yin*, and reduce the fire. Points are mainly selected from the foot Taiyang and Shaoyang meridians, such as Fengchi (GB20), Zanzhu (BL2), Tongziliao (GB1), Hegu (LI4), Taixi (KI3), Sanyinjiao (SP6), Shenshu (BL23), Ganshu (BL18) and Danshu (BL19).

[CLINICAL EXPERIENCE]

1. CONVENTIONAL ACUPUNCTURE

Points: Siguan [i.e., Hegu (LI4) and Taichong (LR3)] and Sihua [i.e., Geshu (BL17) and Danshu (BL19)].

Technique: The Siguan points are performed with reducing needling technique and the Sihua points with even technique. The needling is given once daily with the needles retained for 0.5 to 4 hours during which manipulation is carried out every 10 minutes.

2. LASER THERAPY

Points: Jingming (BL1), Chengqi (ST1), Tongziliao (GB1), Hegu

(LI4) and Taichong (LR3).

Technique: A 3 to 7 mw He-Ne laser is used to irradiate the points, two to three points each time, 5 minutes for each point. The treatment is carried out once daily, or for every other day, 20 sessions forming one course.

3. AURICULAR THERAPY

Points: Eye, liver, Eye₁, Eye₂, Heart, Ear Apex, and Hypertensive Groove.

Technique: Eye, liver, Eye₁, Eye₂ and heart are punctured or embedded with ear seeds while the Ear Apex and Hypertensive Groove are bled. The treatment is given once every other day, 10 sessions in a course. In some cases, with a number of treatments, a decrease of intra-ocular pressure, so it can be regarded that auricular acupuncture is helpful in this regard.

4. COLD MOXIBUSTION

Points: Main points: Taiyang (EX-HN5), Fengchi (GB20), Yintang (EX-HN3), and Yuyao (EX-HN4). Supplementary points: Guangming (GB37), Taichong (LR3), Neiguan (PC6) and Shenshu (BL23).

Technique: Two points are selected each session, and from the second course of treatment, besides a local point, Guangming (GB37) or Taichong (LR3) is combined for excessive liver fire; Neiguan (PC6) for flaring of heart fire; and Shenshu (BL23) for kidney deficiency. The treatment is given once a day, 10 sessions making up one course of treatment. Usually, three courses are given and a re-examination is made after each course. The semi-conductor cold moxibustion apparatus is used in the treatment. In the first course, the temperature of the moxibustion is from –15 to –20°C, 20 minutes for each session and in the second and third courses, the temperature is from –5 to –10 °C, 30 minutes for each session. Altogether, 41 cases were treated with this method, the restoration rate of both eyes was up to 45.26%, and that of a single eye was 43.3%; and the ineffective rate was 11.44%.

5. PRICKING METHOD

Points: The reacting spots on the upper and lower eyelids; and Ganshu (BL18), Danshu (BL19), Xinshu (BL15), and Fengchi (GB20) are combined.

Technique: The pricking method is performed at all the points, two pair of points each session, once every three days. For acute simple glaucoma, five to 10 sessions make up a course of treatment, and for chronic glaucoma, 10 treatments are given. From clinical results, this method is satisfactorily effective for acute simple glaucoma.

6. CUTANEOUS NEEDLING

Points: The running course of foot-Taiyang meridian on the back.

Technique: Tapping the urinary bladder meridian mainly on the back with moderate force, once a day or every other day, 10 sessions making up a course. This method is indicated for the chronic cases.

[REMARKS]

1. Acupuncture claims marked analgesic effect and reduction in varying degrees of the intra-ocular pressure for acute glaucoma. It has been observed that the intra-ocular pressure can be reduced down for 8 to 42 mm Hz, and the reduction can be kept for several to 24 hours. For chronic cases, acupuncture can also be helpful in improving the symptoms.

2. The combined treatment must be given when the intra-ocular pressure is too high during the attack of the acute glaucoma.

TINNITUS AND DEAFNESS

[INTRODUCTION]

Tinnitus and deafness are both the symptoms of hearing abnormality. Tinnitus is characterized by the chief complaint of subjective ringing in the ear, while the deafness chiefly relates to the decrease of hearing or the total loss of hearing. Tinnitus is often preliminary sign of approaching deafness. The two are discussed often together since there is great similarity between them in the aspects of etiology and treatment. As far as the etiology is concerned, it is mainly due to emotional disturbance e.g., rage, fear and fright, leading to wind fire in liver and gallbladder which rises to block the flow of *qi* in the Shaoyang meridians; or the invasion by exogenous pathogenic wind obstructing the hearing orifice; or the accumulation of phlegm-heat misting the hearing orifice; or the deficiency of kidney essence preventing the essential *qi* nourishing the ears. In clinical study, there are two types: excess and deficiency. In the former, there are manifestations of sudden onset of deafness, stuffiness and distention in the ears, and constant ringing in the ear sounding like a cicada or the tide, which cannot be relieved by pressure on the ears. In the latter, the manifestations are chronic deafness, or intermittent tinnitus in a low pitch, which is aggravated by physical exertion and can be relieved by pressure on the ears. The disease is treated by the principle of clearing away the fire in the liver and gallbladder, eliminating the phlegm and reopening the hearing orifice, expelling the wind and dredging the collaterals, reinforcing the kidney and replenishing the essence. The points of the hand and foot Shaoyang meridians, the foot Yangming and foot Shaoyin meridians are mainly selected, such as Yifeng (TE17), Zhongzhu (TE3), Tinghui (GB2), Ermen (TE21), Shenshu (BL23), Ganshu (BL18), Taixi (KI3), and Fenglong (ST40). The reducing technique is performed for the syndrome of excess and the reinforcing technique for the deficiency syndrome. The treatment is given once daily and 10 sessions form a course of treatment.

[CLINICAL EXPERIENCE]

1. CONVENTIONAL ACUPUNCTURE

(1) Treatment According to Excess and Deficiency

Points: Excess syndrome: Tinghui (GB2) and Chimai (TE18). For acute cases, Waiqiu (GB36) and Huizong (TE7), the Xi-Cleft points respectively of gallbladder and Sanjiao (Triple Energizer) meridians are combined; for chronic cases, Riyue (GB24) and Shimen (CV5), the Front-Mu points respectively for the two, are combined. Deficiency syndrome: Ermen (TE21) and Yifeng (TE17). For acute cases, Zhongdu (LR6) and Shuiquan (KI5), the Xi-Cleft points respectively of liver and kidney meridians, are combined; for chronic cases, Qimen (LR14) and Jingmen (GB25), the Front-Mu points respectively for the two, are added.

Technique: Clinically speaking, the excess syndrome is mostly attributable to the disorders of gallbladder and Sanjiao, so the Xi-Cleft and Front-Mu points of both are selected and are punctured with routine reducing technique; the deficient syndrome is involved more with the disorders of liver and kidney, so the Xi-Cleft and Front-Mu points of both are selected and punctured with routine reinforcing needling technique. The needles are retained for 30 minutes. The treatment is given once daily and 10 sessions form a course.

(2) Perpendicular Needling

Points: Fengchi (GB20), Tinggong (SI19), Yifeng (TE17), Gongqiang (an extra point located at the midpoint of the very root of the rear of the auricle) and Hegu (LI4).

Technique: Gongqiang is punctured with needle thrust along the back of the auricle for 0.8 to 1 *cun* and all the other points are needled perpendicularly deep in and out, but no needle-rotating technique is given. The needling is made once a day and 10 sessions form a course. In order to strengthen the effect, the needles can be retained for 30 minutes.

2. MOXIBUSTION

Points: Tinggong (SI19), Ermen (TE21), Tinghui (GB2), Yifeng (TE17), Waiguan (TE5), Shenshu (BL23) and Taixi (KI3).

Technique: Two to four points are selected each time and five to seven moxa cones are performed on each point. On the peri-auricular points, the small cones in the size of a soybean or wheat grain are used, and on other points, the cones are as big as a jujube kernel. The treatment is given once a day or every other day and 10 sessions make a course. This method is indicated for deafness and tinnitus due to the deficiency of kidney essence.

3. ELECTRIC ACUPUNCTURE

Points: Shenshu (BL23), Yifeng (TE17), Waiguan (TE5), Tinghui (GB2) and Tinggong (SI19).

Technique: The even needling technique is applied first and the needling sensation in the peri-auricular points should be conducted to the back of the ear. Then the needles are connected with the electro-acupuncture apparatus for 20 to 40 minutes. Waiguan (TE5) and Shenshu (BL23) are not given the electric stimulation, but just simple needling. The treatment is given once daily, 12 sessions in a course and a two-day break between courses. This method is applicable to sudden deafness.

4. AURICULAR THERAPY

(1) Electric Acupuncture in Auricular Points

Points: Subcortex, Endocrine, Liver and Kidney.

Technique: The ipsilateral or bilateral points are punctured with strong stimulation and then the needles are connected with the electro-acupuncture apparatus for 30 to 60 minutes. The needling is given once a day or every other day, and 15 to 20 sessions form one course.

(2) Auricular Hydro-Acupuncture

Points: External Ear, Internal Ear and Kidney.

Technique: Vitamin B_1 is used for the injection, 0.2 ml for each point, once every other day, and 10 to 15 sessions make up one course.

5. HYDRO-ACUPUNCTURE

Points: Tinggong (SI19), Yifeng (TE17), Wangu (GB12) and Chimai (TE18).

Technique: The 654-2 Injection is used to inject one point from each side, 5 mg for each point; or vitamin B_{12} is injected 0.2 to 0.5 ml in each point; or Angelica Injection and Red-sage Injection is used, 0.5 to 1 ml for each point. The injection is give once every other day and 10 sessions form one course.

6. SCALP ACUPUNCTURE

Points: Bilateral Dizziness-Hearing Zones.

Technique: Horizontal needling is carried out and intermittent needling manipulation is given. The needles are retained for 20 minutes. The needling is performed once a day or every other day. This method is applicable to nervous deafness and tinnitus.

[REMARKS]

1. Acupuncture has a definite therapeutic effect in treating tinnitus and deafness, but it is not fairly effective to treat those caused by organic diseases.

2. In daily life, good living habits should be adopted. Combining moderate physical exertion and rest, avoiding excessive emotional stimulus, and keeping away from over-indulgence in sexual activities. In brief, attention should be paid to self health care.

MENIERE'S DISEASE

[INTRODUCTION]

Meniere's disease is classified in the category of "Dizziness and Vertigo" in traditional Chinese medicine. Its chief complaints are paroxysmal vertigo, severe feeling of rotation of the external environment and the shaking of the body, and inability to sit, all of which are aggravated by a shift of the body position. Tinnitus, decreased hearing and nystagmus are associated. In the view of traditional Chinese medicine, the disease is due to constitutional weakness and excessive activity of thinking and worry, giving rise to deficiency of both the heart and spleen, leading to inadequate generation of *qi* and blood and subsequent malnourishment of the head and eyes; or over-indulgence in sexual coitus leading to the depletion of kidney essence and the emptiness of the "sea of marrow"; or emotional depression or anger harming the liver, bringing on the internal stirring-up of liver wind and liver *yang*; or immoderate consumption of rich and greasy food resulting in the endogenous damp-phlegm which disturbs upward the pure orifices. It should be treated by means of building up the spleen, tonifying the kidney, subduing the liver *yang*, and dissolving the phlegm to reopen the orifices. Points are mainly selected from the hand and foot Shaoyang and hand and foot Jueyin meridians, such as Baihui (GV20), Fengchi (GB20), Shenting (GV24), Neiguan (PC6), Gongsun (SP4), Zusanli (ST36), Fenglong (ST40), Sanyinjiao (SP6), and Taixi (KI3). The reinforcing needling technique is performed for the syndromes of deficiency and the reducing technique for those of excess.

[CLINICAL EXPERIENCE]

1. CONVENTIONAL ACUPUNCTURE

(1) Stressing the Points of Du-Meridian

Points: Shenting (GV24), Shangxing (GV23), Xinhui (GV22), Qianding (GV21), Houding (GV19), Naohu (GV17), Fengchi (GB20), Yanggu (SI), Dadu (SP2), Zhiyin (BL67), Jinmen (BL63), Shenmai (BL62) and Zusanli (ST36).

Technique: All the points of Du-meridian (GV) are punctured each session with even needling technique; among the others, two to three are selected each time in alternation. This method aims to reopen the orifices, regulate the mind, elevate the clarified, and bring down the turbid.

(2) Focusing on Regulating Liver

Points: Taichong (LR3), Ququan (LR8), Zhongdu (GB32), Ligou (LR5), Qimen (LR14), Guangming (GB37), Ganshu (BL18), and Qiuxu (GB40).

Technique: Since it is said in *Internal Classic* that "all the disorders featured by shaking and vertigo resulting from endogenous wind are attributable to the liver," Taichong (LR3) and Ququan (LR8), the Yuan-Primary point and He-Sea point of liver meridian, are prescribed; for a fresh case, the Xi-Cleft point of liver meridian is combined and for a chronic case, the Front-Mu point of liver is added. Alternatively, the combination of Yuan-Primary and Luo-Connecting points is taken i.e., Taichong (LR3) in combination with Guangming (GB37) the Luo-Connecting point of gallbladder. In case tinnitus is associated,

Qiuxu (GB40) the Yuan-Primary point of gallbladder meridian is supplemented in combination with Ligou (LR5) the Luo-Connecting point of the liver meridian. In case, nystagmus is present, Ganshu (BL18) is combined. All the points receive even needling technique, and all the needles are retained for 30 minutes. The treatment is given once daily and 10 sessions form one course of treatment.

(3) Puncturing Point "Ganshen"

Points: Three points of Ganshen (respectively the tender spots at the loci 0.5, 1.5 and 2.5 *cun* lateral to the xyphoid process on the right costal arch).

Technique: After needling, the needles are taken at the handle to sway for 15 to 20 circles and then retained for 30 minutes. The needling is given once daily and 10 sessions make one course. This method was used to treat 19 cases of Meniere's disease, of which seven were cured, eight showed marked effect and four improved.

2. MOXIBUSTION

Points: Baihui (GV20).

Technique: After locating the point, the hair on locus of the point is cut from the root (the area in the size of the nail of the middle finger). The patient takes a sitting position, and a moxa cone as big as a soybean is placed on the point and is ignited from the top and left to burn until there is no more smoke. The physician put off the burning moxa cone by pressing it with a piece of thick paper and the pressing force goes from gentle to heavy. At this moment, the patient should feel comfortable as the heat infiltrates the scalp. Altogether 10 to 15 cones are used. If the patient complains of a burning sensation during moxibustion, this should be borne. Usually the moxibustion causes no suppuration and no special processing is necessary. After two to four weeks there is decrustation and new hair starts to grow. If infection occurs, routine surgical treatment is given. This method is fairly effective in treating an attack of Meniere's disease.

3. PLUM-BLOSSOM NEEDLING

Points: From the 1st to the 4th cervical vertebrae, around the ear, in front of the ear, the depression posterior and inferior to the ear lobe, and the both sides of the lumbosacral spine.

Technique: During the attack, heavy tapping is given, and during remission, moderate tapping is performed. The treatment is given once a day and 10 sessions form a course.

4. HYDRO-ACUPUNCTURE

Points: ① Fengchi (GB20) and Neiguan (PC6) ② Hegu (LI4) and Taichong (LR3). ③ Yiming (EX-HN14) and Sidu (TE9).

Technique: One group of points is selected in each session and three to five ml of 5% or 10% of glucose injection, or 0.5 ml of vitamin B_{12} injection, or 0.5 ml of 0.5% procaine is injected. The above points are alternately injected, once every other day, and five to seven sessions make a course.

5. SCALP ACUPUNCTURE

Points: ① The lower 2/5 of the Sensory Zone and Dizziness and Hearing Zone; ② Thorax Zone and Balance Zone.

Technique: The points are alternated group by group. The treatment is given once every other day and the electro-acupuncture apparatus is connected for 20 to 30 minutes. Ten sessions form a course of treatment, with a three-day break between courses.

6. AURICULAR THERAPY

Points: Kidney, Ear-Shenmen, Occiput, Internal Ear, Subcortex, Sympathetic Nerve, Stomach, Minor Occipital Nerve, Thorax and Endocrine.

Technique: Three to five points are selected each time. After needling, the needles are retained for 30 minutes and embedding follows. Alternatively, 0.3 to 0.5 ml of vitamin B_1 is injected in each point, once every other day and 10 times in a course of treatment.

7. COMBINED TREATMENT

Points: Shangxing (GV23), Baihui (GV20), Shenmen (HT7), 2 *cun* above Sanyinjiao (SP6), and Dizziness and Hearing Zone of scalp

454

acupuncture.

Technique: Penetrating from Shangxing (GV23) with rotating needling technique; Shenmen (HT7) and 2 *cun* above Sanyinjiao (SP6) are punctured perpendicularly with needles retained for 30 minutes. Mild moxibustion with moxa stick is performed over Baihui (GV20) for 20 minutes. To the severe cases Dizziness and Hearing Zone is combined and the needle is connected with electro-acupuncture apparatus for 20 minutes. The treatment is given once daily and 10 sessions make a course of treatment.

[REMARKS]

1. Meniere's disease can be usually relieved by acupuncture for its attack of vertigo and the accompanied tinnitus can also be eased in most cases.

2. The patients should keep in a good mood. Meanwhile the low-salt, low-fat and moderate carbohydrate diet is apt to the patients. Cigarette-smoking and drinking of alcohol, strong tea and coffee are prohibited during the attack.

OTITIS MEDIA SUPPURATIVA

[INTRODUCTION]

Otitis media suppurativa, either acute or chronic, is mostly caused by inflammation in the nasal cavity and the pharynx entering the middle ear via the auditory tube. In children since their auditory tube is shorter and thicker, the possibility of the disease is increased. Clinically, the chief manifestations are pain in the ear, purulent discharge, and decreased hearing. It is mostly due to the invasion of exogenous wind-heat toxins; or to fire in liver and gallbladder stagnating in the ear orifice leading to the rotting of blood and flesh and creation of pus; or to the weakness of the spleen causing dysfunction of transformation, which results in the retention of turbid dampness accumulating in the ear. It is treated on the principle of expelling the wind-heat, building up the spleen and stomach, and dissolving the turbid dampness. Points are mainly selected from the hand and foot Shaoyang and Yangming meridians, such as Yifeng (TE17), Waiguan (TE5), Ermen (TE21), Xingjian (LR2), Fengchi (GB20), Yinlingquan (SP9), Sanyinjiao (SP6) and Hegu (LI4). Reinforcing technique is performed for the syndromes of deficiency and the reducing one for those of excess. The treatment is given once daily and the needles are retained for 30 minutes.

[CLINICAL EXPERIENCE]

1. CONVENTIONAL ACUPUNCTURE

(1) Treatment According to Different Stages

Points: ① Tinghui (GB2), Hegu (LI4) and Jiache (ST6). ② Hegu (LI4), Yifeng (TE17) and Ermen (TE21).

Technique: The first group of points is used for the redness swelling and pain of the ear. Tinghui (GB2) is penetrated 0.2 *cun* and the needle is rotated and retained for one minute; Hegu (LI4) is penetrated for 0.4 *cun* and the needle is rotated and retained for one minute; and Jiache (ST6) is penetrated for 0.3 *cun* and the needle is rotated and retained for two minutes. The second group of points is used for the purulent discharge in the otitis media suppurativa. Hegu (LI4) is penetrated 0.3 to 0.4 *cun* and the needle is rotated and retained for one minute; Yifeng (TE17) is penetrated 0.3 *cun* and the needle is rotated and retained for one minute; Ermen (TE21) is also penetrated 0.3 *cun* and the needle is rotated and retained for one minute. The needling is given once a day and 10 sessions make up one course of treatment.

(2) Prescribing Points According to Syndrome-Differentiation

Points: Primary points: Penetrating from Ermen (TE21) to Tinggong (SI19), Yifeng (TE17), Zhongzhu (TE3) and Zulinqi (GB41). Quchi (LI11) and Dazhui (GV14) are for fever, and Taiyang (EX-HN5) and Fengchi (GB20) for headache.

Technique: The patient is required to grit a chopstick transversely in the mouth, while Ermen (TE21) is penetrated toward Tinggong (SI19) 1 to 1.5 *cun* at an angle of 30° and the needle-rotating and handle-scraping techniques are performed. Yifeng (TE17) is punctured perpendicularly 1 to 1.5 *cun* and the handle-scraping technique is also performed. Both Zhongzhu (TE3) and Zulinqi (GB41) are punctured 0.3 to 0.5 *cun* perpendicularly and the needle-rotating technique is performed. All the needles are retained for 30 to 60 minutes, with manipulation every 15 minutes. The treatment is given once a day. If the medicinal powder can be blown into the ear, the effect is more satisfactory. Nine g of baked snake slough are ground into a very fine powder; when there is purulence in the ear, a disinfected cotton ball is used to clean the pus and the medicinal powder is blown into the ear, 0.5 g each time, two or three times a day. If it is very dry in the ear, the powder can be mixed with sesame oil, made into cream, and applied two or three times a day.

2. MOXIBUSTION

Point: Yifeng (TE17).

Technique: Before moxibustion, the pus in the external auditory canal should be cleaned out by a disinfected cotton stick; the irrigation is made with a hydrogen dioxide solution, the external auditory canal being cleaned again with the disinfected cotton stick. Then, mild moxibustion is performed with moxa stick until a local skin flush appears, and the burning heat sensation (avoid blistering). Usually, moxibustion is performed for about one minute. Afterwards, the drainage tissue is put in the external auditory canal so as to facilitate drainage of pus. The moxibustion is given once daily and five sessions form a course of treatment.

3. AURICULAR THERAPY

(1) Puncturing the Auricular Points

Points: Ear, Internal Ear, Kidney, Endocrine, and root of auricular vagus nerve.

Technique: All the points are punctured with strong stimulation and the needles are retained for one hour. The needling is once daily and five to seven sessions make up a course of treatment. The method was used to treat 51 cases of otitis media suppurativa, of which 21 were cured, 13 showed marked improvement, and 10 had some improvement (total effective rate being 86.3%). The authors also feel that auricular acupuncture has an analgesic and secretion-decreasing effect for some types of catarrhal otitis media and otitis media suppurativa, probably because the needling at the Root of Auricular Vagus Nerve can open the obstructed auditory tube.

(2) Embedding of the Intradermal Needle

Points: Mouth, Supratragus, middle of the cymba concha, and Internal Ear.

Technique: After routine sterilization, intradermal needles are thrust in the above points for three to five mm and then are fixed with adhesive plaster. Patients are required to press the Mouth and Supratragus three to five times a day, for one to two minutes each time. Usually, after two to three sessions the pus in the ear disappears, but three more sessions should be given to consolidate the therapeutic effect.

(3) Bleeding Method

Points: Kidney, Internal Ear, External Ear, Endocrine, and the 2nd blood vessel on the back of the auricle.

Technique: The 2nd blood vessel on the back of the auricle is pricked with a one-*cun* needle (Size: No.28) for bleeding of one to three drops of blood, and then the other points are punctured with needles that are retained for 20 minutes. The treatment is given once a day and is applicable for acute otitis media.

4. ELECTRIC ACUPUNCTURE

Points: ① Yifeng (TE17) and Ermen (TE21). ② Wangu (GB12) and Tinggong (SI19).

Technique: The points are alternated in needling, and the needles are connected with the impulse electric current. Treatment is given once a day, 20 minutes each time, and 10 sessions form one course.

[REMARKS]

1. Acupuncture has fairly good effect in treating this disease. For acute otitis media, a couple of sessions can cure before suppuration.

After suppuration, the blowing of medicinal powder into the ear (as mentioned above), or using a cotton stick soaked with white vinegar (white vinegar and cold boiled water, half and half) or with 3% hydrogen dioxide solution to irrigate the pus, and ear drops of coptis root solution can also obtain satisfactory effect. Heavy moxibustion is needed for chronic otitis media.

2.   If high fever, headache, vomiting, unconsciousness, delirium, and convulsion are present, it is a critical syndrome caused by the transmission of the pathogenic toxin to the brain, the equivalent of "otogenic meningitis." Attention must be paid to treating this with combined traditional Chinese and Western medicine.

DEAF-MUTISM

[INTRODUCTION]

The majority of patients have mutism resulting from deafness. In modern medicine, the disease is divided into two types: congenital and acquired. The former is due to the underdevelopment or even non-development of the auditory organs during the embryonic period, the misuse of medication during pregnancy, and labor injury; the latter is caused by other diseases e.g., otitis media and is characterized by semi-deafness, but rarely complete deafness. Drug intoxication, such as, streptomycin, can severely damage the acoustic nerves, thus leading to deafness. Hence sounds and the voice cannot be transmitted to the high nerve center, so there is no chance of imitating language, so that the deafness eventually results in mutism. Traumatic injury can also be a causative factor. In traditional Chinese medicine, it is understood that the etiology and pathogenesis of the disease involves the innate insufficiency of both liver and kidney; or invasion of epidemic febrile-toxin which stagnates in the meridians and collaterals obstructing the pure orifice, so that there is loss of hearing in young childhood and subsequently the inability to pick up language; or traumatic injury or the extraordinary high sound disturbing the flow of *qi* in meridians and collaterals, leading to stagnation of *qi* and blood obstructing the ear orifice. The treatment serves to dredge the meridians and collaterals, reopen the obstructed orifices, and regain the ability to pronounce. Points are mainly prescribed from the hand and foot Shaoyang and Taiyang, and Du meridians, such as Tinghui (GB2), Yifeng (TE17), Zhongzhu (TE3), Hegu (LI4), Yamen (GV15), Lianquan (CV23), Waiguan (TE5), Yangchi (TE4), Zulinqi (GB41), Tongli (HT5), Jinmen (BL63) and Zusanli (ST36). Even needling technique is performed. Usually, the deafness is treated first and, when the hearing is restored, the mutism is dealt with along with linguistic training. The treatment is given once a day, and the treatment course should be fairly long.

[CLINICAL EXPERIENCE]

1. CONVENTIONAL ACUPUNCTURE

(1) Puncturing Extra Points

Points: Erlingxue [posterior and inferior to the mastoid process i.e., 0.5 *cun* anterior and superior to the point Fengchi (GB20)], in combination of Yifeng (TE17), Tinggong (SI19) and Lianquan (CV23).

Technique: Erlingxue is penetrated obliquely toward the ear 0.5 *cun* deep with strong stimulation to conduct the needling sensation to the ear. Yifeng (TE17) and Tinggong (SI19) are punctured perpendicularly 0.8 *cun* and Lianquan (CV23) is needled obliquely upward for 0.5 *cun*. Moderate stimulation is performed for the combined points. All the needles are retained for 30 minutes. The treatment is given once daily and seven sessions are taken as a course of treatment.

(2) Point-Grouping Treatment

Points: ① Yifeng (TE17), Ermen (TE21), Tinggong (SI19), and Tinghui (GB2), combined with Zhongzhu (TE3), Houxi (SI3) and Zhilong (in the postauricular depression, at the level of the tragus). ② Penetrating from Tinghui (GB2) to Yifeng (TE17), Chimai (TE18), and Zhilong$_2$ [0.5 *cun* superior to Yifeng (TE17)], combined with Tianrong (SI17), Zhongzhu (TE3) and Ermen (TE21). ③ Yamen (GV15), Tiantu (CV22), penetrating from Tinghui (GB2) to Yifeng

(TE17), Tingling [between Tinghui (GB2) and Tinggong (SI19), 0.2 cm more posterior], Tianting [0.5 *cun* inferior to Anmian (EX)], combined with Waiguan (TE5), Hegu (LI4) and Zhilong$_3$ [between Ermen (TE21) and Tinggong (SI19), 0.2 cm more posterior]. ④ Yamen (GV15), penetrating from Tinggong (SI19) to Tinghui (GB2), Zhilong$_4$ (at the lower border of the ear lobe), Zengyin [the midpoint of the line connecting the Adam Apple and the submandibular angle, anterior and superior to Renying (ST9)], combined with Jinjin (EX-HN12), Yuye (EX-HN13), Renying (ST9) and Tongli (HT5).

Technique: In each session a group of points is selected, and the needling is given once daily, 10 sessions forming one course of treatment with a two-day break between courses. If the hearing is improved after needling, other points for mutism can be combined, e.g., Yongquan (KI1) for the slurring of speech, Tiantu (CV22) and Lianquan (CV23) for the inability to pronounce guttural sounds, Dicang (ST4) for the inability to pronounce labial sound and Zhigou (TE6) for mispronunciation. If no improvement is obtained with all these methods, Baihui (GV20), Sishencong (EX-HN1) and Yintang (EX-HN3) are combined.

(3) Etiological and Symptomatic Treatment

A. Congenital Deaf-mutism

Points: Primary points: Ermen (TE21), Yifeng (TE17), Yamen (GV15), Zhongzhu (TE3) and Waiguan (TE5). Secondary points: Yiming [EX-HN14, 1 *cun* posterior to Yifeng (TE17)], Quchi (LI11), Baihui (GV20), Renzhong (GV26), Jisanxue [altogether 3 points respectively located at 1 *cun* inferior to Yamen (GV15), to the spinous process of the 1st thoracic vertebra, and to that of the 5th lumbar vertebra].

Technique: In each session, the primary points are mainly selected. Ermen (TE21) is penetrated to Tinghui (GB2), Yifeng (TE17) and Yamen (GV15) are punctured with routine technique, and Zhongzhu (TE3) and Waiguan (TE5) are alternated for needling. One or two secondary points can be used when necessary. Moderate stimulation is performed and needles are retained for 20 to 30 minutes. The treatment is given once daily and 10 sessions form one course.

B. Traumatic Deaf-mutism and Decrease of Hearing

Points: ① Ermen (TE21), Yamen (GV15) and Zhongzhu (TE3). ② Xiaguan (ST7), Yifeng (TE17) and Lianquan (CV23).

Technique: The two groups are alternated. Ermen (TE21) is penetrated to Tinghui (GB2); Xiaguan (ST7) is punctured first perpendicularly, and then pull the needle up to the subcutaneous layer and change the angle to penetrate obliquely backward to Tinggong (SI19) for 1.5 to 2.5 *cun*. The other points are punctured with the routine method. Dazhui (GV14), Zhongchong (PC9), Quchi (LI11), Shenmen (HT7), Shenshu (BL23) and Zusanli (ST36) are combined if tinnitus is present.

C. Drug-Intoxicating Deaf-mutism

Points: ① Ermen (TE21), Yifeng (TE17), Zhongzhu (TE3) and Waiguan (TE5). ② Chimai (TE18), Yamen (GV15), Sidu (TE9) and Lingxia [2 *cun* below Yanglingquan (GB34)]. ③ Sidu (TE9), Zhongzhu (TE3), Xiaguan (ST7), Jiaosun (TE20) and Yiming (EX-HN14).

Technique: The above three groups of points are alternated for the needling, one group a day. Or the 654-2 injection can be injected in the points, 0.5 ml for each. To do acupuncture, the needles are retained for 15 to 30 minutes and 10 sessions make a course of treatment.

D. Deaf-mutism Caused by Otitis Media

Points: Yamen (GV15), Ermen (TE21), Yifeng (TE17), Zhongzhu (TE3) and Waiguan (TE5).

Technique: Yamen (GV15) can be excluded for those with semi-deaf-mutism or decreased hearing. Xiaguan (ST7) is added when there is otopiesis. If there is tinnitus, Dazhui (GV14), Quchi (LI11) and Zusanli (ST36) are used instead of Waiguan (TE5). When there is suppuration, acupuncture is combined with moxibustion at Yifeng (TE17). The treatment is given once a day and 10 sessions make up one course.

E. Deaf-mutism (including complete deaf-mutism, semi-deaf-mutism, and simple deafness) Caused by Infectious Disease (measles, epidemic meningitis, typhoid, high fever, convulsions, etc.)

Points: Yifeng (TE17) and Yamen (GV15), or Xiaguan (ST7),

Chimai (TE18), and Dazhui (GV14).

Technique: Xiaguan (ST7) is penetrated to Tinggong (SI19), and the others are needled with routine technique. If it is only a case of decreased hearing, Ermen (TE21), Yifeng (TE17), Zhongzhu (TE3), and Waiguan (TE5) can be used. If tinnitus is associated, Xiaguan (ST7), Fengchi (GB20), Jiaosun (TE20) and Baihui (GV20) are recommended. After the arrival of *qi,* the needles are retained for 10 to 20 minutes. The treatment is give once daily, 10 sessions forming a course.

(4) Single-Point Needling
Point: Fuliu (KI7).

Technique: The point is punctured and manipulation performed to conduct the needling sensation to the knee. The needle is retained for 30 minutes. This method is indicated for deafness due to auditory tube inflammation.

2. ELECTRIC ACUPUNCTURE

Points: ① Ermen (TE21) and Yifeng (TE17). ② Tinghui (GB2) and Chimai (TE18). ③ Xiaguan (ST7) and Yiming (EX-HN14).

Technique: One group of points is selected in each session and three groups are alternated. After the arrival of *qi,* the electro-acupuncture apparatus is connected with the points for 10 to 15 minutes with a frequency of 180 to 240 beats per minute. Needling is given once a day and 10 sessions form one course.

3. CATGUT-EMBEDDING IN ACUPOINTS

Points: Sidu (TE9), Yifeng (TE17) and Yiming (EX-HN14).

Technique: One point is used each time and all the points are alternated. A trocar is used to embed the catgut into the point. The embedding is given once a week and it can be made continuously for three to 20 sessions.

4. CUPPING METHOD

Points: Yifeng (TE17), Fengchi (GB20) and Yamen (GV15).

Technique: Acupuncture is given first. After the arrival of *qi,* the needles are removed. Then the cupping is performed for 5 to 15 minutes each point, once daily. Ten sessions are taken as a course of treatment.

[REMARKS]

1. From the clinical view, acupuncture has certain effect in treating this disease, but only the symptoms are improved. It is difficult to make a complete cure. To those with complete loss of hearing, it is very difficult to obtain any effect.

2. To puncture Yamen (GV15), the depth of insertion should be appropriate in order to avoid the injury of the medullar bulb, giving rise to paralysis.

3. The deafness is treated first and then the mutism. When the patient starts to have the recovery of hearing, the linguistic training should be combined.

RHINITIS

[INTRODUCTION]

Rhinitis is classified into acute and chromic types. Clinically, the former results from recurrent common cold in which the germs invade the nasal mucosa, whereas the latter is often the consequence of frequent reoccurrence of acute rhinitis, or the result of long-term constant irritation of the nose by harmful gases. Rhinitis is marked by nasal obstruction and nasal secretion (mucosa, clear nasal discharge or thick, foul, yellow discharge); the acute variety may be associated with fever, headache, etc. According to traditional Chinese medicine, rhinitis is either induced by the attack of the human body launched by exogenous wind-cold or wind-heat, which causes dysfunction of lung *qi* in dispersing; or improper diet that weakens the body resistance (anti-pathogenic *qi*) and impairs lung *qi*, resulting in the functional abnormality of the nasal cavity. Treatment is directed toward eliminating pathogenic wind, promoting the lung's function in dispersing *qi*, and opening the nose. Points applied in the treatment are mainly the points of Hand Yangming meridian and Hand Taiyin meridian, e.g., Dazhui (GV14), Shangxing (GV23), Yingxiang (LI20), Quchi (LI11), Lieque (LU7) and Hegu (LI4). If the condition is attributable to deficiency type, the reinforcing method is applied, for that of excess, reducing technique is adopted.

[CLINICAL EXPERIENCE]

1. CONVENTIONAL ACUPUNCTURE

(1) Puncturing the Extra Point

Point: The front part of the inferior nasal conchae, unilateral Hegu (LI4) is combined.

Technique: Enlarge the nostrils with a nasoscope, and insert a sterilized two-*cun* needle into the front part of inferior nasal conchae 2-3 mm deep. Retain the needle in the point for 15-30 minutes, during which slightly twist the needle to enhance stimulation. Upon the removal of the needle, use a cotton ball to press the point for three to five minutes to prevent bleeding. Conduct the treatment once a day. Five sessions constitute one course. This method has been applied in 53 cases over one or two courses, and 22 were cured, 17 remarkably improved, and 11 improved, while three showed no effect.

(2) Puncturing Yingxiang (LI 20) as Principal Point

Points: Main points: Yingxiang (LI20). Supplementary points: Hegu (LI4) is added if pain is felt. Tongtian (BL7) for hyposmnia, Zuanzhu (BL2) for dizziness, Sanyinjiao (SP6) for dream disturbed sleep, Suliao (GV25) for nasal obstruction.

Technique: Puncture Yingxiang (LI 20) deeply, 0.5-1.0 *cun*, until the patient feels pain with tears, retain the needle in place for 30 minutes. Puncture other points in the conventional way in accordance with the manifestations. Give the treatment once daily, five sessions constituting one course.

(3) Puncturing Biyanxinxue (the stigma in the nasal cartilage where the trigeminal nerve passes through, a sensitive spot)

Technique: Puncture the point and conduct twisting manipulation;

and retain the needle for 20 minutes. Apply the treatment once a day, 10 sessions forming one course. Additional points may be added based on the manifestations.

2. MOXIBUSTION

Points: Xinhui (GV22) and Juegu (GB39)

Technique: Apply indirect moxibustion on the two points insulated respectively with a ginger slice (0.1-0.2 cm thick, the size of a big coin), with a moxa cone as big as a date-core. The treatment normally uses four to five cones until the ginger slice turns gray-brown. Apply moxibustion once a day, first on Xinhui (GV22) for three to five days; if there is no effect, treat Juegu (GB39).

3. BLEEDING

Points: Shangyingxiang (extra point above LI20) and Tongtian (BL7)

Technique: Prick Shangyingxiang with a needle to cause bleeding; needle Tongtian (BL7) with the reducing twisting method to direct the needling sensation to the nostrils, and retain the needle for 30 minutes. Treatment is given once a day, with five treatments in one course.

4. AURICULAR THERAPY

Points: Internal Nose, External Nose, Endocrine, Adrenal and Lung.

Technique: Conduct ear acupuncture once a day or once every other day (five sessions equal one course). Semen Vaccaria may be adopted instead of a needle, and applied once for three to five days in winter and one to two days in summer. Five sessions constitute one course.

5. EMBEDDING THERAPY

Points: Yingxiang (LI20), Hegu (LI4), Shangxing (GV23) and Baihui (GV20)

Technique: Needle Yingxiang (LI 20) 0.5-1.0 *cun* deep. After the arrival of the needling sensation, remove the needle and embed an intradermal needle into the point and fix with adhesive tape to prevent it falling off. The needle is embedded for four days. During this time, if the needle sensation disappears, press the point to enhance it. Other points are then treated by needling. Usually, after two or four treatments with embedding, the symptoms may disappear completely or are alleviated.

6. CUPPING THERAPY

Points: Dazhui (GV 14), Fengmen (BL 12) and Feishu (BL 13).

Technique: Apply stationary cupping for 10 minutes on each point or conduct sliding cupping 15-20 times from Dazhui (GV 14) to Feishu (BL 13). Give treatment once a day, five sessions in a course. This method is suitable for acute rhinitis.

[REMARKS]

Rhinitis should be managed in a timely way, even though the symptoms may be relatively mild. If nasal infection spreads or improper squeezing of the nose induces nasosinusitis, otitis media, pharyngitis, pneumonia, acupuncture treatment usually exerts a satisfactory effect.

ALLERGIC RHINITIS

[INTRODUCTION]

Allergic rhinitis IS clinically manifested mainly as paroxysmal watery nasal discharge and sneezing encountered in any age of patient. It is often seen in the transition from summer to autumn, or from autumn to winter, or in spring. It may also occur all the year round in some patients. If it is protracted, it may be complicated with nasal polyp. According to TCM, it is due to weakness of lung *qi,* so that the defensive *qi* is not strong enough to guard the superficial portion of the body, which gives rise to an attack of pathogenic wind and cold. Secondly, spleen *qi* or kidney *qi* deficiency may affect lung function, inducing the condition. As the kidney is known as the root of *qi,* a deficiency of kidney *qi* leads to its dysfunction in taking in the respiratory *qi*; failure of descending of *qi* results in retention of lung *qi*; spleen *qi* deficiency leads to insufficiency of the acquired *qi,* which causes poor nourishment of lung *qi*. Thus the latter becomes deficient. The principle of treatment is to reinforce the lungs to eliminate pathogenic factors, strengthen the spleen and replenish the kidneys. Points may be chosen mainly from the Hand Taiyin Meridian, and both Hand and Foot Yangming Meridians, e.g., Yingxiang (LI 20), Yintang (EX-HN3), Feishu (BL 13), Hegu (LI 4), Lieque (LU7), Taiyuan (LU 9) and Zusanli (ST 36). Even movement of needling technique is applied, and the needles are retained in the points for 30 minutes. Treatment is applied once a day and 10 treatments constitute one course.

[CLINICAL EXPERIENCE]

1. CONVENTIONAL ACUPUNCTURE

(1) Deep Puncture

Point: Yintang (EX-HN3)

Technique: Pinch the point, then insert a 1.5-*cun* needle (Size: No.30) into the point 0.2 *cun* deep. After the arrival of *qi,* guide the needle slowly and cutaneously downward about 1 *cun* inside, and then apply twisting, lifting and thrusting manipulation to induce the needling sensation exteriorly to the head and interiorly to the nasal cavity. Retain the needle for 20 minutes, re-manipulating it once every five minutes. Conduct the treatment once a day or once every other day, 10 sessions in one course.

(2) Blood Circulation Invigorating Method

Point: Yingxiang (LI 20), Yintang (EX-HN3), Geshu (BL 17) and Xuehai (SP 10)

Technique: Puncture Yingxiang (LI 20) 0.2-0.5 *cun* deep obliquely upward and puncture Yintang 1.0 *cun* deep transversely downward. With these two needles inserted, a heavy sensation is induced in the local area, and the needling sensation should radiate to the nose. Puncture Geshu (BL 17) 0.5 *cun* obliquely to cause heaviness and distending sensation. Apply the treatment once a day, 10 treatments constituting one course of treatment. This method is suitable for intractable allergic rhinitis.

(3) Puncturing "Liao" Points

Points: Juliao (ST3), Suliao (GV 25), Heliao (LI 19), Jiabi (located at the junction of the nasal bone and the cartilage at the lateral side of the nose), Dazhui (GV 14), Zusanli (ST 36) and Hegu (LI 4).

Technique: Needle all the points with prolonged stimulation, i.e., twist the needle for 10 minutes, then retain it for 20 minutes. Apply the treatment once daily, 10 sessions in one course.

(4) Puncturing Extra Points

Point: Biqiu (located at the nasal concha attached border) and Xiabijia (below Biqiu)

Technique: Insert a two-*cun* filiform needle from the anterior superior aspect of the nasal concha attached border (Biqiu) to the mucus, 0.2-0.3 *cun* deep, then to the Xiabijia for 0.2-0.3 *cun*, removing immediately. Acupuncture may induce a sneeze, nasal discharge or cough. After the removal of the needle, the symptoms should disappear. Apply the treatment once every other day.

2. MOXIBUSTION

(1) Mild Warmth Moxibustion

Points: Feishu (BL 13), Yingxiang (LI 20), Yintang (EX-HN3), Hegu (LI 4) and Dazhui (GV 14).

Technique: In each session, select two to four points and apply moxibustion on each point for 15-20 minutes. Give the treatment once or twice a day, 10 sessions in one course.

(2) Moxibustion with Moxa Cone

Points: Xinhui (GV 22), Shangxing (GV 23) and Fengmen (BL 12).

Technique: First puncture holes on a ginger slice (0.1-0.2 cm thick in the size of a five-fen coin), then place it on Xinhui (GV22), and add a moxa cone in the size of a date core. Treat the point with more cones until the ginger slice becomes brown, then apply the same treatment to the other two points. Moxibustion is applied once every other day, 10 sessions in one course.

3. AURICULAR THERAPY

Points: Inner Nose, External Nose, Lung, Spleen, Kidney, Pingjian, Xiajiaoduan, Allergic Area and Adrenal.

Technique: In each treatment, select three to five points. Needle the points with a short filiform needle. The needling is done with an even movement, with retention for 30 minutes. Give the treatment once daily, and 10 treatments form one course. It is also possible to apply the treatment with seeds (Semen Vaccaria) instead of needle.

4. CUPPING

Points: Dazhui (GV 14), Feishu (BL 13), Gaohuangshu (BL 43) and Shenshu (BL 23).

Technique: Apply cupping on the above points, and leave the cups on the points for 10 minutes. Apply the treatment once daily, 10 sessions in one course. This method is suitable and effective for weak patients who suffer from the illness for a long period of time and have a fear of the needle.

5. LASER ACUPUNCTURE

Points: Zusanli (ST 36), Yingxiang (LI 20) and Fengchi (GB 20). Supplementary points: Hegu (LI 4), Fengmen (BL 12), Gaohuangshu (BL 43) and Pishu (BL 20).

Technique: Use a Hi-Ni laser optical fiber to give laser radiation to the points, each one for three to five minutes. One treatment should not last more than 30 minutes. Apply the treatment once a day, 10 sessions in a course, allowing a three to five-day break between courses. For Epistaxis, or nasal discharge stained with blood, add Shangxing (GV23); for severe nasal blockage, add Bitong (Extra); and for hyposmia, add Tongtian (BL7). This method was applied in 50 cases, 22 being cured, 27 showing improvement and one case without improvement.

6. WRIST ACUPUNCTURE

Point: Upper point bilaterally

Technique: Insert the needle from the upper point (in the depression between the medial border of the ulna and the ulnar side of wrist flexion tendon) level with Neiguan (PC6). The needle is inserted 1.4 *cun* subcutaneously toward the elbow. Retain for 30-60 minutes. Apply the treatment once a day or once every other day. Ten treatments form one course. This treatment was applied in six cases and only one showed no effect.

[REMARKS]

1. Acupuncture has good effect for acute attack of allergic rhinitis, but it needs a longer period of treatment for chronic cases.

2. Acupuncture has the effect of regulating the immune system of patients with allergic rhinitis. It has been observed that application of white pepper powder to the points has an effective rate of 95%, and, after treatment, the IgG in the serum and nasal discharge increased obviously while IgE in the nasal discharge decreased obviously.

PARASINUSITIS

[INTRODUCTION]

Parasinusitis refers to the inflammation of the membrane of the parasinuses. The main symptoms include constant running nose, headache and nasal obstruction. Rhinorrhea is so named because of constant nasal discharge. The incomplete curing of an acute case will make it a persistent chronic one. Chinese medicine views the disease as mainly caused by wind cold or wind heat attacking the lung, resulting in retention of excessive heat there. And it is also due to pathogenic heat burning the nose along the meridian, or overeating greasy and sweet food that produces damp in the interior; or emotional factors leading to impairment of the free flow of liver *qi* and fire produced because of stagnation. As a result, the liver and gallbladder fire attacks the upper clear orifice. The treatment principle is to eliminate wind, disperse heat, benefit lung and open the orifice and clear away the liver and gallbladder fire. The points are mainly selected from the lung meridian of Hand-Taiyin, Hand and Foot-Yangming meridians, Governor Vessel and Foot-Jueyin meridian, i.e., Shangxing (GB23), Yintang (Ex-HN3), Fengchi (GB20), Lieque (LU7), Hegu (LI4) and Xingjian (LR2). Reducing needling technique is applied.

[CLINICAL EXPERIENCE]

1. CONVENTIONAL ACUPUNCTURE

(1) Deep Puncturing Method

Point: Yingxiang (LI20)

Technique: A three-*cun* needle (Size: No.28) is inserted on the point, 1 to 1.5 *cun* deep. The needle is inserted at first 0.2 to 0.5 *cun* deep, then it goes to the anterior upper end of the inferior nasal concha obliquely 35 to 40° and no any reinforcing and reducing manipulation is given. The treatment is given once a day, the needle is retained for 40 minutes and five treatments make one course. The second course of treatment starts one week later if the case is not cured. Several drops of blood happen after inserting the needle, but it is not necessary to stop bleeding and at same time, severe running nose and sneezing are associated.

(2) Puncturing Acupoint

Point: Zanzhu (BL2)

Technique: To detect the tenderest point at the inner end of the eyebrow, and then insert a one-*cun* filiform needle swiftly and subcutaneously with the tip of the needle pointing downward slightly (about 80°). The needle is inserted with rotation to a suitable depth (about 0.5 *cun*) until the patient feels soreness and distention and the nasal obstruction is much relieved. Then, the needle is rotated gently to induce the sensations of soreness and distention radiating to the forehead and orbital region. Three to five rotations are required each time for three applications. The technique is effective for rhinogenous headache. The treatment is given one to two times a day and five treatments make up one course.

(3) Adjacent Puncturing

Points: Shangyingxiang (Ex-HN8), Tongtian (BL7) and Fengchi

(GB20).

Technique: Even needling with rotation is applied on all points and a radiating sensation is required to the nasal cavity during manipulation to benefit lung *qi* and open the orifice. Needles are retained for 30 minutes and manipulated once every 10 minutes. The treatment is given once a day and 10 treatments make up one course.

2.   MOXIBUSTION

Points: Xinhui (GV22), Juegu (GB39) and Baihui (GV20).

Technique: Indirect moxibustion isolated with ginger (about 0.1 *cun* thick) is applied with a moxa cone in the size of date kernel. Moxibustion is given until the ginger turns gray-brown. Generally, four to five cones are required, once a day. Xinhui (GV22) is stimulated for three to five times and Juegu (GB39) is replaced if there is no effect. *Plain Question* records that: "Nasal discharge happens if the gallbladder heat is transported into the brain." Juegu (GB39) is the major Luo-connecting point in the three *yang* meridians of foot, and the Governor Vessel enters the brain, which is why moxibustion is applied on Juegu (GB 39). Xinhui (GV 22) can reduce the pathogenic heat in the gallbladder meridian and clear the heat from the brain marrow so as to cure nasal discharge. Therefore, when the first two points have no effect, moxibustion on Baihui (GV20) is given for 10 to 20 minutes.

3.   ELECTRIC ACUPUNCTURE

Points: Fengchi (GB20), Hegu (LI4), Neiguan (PC6), Zusanli (ST36) and Neiting (ST44).

Technique: No deep puncture is applied, but only with gentle manipulation. After the arrival of *qi,* the negative electrode is attached to Fengchi (GB20) and the positive one to the points on the upper limb. The points are stimulated with continuous wave, 4 to 4 Hz for 60 to 90 minutes. The treatment is given once a day or once every other days, and 10 treatments make up one course. A seven-day rest is required between two courses, and one to two more courses of treatment are required after the improvement of the symptoms to consolidate the therapeutic effect.

4. AURICULAR THERAPY

Point: External Nose, Internal Nose, Forehead, Tragus, Lung, Infer-tragic Apex and Endocrine.

Technique: A filiform needle is inserted with reducing technique. The needle is retained for an hour. The treatment is given daily and on both ears alternately. The embedding-needle method and seed-pressing technique are also applicable. Ten treatments make one course.

5. LASER THERAPY

Points: Yintang (Ex-HN3), Yingxiang (LI20) and Hegu (LI4).

Technique: He-Ne laser is applied on each point for five minutes, 3 to 25mW. The treatment is given once daily.

[REMARKS]

1. Although acupuncture can achieve good therapeutic effect for rhinorrhea, comprehensive therapy should be applied, like taking Huodan Pills and Cangerzi Powder, to try to cure the disease in the acute stage. If the disease develops to the chronic stage, treatment will be very difficult.

2. For chronic, repeated attack cases, a special examination is given to avoid tumor.

EPISTAXIS

[INTRODUCTION]

Epistaxis may be induced by an attack of exogenous pathogenic wind-cold, which results in dysfunction of the lung in dispersing, along with accumulation of heat impairing the vessels and forcing blood to flow abnormally out of vessels and nose; or it may be due to indulgence in sweaty, greasy and highly-flavored food, which create heat in the stomach, damaging the vessel and making the blood flow upward and out of the nose. It may also be caused by *yin* deficiency of the liver and kidney, with fire of deficiency type flaring upward, damaging vessels so that blood flows out of nose. The treatment principle involves activating the lung's function, dispersing, clearing heat from the stomach, reducing fire and replenishing *yin* respectively, so as to stop the bleeding. Points are mainly selected from the lung meridian and stomach meridian, i.e., Yingxiang (LI20), Suliao (GV25), Shangxing (GV23), Renzhong (GV26), Yintang (EX-H3), Fengchi (GB20), Dazhui (GV14), Lieque (LU7), Kongzui (LU6), Quchi (LI11), Shousanli (LI10), Hegu (LI4), Weizhong (BL40), Neiting (ST44) and Zusanli (ST36). In each treatment, choose one or two adjacent points and apply mild stimulation. In addition, needle one or two distal points with strong stimulation. Treatment is applied once daily, although for severe cases, two or three treatments can be given.

[CLINICAL EXPERIENCE]

1. CONVENTIONAL ACUPUNCTURE

(1) *Reducing Method of Twisting Manipulation*
Point: Dazhui (GV 14)

Technique: Puncture the point with a 1.5-*cun* needle inserted perpendicularly to a depth of 0.5 *cun*; the needle is then inserted obliquely upward 1 *cun*. After the arrival of *qi,* apply twisting manipulation in reducing technique to cause a sensation to the forehead. Retain the needle for 15 minutes, during which time, re-manipulate the needle every three to five minutes.

(2) *Puncturing the Ying-Spring Point*
Point: Xingjian (LR2)

Technique: Puncture the point on the right side if bleeding appears from the left nostril, and vice versa. If bleeding comes from both nostrils, needle the point bilaterally. Use a 1.5-*cun* needle, (Size: No.30) to puncture the point to a depth of 1 *cun*. Needling is in the reducing method of twisting, and should be retained for three to five minutes.

(3) Puncture Local Point

Point: Yingxiang (LI 20)

Technique: Puncture the point of the affected side obliquely upward toward the middle, 0.3-0.4 *cun* deep; retain the needle for 15-30 minutes. Manipulate every three to four minutes with lifting-thrusting and twisting. If the result of the treatment is not good, needle the point bilaterally. If the patient also suffers from hypertension, cardiac diseases or has a weak constitution, apply weak stimulation in the needling. This method has been applied in 50 cases, with 45 cases (treated three to four times) cured, three cases improved, and two proving ineffective.

(4) Selection of Points According to the Differentiation of Syndromes

Points: ① Neiting (ST44), Shangjuxu (ST37) and Lidui (ST45). ② Taichong (LR3), Xiaxi (GB43) and Dadun (LR1). ③ Feishu (BL13), Chize (LU5), Yuji (LU10), Fenglong (ST40) and Shaoshang (LU11). ④ Lieque (LU7), Quchi (LI11) and Hegu (LI4). ⑤ Taixi (KI3), Sanyinjiao (SP6), Xingjian (LR2) and Fengchi (GB20). ⑥ Shangxing (GV23), Yingxiang (LI20), Hegu (LI4), Taichong (LR3) and Neiguan (PC6).

Technique: For the flaring up of stomach fire, needle Neiting (ST 44), Shangjuxu (ST 37) in the reducing method, manipulating the needle continuously for five minutes; bleed Lidui (ST 45) with a three-edged needle. For flaring up of liver fire, puncture Taichong (LR3), Xiaxi (GB 43) with reducing method, manipulating the points continuously for five minutes; prick Dadun (LR1) to let out blood. For accumulation of heat in the lungs, puncture Chize (LU5), Yuji (LU10) and Fenglong (ST40) and manipulate the needle continuously for five minutes with reducing technique; prick Shaoshang (LU11) with a three-edged needle to let out blood. For wind heat damaging the collaterals, puncture Lieque (LU7), Quchi (LI 11) and Hegu (LI 4) with the reducing method and manipulate the needle for five minutes. For *yin* deficiency with hyperactivity of *yang*, needle Taixi (KI3) and Sanyinjiao (SP6) with the reinforcing method, and puncture Xingjian (LR2) and Fengchi (GB20) with even movement. If epistaxis is due to trauma, needle Shangxing (GV23), Yingxiang (LI20) with even movement and Hegu (LI4), Taichong (LR3) Neiguan (PC6) with the reducing method. The treatment is applied once a day, five sessions constituting one course.

(5) *Principal Point Combined with Supplementary Point*

Point: Main points: Yingxiang (LI20 bilateral) and Shuigou (GV26). Supplementary points: Hegu (LI4).

Technique: Apply conventional needling with the reducing method at these points. Usually, after the needles are inserted into the points for 10 minutes, bleeding stops. This method is effective for stubborn cases.

(6) *Puncturing the Extra Point*

Point: Zhiniuxue (located in the middle point of the distal transverse crease of middle finger on the palm side), Yingxiang (LI20) and Kongzui (LU6).

Technique: First bind bilateral Zhiniuxue tightly with thread, and then needle Yingxiang (LI20) bilaterally to cause contraction of the vessel at the side of the nose. Afterwards, puncture Kongzui (LU6) bilaterally; following the arrival of *qi,* apply the reinforcing method at the point. In general, after one or two treatments, bleeding may stop.

2. MOXIBUSTION

Points: ① Shangxing (GV23). ② Fengfu (GV16). ③ Yongquan (KI1). ④ Xinhui (GV22).

Technique: In each session, treat one of the above points with moxa stick over the point for 30 minutes. Nasal bleeding will gradually stop. If after one session of treatment, the bleeding does not stop, a second session may be conducted eight to 10 hours after the first. If the bleeding is heavy and not brought under control, apply direct moxibustion with three cones on the extra point Dagukong (located on the thumb). Treat the point on the right side if bleeding appears in the left nostril, vice versa.

3. AURICULAR THERAPY

Points: Inner Nose, Lung, Shenmen and Adrenal Gland

Technique: Embed intradermal needle into the points. Fix the points with adhesive plaster, and change the needle once every three to four days. This method was applied for 36 cases, and after one of two sessions, the bleeding stopped in 20, abated in six cases. There were five ineffective cases and no result is known in the remaining five.

4. PRICKING METHOD

Points: Dadun (LR1) and Shaoshang (LU11)

Technique: Prick the two points with a three-edged needle to let out blood. In general, the bleeding stops after the point has been pricked. This method is suitable for the condition precipitated by heat in the liver and lung.

5. MEDICAL APPLICATION ON ACU-POINT

Point: Yongquan (KI1)

Technique: Take one or two pieces of garlic and smash them into a paste. Turn the paste into a 5-fen coin-sized cake, 3-5 mm thick, and apply onto the point of the affected nostril side; if both nostrils are bleeding, treat the points bilaterally. Wrap the point with oily gauze. When there is a burning pain in the local region, remove the garlic. Generally, 10 minutes after the application, bleeding subsides and finally stops after a further 20 minutes.

6. LASER THERAPY

Points: Shangxing (GV23), Yingxiang (LI20), Hegu (LI4) and Nasal Mucosa

Technique: Use 3-7mW Hi-In laser radiating the above points directly with optical fiber tube, five minutes for each point. Apply the treatment once a day. Five sessions constitute one course.

7. COMBINED TREATMENT

Points: Weizhong (BL40), Shangxing (GV23) and Zusanli (ST36)

Technique: First prick the superficial vein of Weizhong (BL40) with a three-edged needle to let out blood, and then needle Shangxing (GV23) and Zusanli (ST36); needle Shangxing (GV23) transversely toward Shenting (GV24), 0.3-0.5 *cun*; puncture Zusanli perpendicularly, 1.5-2 *cun* deep. The latter two points are treated with twisting manipulation continuously for five to 10 minutes. Treatment is applied once a day.

[REMARKS]

1. During the treatment, cold compression with a moist towel is applied to the forehead, and the nostrils are plugged.

2. If acupuncture and moxibustion are not satisfactory for continuous heavy bleeding, comprehensive measures should be taken in a timely way in order to prevent much loss of blood and further adverse effects.

3. Although the majority of the cases of epistaxis are attributable to heat syndrome, moxibustion may exert the effect of dispersing heat. Hence it is also applicable for this condition.

4. If the nose bleeds continuously resulting from trauma, finger pressure serving as a needle is an effective method and may be applied, i.e., pressing Kunlun (BL60), and Taixi (KI3) with thumb and index fingertips toward each other. Treat the bilateral point with both hands.

SORE THROAT

[INTRODUCTION]

Sore throat, consisting of acute syndrome and chronic syndrome, is a common disorder of the throat; in severe cases, dysphagia and difficulty in breathing can be seen. According to traditional Chinese medicine, it relates to the accumulated heat in the lung meridian or to wind-heat attacking the lung, the pathogenic heat thus affecting the lung system; or it is due to overeating hot spicy and deep fried foods, which induce heat and fire of the lung and stomach flaring upward, affecting the throat. It may also result from long-term exposure to toxic, abnormal gases or dusts; or extended vocal activity, or indulgence in sexual activities. Alternatively, the remaining pathogenic heat, in the case of febrile diseases, impairs the essence of the lung and kidney so that the *yin* fluid cannot moisten the throat, but the fire of the deficiency type flares to the throat causing soreness. Treatment is directed toward dispersing wind, clearing the heat from the stomach, activating lung *qi,* nourishing kidney *yin* and easing the throat. For excessive heat syndrome, points are mainly selected from the Yang-ming meridians of hand and foot; for deficiency syndrome, points are selected mainly from the Shaoyin meridian of foot, such as Chize (LU5), Shaoshang (LU11), Hegu (LI4), Taixi (KI3), Zhaohai (KI6), Taiyuan (LU9), Feishu (BL13), etc. The excess syndrome is treated with the reducing method and *yin* deficiency syndrome is managed with even movement, needles are retained in place for 15-20 minutes. Treatment is applied once or twice daily, 10 sessions constitute one course of treatment.

[CLINICAL EXPERIENCE]

1. CONVENTIONAL ACUPUNCTURE

(1) Puncturing Single Point
Point: Tianzhu (BL 10)

Technique: Insert the needle obliquely from the lateral in a depth of 1.0-1.3 *cun.* Sometimes the distending and numb sensation may disperse to the head and shoulder. Then apply needle stimulation in moderate degree with lift-thrust manipulation for one minute. Retain the needle in the point for 30 minutes and during this period, re-manipulate the needle once every 10 minutes, 5 sessions constitute one course of treatment. This method was applied for 59 cases of acute pharyngitis, the effective rate being 96%. In most cases the white blood cell account was markedly drooped down the next day after acupuncture treatment. In general after 3-day treatment the condition was cured or remarkably alleviated.

(2) Puncturing the Empirical Point
Point: Liyanxue

Technique: Patient sit erect with shoulder drooped, eyes looking forward. The point is located in the depression posterior to the midpoint between the ear lobe and the angle of the mandible. Puncture the point toward the throat 0.8-1.2 *cun* deep, apply the manipulation of scraping the handle of the needle, retain the needle 30-60 minutes, and re-scrape the needle handle every 10-20 minutes during the retention period. If the patient has high fever, Dazhui (GV 14), Shaoshang (LU 11) or Hegu (LI 4) may be combined in the treatment treated with reducing technique, and the needles are not retained in the points. Apply the treatment once daily, 5 treatments constitute one course.

(3) *Puncturing Luozhen Point*

Points: Main points: Luozhen (located in the center of the loops of the index finger). Supplementary points: Hegu (LI4), Tianrong (SI17) and Tiantu (CV22),

Technique: Puncture Luozhen point perpendicularly 0.2-0.3 *cun*, and after needle sensation is obtained, squeeze out a little blood. Puncture the supplementary points with the reducing method. Apply the treatment once a day, and after three to five treatments the problem is usually cured. This method is suitable for acute and chronic laryngitis & pharyngitis and tonsillitis.

2. MOXIBUSTION

Point: Hegu (LI 4)

Technique: Take a garlic slice (0.1-0.2 *cun* thick, as large as a 5-fen coin) and place it onto the point; apply moxibustion at the point with three to five cones in the size of a date core. Conduct the treatment once daily, three sessions constituting one course. The patient should be offered an empirical prescription of herbal therapy, the prescription consisting of Shengdi (Radix Rehmanniae) 20 g, Wuweizi (Cortex Acanthopanacis), 20 g, Gongying (Herba taraxaci), 15 g, Niuxi (Radix Achyranthis bidentatae), 10 g, Chishao (Radix Paeoniae Rubra)10 g, Taoren (Semen Persicae) 7.5 g, Chaihu (Radix Bupleuri) 5 g, Jiegeng (Radix Platycodi) 5 g, Honghua (Flos Carthami) 5 g, Shenggancao (Radix Glycyrrhizae) 5 g, Rougui (Cortex Cinnamomi) 3.5 g. One decoction is taken orally every day. This method has been applied in over 300 cases, and the majority were cured after one session of moxibustion and four days of herbal treatment.

3. BLEEDING METHOD

Points: Shaoshang (LU11) and Shangyang (LI 1).

Technique: Prick the points with a three-edged needle to let out a few drops of blood. It is suitable for acute pharyngitis and laryngitis.

4. AURICULAR THERAPY

Points: Throat, Trachea, Lung, Anti-apex, Brain, Neck, Kidney and Sympathetic.

Technique: For acute pharyngitis and laryngitis, puncture the points with a filiform needle with moderate or strong stimulation. Conduct the treatment once or twice daily. When the acute symptoms are under control, put seeds onto the points, rather than needling. The seed method is also used for chronic pharyngitis and laryngitis.

5. ELECTRIC CONDUCTION METHOD

Points: Fengchi (GB20), Neck triangular area, Tiantu (CV22), Dazhui (GV14) and Futu (LI18).

Technique: Use 2 plate-electrodes in 5-7V induction of DL-3 698 Electro-apparatus on bilateral Fengchi (GB20). Move the electrodes laterally downward, and when they are being moved to both sides of the neck, increase the intensity of the stimulation to induce a running water-like sensation in the entire throat, and both a shrinking feeling and a comfortable sensation. Apply continuous chopping stimulation for two to four minutes. Lay the negative electrode, which is 3-4V, to Tiantu (CV22), and the positive electrode to Dazhui (GV14), and apply continuous chopping stimulation for two to four minutes. Then put the negative electrode to the bilateral Futu (LI18) respectively to stimulate the point for one or two minutes. Apply the treatment once daily. Five treatments constitute one course, and the treatment should cover two or three courses.

6. FINGER ACU-PRESSURE

Points: Find the tenders spots on the back, and then choose the relevant points on the four limbs according to the principle of selecting the points from the meridian, which is in relation with the tender spots. With the patient in a prone position, the practitioner uses the thumb to knead the sides of spine (along the course of the bladder meridian) so as to find the tender spot. If the tenderness appears at Feishu (BL13, the Back-shu point of the Lung), Yuji (LU10), Chize (LU5), Shousanli (LI10), Quchi (LI11) are treated; if the tender spot at the Xingshu (BL15, the Back-shu point of the heart), Shenmen (HT7), Tongli (HT5), Jianzhen (SI 9) and Houxi (SI3) are chosen; if the tender spot is at Ganshu (BL18, the Back-shu point of the liver), Taichong (LR3) is selected; if the tender spot is at Pishu (BL20), Sanyinjiao (SP6) is treated; for the tender spot at Weishu (BL21), Zusanli (ST36), Neiting (ST44) and Renying (ST9) are treated; and for Shenshu (BL23), Yongquan (KI1) and Zhaohai (KI6) are treated.

Technique: Use the palm side of the thumb, index finger or middle finger to press the tender spot on the back, and then the points on the four limbs. Press each point for one or two minutes, and then use the thumb and index finger to press the tissue at the side of the thyroid cartilage for three or four minutes. This method has been applied in 50 cases of irritable throat, and each case achieved a satisfactory result after one to three sessions.

7.   MEDICINAL APPLICATION ON ACU-POINT

Point: Tiantu (CV 22)

Technique: Put 2 × 2 cm medicinal plaster for rheumatic pain on the point, changing the plaster once everyday over a five-day period. This method has been applied in 100 cases, resulting in 55 cases asymptomatic with improvement of throat congestion and, 16 cases asymptomatic without change of the throat; and 10 cases saw an improvement of the symptoms.

[REMARKS]

1.   For patients with a long-term condition, or with little therapeutic effect, examination by the ear-nose-throat department should be made so as not to delay necessary treatment.

2.   It is suggestive to add Liu Shen Wan (patent Chinese medicine) in combination with the treatment mentioned above.

3. It is advisable for the patient to take lightly-flavored food, and avoid spicy food, tobacco and alcohol.

TONSILLITIS

[INTRODUCTION]

Tonsillitis is caused by inflammation of pharyngeal tonsil by the invasion of streptococcus and staphylococcus, and it is marked by congestion, swelling and pain of tonsil, and may accompanied by fever and headache. This problem is also called "moth of throat" for the swollen tonsil looks like silkworm moth. Throat is what the lung and stomach pertains to, and connects with stomach via esophagus and lung via trachea. This problem can be invasion of wind-heat to the lung, and burning of lung by heat; or by overeating spicy and greasy food, leading to disturbing stomach fire to condense the body fluid into phlegm and then phlegm fire accumulation in the throat; or by deficiency of kidney *yin* and upsurge of deficient fire to the throat. The principle of treatment is to disperse lung *qi,* clear stomach heat, benefit throat and nourish kidney *yin*. The points of Hand Taiyang, Hand Foot Yangming and foot Shaoyin are selected as the main points such as Shaoshang (LU11), Chize (LU5), Hegu (LI4), Quchi (LI11), Neiting (ST44) and Taixi (KI3). And reinforcing technique is used for deficiency syndrome, reducing technique for excess syndrome. The needle is retained for 30 minutes, once daily, 10 times constitute one course.

[CLINICAL EXPERIENCE]

1. CONVENTIONAL ACUPUNCTURE

(1) Puncturing Jing-well Point

Points: Main points: Shaoshang (LU11), Shangyang (LI1), Guan-chong (SJ1) and Dadun (LR1).

Supplementary points: Tianrong (SI11), Hegu (LI4), Neiting

(ST44) and Quchi (LI11).

Technique: Two main points and two supplementary points are selected, and all the points are used in turn. Jing-well points are punctured by one-*cun* needle (Size: No.28), and then two to three drops of blood are squeezed out. The supplementary points are punctured by No.30 needle. The needle is retained for 10 to 20 minutes. They are manipulated a few times. The treatment is given once a day, and 5 times constitutes one course.

(2) Penetrating Technique

Points: Lieque (LU7) to Pianli (LI6) and Hukou (Extra) to Hegu (LI4).

Technique: The contralateral points or both sides of points are punctured. Penetrating technique is used from Lieque (LU7) to Pianli (LI6) and Hukou (midpoint of thumb web). The needle is inserted 1 *cun* deep. Strong stimulation is performed without retention of needle. The treatment is given once a day, and 10 times constitutes one course.

(3) Puncturing the Affected Area

Point: Tonsil

Technique: Inserting a 1.5-*cun* (Size: No.30) needle from a point along the inferior medial border, 0.5 *cun* anterior to the mandible into the tonsil 0.8 to 1.2 *cun* deep. Manipulating the needle by rotating technique until the patient feels sore and distension in the throat and less pain in the local area. Retaining the needle for 15 to 20 minutes, and manipulating once every 5 minutes. The treatment is given once a day and 5 times constitutes one course. Quchi (LI11) is used for excessive heat, Taiyang (extra) is used for headache, and Fengchi (GB20) is used for exterior syndrome.

(4) Puncturing Shu-Stream Point

Point: Zhongzhu (SJ3)

Technique: Zhongzhu (SJ3) is Shu-stream point of Sanjiao Meridian of Hand Shaoyang. It is punctured 0.5 *cun* deep with strong stimulation. Retaining the needle for one hour, meanwhile, manipulating the needle three to five times. In case of severe condition, penetrating heaven-coolness is applied. It is given once a day and ten times is one course.

(5) Round Needle Technique

Point: Swollen tonsil.

Technique: A round needle is twined tightly on a stick with thread, asking the patient to open the mouth, and pressing his tongue by tongue depressor. Inserting the stick and puncturing the swollen tonsil quickly in one to three places to see bleeding. It is given once a day and three times are one course.

(6) Puncturing the Experience Point

Points: Liyang Point [0.8 *cun* lateral to Tianding (LI17)]

Technique: The needle is inserted 0.5 to 1 *cun* deep and manipulate the needle by rotating technique with even movement, retaining the needle for 30 to 60 minutes and manipulating it once every 10 minutes. It is given once a day and three times are one course. In most cases, pain is much less one hour later, and it is cured 5 to 6 hours later. This point is called Liyang point for it can benefit throat. To strengthen the therapeutic effect, Tiantu (CV22), Neiguan (PC6), and Hegu (LI11) are added.

(7) Puncturing Jing-River Point

Points: Tianzhu (BL10) and Hegu (LI11).

Technique: Tianzhu is punctured 1 *cun* deep with needling sensation toward the throat, retaining the needle for 30 minutes and manipulating the needle once every 5 minutes. Hegu (LI4) is punctured rapidly with reducing technique without retention of needle after the arrival of *qi*. It is given once a day and 10 times is one course.

2. MOXIBUSTION

Point: Jiaosun (SJ20).

Technique: Apply some vegetal oil on Dengxincao, igniting it and performing moxa over the point. It is better to hear a sound "pa." It is given once a day, and three times are one course.

3. THREE-EDGED NEEDLE TECHNIQUE

(1) Spot Pricking Method

Points: Shaoshang (LU11) and Shangyang (LI1).

Technique: After the sterilization, prick the above points by a three-edged needle to cause a few drops of blood out. More blood can be squeezed out if there is less blood. Both sides of points are used. It is given once a day. Usually, it can be cures by one to three times of treatment. A total of 15 cases of tonsillitis have been treated and all of them are cured.

(2) Puncturing Extra Point
    Point: Taiyang (Extra).

Technique: After sterilizing the point, prick the point by three-edged needle to cause a few drops of blood out. The treatment is given once a day and three times are one course. The swelling and pain of throat can usually be alleviated by this treatment.

4. AURICULAR ACUPUNCTURE

(1) Bleeding Therapy
    Point: Veins on the back of ear.

Technique: Massaging the back of ear to make the veins congested. After the routine asepsis, use No.6 or 7 syringe needle or a three-edged needle to prick and cause five to seven drops of blood out. The same side of the ear to the affected is used. The treatment is given once a day and three times form one course. When the throat is red and swelling, the veins on the back of ear can be clearly seen.

(2) Needling Technique
    Point: Detecting tenderness on the tragus or on the lower portion of scapha in some cases.

Technique: Apply strong stimulation, retaining the needle for 30 to 60 minutes. It is given once a day. Usually, inflammation can be relieved by two to three times of treatment. A total of 304 cases of acute tonsillitis are treated, and the total effective rate is 90.1%.

(3) Embedding Seeds on the Ear Points
    Point: Throat, Tonsil, helix 1 to 6, Shenmen and Adrenal.

Technique: Four to 6 points are selected, Wangbuliuxing seeds are fixed on them. The seeds are retained for two days in summer and three days in winter. Three times is one course. This method is more indicated for chronic tonsillitis.

5. FINGER ACUPUNCTURE THERAPY

Point: Jiaosun (SJ20)

Technique: Let the patient keep a sitting position. The practitioner put his thumb on one side or both sides of points and apply pressing technique by rotation from the mild force to the heavy force, then plucking technique, and finally pushing technique. Ask the patient to swallow. The process last one to five minutes, and it is given once a day.

6. LASER THERAPY

Points: Swollen tonsil, Hegu (LI4) and Shaoshang (LU11).

Technique: Radiating the above points by 3 to 7 mv He-Ne laser tube with 5 minutes on each point. The treatment is given once a day and 5 times constitute one course.

7. CUPPING

Point: Dazhui (CV14).

Technique: Insert the needle quickly into the point 0.5 *cun* deep, and manipulate the needle quickly for one minute after the arrival of *qi* without retention of needle. Put something, which is not easy to conduct heat like orange peel or potato peel, on the point with alcohol cotton ball on it. Ignite the cotton ball and put cup on it. Retain the cup for 10 to 15 minutes and repeat it two times. The result is that the patient can feel comfort and clear sensation in the throat in the first treatment.

8. MEDICINAL APPLICATION ON THE POINT

Point: Yongquan (KI1).

Technique: Grind three portions of Huanglian (goldthread rhizome) and two portions of Wuzhuyu (Chinese cubeb) together into powder. During the treatment, mix rice vinegar with a certain mount of powder into the paste. Apply it on both sides of Yongquan (KI1), covering them by paper and fixing them by the plaster. On the next morning, remove them. It is given once a day and three times are one course.

9. PLUM-BLOSSOM NEEDLE THERAPY

Points: The lateral sides of vertebra, Shangyang (LI1), Hegu (LI4), the nape, the lateral side of the neck, the front of neck and throat, the triangular area of lower jaw.

Technique: Prick the above areas by plum-blossom needle until the skin turns red. It is given once or twice a day and three times are one course.

[REMARKS]

1.   Acupuncture can effectively reduce fever, subdue the swelling, and stop pain in both acute and chronic conditions.

2.   During the period of illness, it is better to eat light food, but not greasy, sweet, and pungent food.

3.   In case that the swollen tonsil can not be relieved by long time of treatment or it repeatedly occurs, the tonsil operation should be considered. This is because many other ailments like nephritis and arthritis are closely related with tonsil infection.

RECURRENT ULCERATIVE STOMATITIS

[INTRODUCTION]

Oral ulcer is mainly manifested by yellowish and whitish ulcerative spots as big as a bean on the oral membrane or on the tongue. Because it is characterized by periodical recurrence, it is also called recurrent oral ulcer. Modern medicine thinks that the real reason for it is unknown, but is probably induced by poor digestion, dysfunction of the endocrine system, mental stress, lack of vitamins and sleep. TCM holds that it can be caused by invasion and flaring upward of external wind-heat, or by overeating greasy and fat food, or by an unclean mouth leading to accumulation of heat in the heart and spleen, or by over-thinking leading to deficiency of the heart and spleen, or by constitutional *yin* deficiency or consumption of kidney essence leading to flaring up of deficient fire. The principle of treatment is to eliminate wind and heat, nourish *yin* and stop pain. The points of Hand and Foot Yangming and Foot Shaoyin are selected as the main points as Hegu (LI4), Jiache (ST6), Yingxiang (LI20), Zusanli (ST36), Neiting (ST44), Lianquan (CV24) and Taixi (KI3). Reinforcing technique is used for deficiency and reducing technique is used for excess. The needle is retained for 30 minutes, and 10 times constitute one course.

[CLINICAL EXPERIENCE]

1. CONVENTIONAL ACUPUNCTURE

(1) Puncturing Single Point
Point: Tianying point (local ulcerative area)

Technique: Ask the patient to wash out the mouth, and then sterilize the ulcerated area with Mercurochrome. Then, insert the needle until there is bleeding. Usually, only puncturing the small ulcer once is enough, but large ones, more than 0.3 cm, need two to four treatments once a day.

(2) Puncturing the Main and Supplementary Points
Points: Main points: Dicang (ST4) and Chengjiang (CV24). Supplementary points: Hegu (LI4), Quchi (LI11), Zusanli (ST36) and Sanyingjiao (SP6). For ulcer on the tongue, add Jinjin (Extra) and Yuye (Extra); for ulcer on the upper lip and membrane on the cheek, add Yingxiang (LI20).

Technique: Prick Jinjin (Extra), and Yuye (Extra) after sterilizing with Mercurochrome. Prick the points, and then ask the patient to wash out the mouth. After the bleeding stops, sterilize the area again, and puncture other points with even technique. After the needling sensation is achieved, retain the needle for 10 to 20 minutes. It is given twice to three times a week and 10 times treatments form one course. Only puncture the points on the tongue twice in one course.

(3) Shallow Puncture
Points: Chengjiang (CV24), Shuigou (GV26), Hegu (LI4), Jinjin (extra), Yuye (extra), Weizhong (BL40) and Houxi (SI3).

Technique: Puncture Chengjiang (CV24) 0.2 *cun* deep, retaining and rotating the needle for three minutes; puncture Shuigou (GV26) 0.2 *cun* deep, retaining and rotating the needle for two minutes; puncture Hegu (LI4) and retain the needle for two minutes; prick Jinjin (extra) and Yuye (extra) and cause bleeding, and then stop; puncture Weizhong (BL40) 0.4 to 0.5 *cun* deep, retaining and rotating the needle for two minutes; puncture Houxi (SI3) 0.3 to 0.4 *cun* deep, retaining and rotating the needle for two minutes. It is given once a day, and 10 treatments constitute one course.

(4) Nourishing Water and Reducing Fire Method

Points: Yongquan (KI1) and Laogong (PC8).

Technique: Puncture the points 0.5 *cun* deep, retaining the needle for 30 minutes; meanwhile, manipulate the needle three times. It is given once a day, and five treatments constitute one course. A total of 36 case of aphthae were treated, and 28 were cured.

(5) Regulating Yangming

Points: Quchi (LI11), Zusanli (ST36) and Hegu (LI4).

Technique: Select two points each time, lifting and thrusting the needle gently with small amplitude until there is a slight traveling feeling. Retain the needle for five minutes, manipulate once, and then retain it for another 10 minutes. Treatment is given three times a week, 10 sessions in one course. This method is indicated in ulcerative stomatitis ulcer due to accumulation of heat caused by spleen deficiency.

2. BLEEDING

(1) Puncturing Empirical Point

Points: Take Dazhui (GV14) as the core, two to three points 1.5 to 2 cm left and right to it, ordered in arc.

Technique: After sterilization, use a three-edged needle to puncture Dazhui (GV14) perpendicularly with the tip downward. The needle passes through the skin to break two to three subcutaneous fibers. Then, prick other points on the left and right of Dazhui (GV14) with the same method. After pricking five to seven points, squeeze the needle holes to obtain three to five drops of blood. Stop the bleeding by pressing. Sterilize the skin, and apply Yushizhi paste externally. It is given twice a week. A total of four cases were cured.

(2) Puncturing the Points Bilaterally

Points: Sifeng (Extra) bilaterally

Technique: Prick the points with a three-edged needle or thick needle and let some blood or yellowish white fluid out. It is given once a week. This method has been used to treat stomatitis in children, and usually it can be cured by one or two treatments.

3. FINGER ACUPUNCTURE TECHNIQUE

Points: Xiaguan (ST7), Jiache (ST6) and Renzhong (GV26).

Technique: Press Xiaguan (ST7) bilaterally with both index fingers, and Jiache (ST6) bilaterally by both middle fingers; press heavily on Renzhong (GV26) with both thumbnails in turn, up and down. One minute is used for each point and treatment is given once in the morning and again in the evening.

4. AURICULAR THERAPY

Points: Main points: Shenmen, mouth, tongue, sympathetic added for the invasion of seasonal factors; heart, liver, and small intestine added for liver fire; liver, spleen, stomach, large intestine added for stagnation of liver and spleen deficiency; heart, kidney, sympathetic, and adrenal added for *yin* deficiency of heart and kidney.

Technique: Select the points according to differentiation of syndrome; only one ear is treated each time. Insert the needle rapidly, manipulating gently. Retain the needle for 30 minutes. It is given once a day and the two ears are treated in turn. Five treatments form one course. After withdrawal of the needle, an embedded needle can be used to consolidate the effect.

5. LASER THERAPY

Points: Lung, Heart, Mouth and Sanjiao.

Technique: Radiate the points with laser apparatus for five minutes on each ear. It is given once a day, five treatments in one course.

6. MEDICINAL APPLICATION ON ACUPOINT

(1) Wuzhuyu Powder

Point: Yongquan (KI9)

Technique: Prepare equal amounts of Wuzhuyu and Dilong powder, 15 to 20 g each time, and mix them with an appropriate amount of flour and vinegar into paste. Apply on Yongquan (KI1) and fix with a bandage. Treatment is given once every other day, three to five treatments constituting one course.

(2) Aphthae Paste

Point: Shenque (CV8)

Technique: Grind 30 g of Xixin into fine powder and mix with an appropriate amount of vinegar into a paste, which is applied on the point and fixed. It is given once a day. This method is indicated in aphthae in children.

7. ACUPUNCTURE AND MOXIBUSTION

Points: Hegu (LI4), Xiaguan (ST7), Dicang (ST4), Jiache (ST6), Quchi (LI11), Zusanli (ST36), Sanyinjiao (SP6), Chengjiang (CV24), Shaoshang (LU11) and Yanglao (SI6)

Technique: Apply the bleeding method on Chengjiang (CV24) and Shaoshang (LU11); apply moxibustion with moxa stick on Yanglao (SI6) for five to 10 minutes; apply acupuncture on the rest of the points with even needling technique, with the needles retained for 20 minutes. The treatment should be given everyday and 10 treatments form one course. The method is good to treat intractable neurological ulcer of the mouth.

[REMARKS]

1. The recurrent ulcer of the mouth is a kind of mouth disease normally seen in the clinic. There is no special effective method to treat it at present, but acupuncture treatment does have a certain effect.

2. Washing the mouth with herbal tea can be also combined with the acupuncture treatment in order to improve the effect. For example, the herbs can be: Wumei 30 g, Shenggancao 20 g.

3. No spicy and rich foods should be eaten; more vegetables and fruit should be eaten; work and rest should be properly balanced.

TOOTHACHE

[INTRODUCTION]

Toothache is the commonly seen symptom in the clinic. It occurs usually with pulpitis, peridentitis, dental caries and so on. The Hand and Food Yangming meridians enter the upper and the lower teeth respectively. The kidney dominates the bone and the teeth are the remainders of the bone; therefore, toothache is closely related to the stomach, large intestine and kidney. For examples, if the patient likes eating greasy, spicy, or rich food, excessive heat will be produced in the stomach and intestine, and the pathogenic heat and fire will go upward along the meridians; or if the patient has constitutional excessive Yang and is attacked by the pathogenic wind, so the wind and fire accumulate in the Yangming meridian, it will eventually attack upward along the meridian; or if the patient has kidney *yin* deficiency, the deficient fire will flare up; or if the patient has an unclean mouth with food particles retained for a long time until they rot, and the dental corona becomes decayed; then toothache will ensue. The treatment principle is to clear the heat, nourish *yin* and relieve the pain. The points should be mainly selected from the Hand and Foot Yangming meridians. Apply reducing or reinforcing needling technique according to the differentiation of the syndromes. Points can be: Xiaguan (ST7), Jiache (ST6), Hegu (LI4), Neiting (ST44), Taixi (KI3), Shenshu (BL23) and so on. The needles should be retained for 30 minutes, with five treatments in one course.

[CLINICAL EXPERIENCE]

1. CONVENTIONAL ACUPUNCTURE

(1) Selecting the Points on the Lower Part of the Body for Treating Diseases of the Upper Body.
Point: Zusanli (ST36)
Technique: Puncture Zusanli (ST36) of the healthy side; the needling sensation is required to reach the teeth. After apply reducing

needling technique for three to five minutes, the needles should be retained for an hour. Xiaguan (ST7) can be added for treating upper jaw toothache; and Jiache (ST6) or Jueyinshu (BL14) of the affected side can be added for treating lower jaw toothache. The treatment is given once or twice a day.

(2) Selecting Neighboring Points

Points: Yifeng(TE17) of the affected side.

Technique: Select Yifeng (TE17) of the affected side, puncturing 1.0 *cun* perpendicularly. Apply lifting, thrusting, twisting and rotating needling technique to make the sensation radiate to the affected area. The needles should remain for 60 minutes and be manipulated every 10 minutes. Puncture the bilateral side for treating toothache on both sides of the mouth. No matter whether upper or lower jaw toothache, as long as there is inflammation of the dental neck, this method will always have special effect.

(3) Modification of the Points According to the Differentiation of the Syndromes

Points: Main point: Hegu (LI4). Supplementary points: Xiaguan (ST7), Siba (ST2), Quanliao (SI18), Renzhong (GV26), Jiache (ST6), Chengjiang (CV24), Jiachengjiang (Ex), Tianrong (SI19), Taiyang (Ex) and Touwei (ST8).

Technique: Hegu (LI4) should be selected every time. Xiaguan (ST7) is added for treating upper jaw toothache; Siba (ST2) or Quanliao (SI18) is added for treating upper front toothache; Xiaguan (ST7) and Jiache (ST6) are added for treating lower jaw toothache, while Chengjiang (CV24) or Jiachengjiang (Ex) can also be added sometimes. For treating acute peridentitis, Xiaguan (ST7) and Tianrong (SI17) should be added; Taiyang (Ex) and Touwei (ST8) should be added for treating headache. Puncture all the points as usual with the reducing method. The needles are retained for 60 minutes and manipulated three to five times intermittently.

(4) Puncturing Jing-well Point

Point: Kunlun (BL60)

Technique: Puncture the point with the tip of the needle toward the anterior aspect of the inner malleolus to a depth of 0.3-0.5 *cun*.

The technique is based on the theory of "tonifying method for deficient syndrome and reducing method for excessive syndrome." Retain the needle for 30 minutes, manipulating every five minutes.

(5) Penetrating Puncture

Points: Taiyang (Ex) penetrating to Xiaguan (ST7) of the affected side.

Technique: Puncture Taiyang (Ex) penetrating to Xiaguan (ST7) of the affected side; the needles are retained for one hour with a single manipulation. Reducing needling technique should be applied. If the pain cannot be relieved after one hour, then the time of needle retention can be extended. From clinical observation, this method has the best effect of treating toothache due to wind and fire of the stomach.

2. MOXIBUSTION

(1) Moxibustion with Moxa Cone on Garlic

Points: Hegu (LI4), Jiache (ST6), Xiaguan (ST7), Neiting (ST44), Sanjian (LI3), Taixi (KI3) and Ermen (TE21)

Technique: Select two to four points each time and apply five to seven cones on every point each time. The size of the moxa cone should be the same as a date kernel or a soybean. The treatment is given once or twice a day, and mostly is given when the pain is present. Moxa cone can be also applied with ginger.

(2) Moxibustion with Moxa Cone on the Skin

Points: Neiguan (PC6), Waihuaijian (EX), Yangxi (LI5), Yuji (LU10), Lieque (LU7), Hegu (LI4), Taixi (KI3), Ermen (TE21) and Jianjing (GB21)

Technique: Selecting two to three points every time and apply three to five cones for each point every time; the size of the moxa cone should be the same as soybean or the wheat grain. The treatment is mostly given when the pain comes. The pain will be relieved or stopped normally after the moxibustion treatment; otherwise it can be applied again after three hours. Five treatments form one treatment course. The effect of all the points mentioned above has been proved by the experiences of ancient famous doctors. Mild moxibustion with moxa stick can also be applied.

3. ELECTRIC ACUPUNCTURE

Points: Main points: Xiaguan (ST7) and Jiache (ST6). Supplementary points: Hegu (LI4) and Zusanli (ST36)

Technique: Puncture Xiaguan (ST7) perpendicularly to a depth of 0.5-1 *cun*, apply the lifting, thrusting, twisting and rotating needling technique. The needles should be manipulated continually until the pain is relieved. Puncture Jiache (ST6) penetrating to Dicang (ST4), 1.5–3 *cun* deep, with the scraping and rotating needling technique. Puncture Hegu (LI4), 0.5-1 *cun* deep, for treating upper jaw toothache, and Zusanli (ST36) perpendicularly about 1.5-2 *cun* deep for treating lower jaw toothache. Apply the lifting, thrusting, rotating and twisting needling technique and combine the therapeutic instrument G6805, frequency 2-4 HZ, connecting to the electricity for 15 to 30 minutes. The treatment should be given everyday, with three treatments in one course.

4. AURICULAR THERAPY

(1) Puncturing New Points

Points: Cuimianxue (located on the inner side of the ear lobe, below the Intertragic notch, the mid point of the junction of the ear lobe and the face)

Technique: Puncture the point of the affected side. After sterilization, puncture 0.5-1 *cun* deep perpendicularly with a one-*cun* needle. Strong stimulation should be applied for three to five minutes after *qi* arrives. The treatment is given everyday.

(2) Quick Puncturing

Point: Face, Tragus, Houya, Ear-Shemen

Technique: Select two to three points bilaterally each time. After local sterilization, use 0.5-*cun* needles to puncture the points 0.5-0.1 *cun* deep. Rotate the needle rapidly (2-3 times/second). They are retained for 30-60 minutes and manipulated once every 10-20 minutes.

(3) Seed-pressing Method

Points: Main points: Sensitive point and reactive point. Supplementary points: toothache point, anesthesia point, ear-Shenmen and sub-cortex. Stomach and large intestine should be added for treating toothache due to the stomach fire; face and internal ear should be added to treat toothache due to the wind fire; and kidney should be added for toothache due to deficient fire.

Technique: Select one side of ear points, adding two or three associated points apart from the main point. Fix Wangbuliuxing seeds or mung beans on the points with plaster.

5. CHINESE MASSAGE

Point: Zhongchong (PC 9)

Technique: The pain can be relieved or stopped by applying massage on Zhongchong (PC 9) of the affected side for one or two minutes. This method is used for treating the emergent case under bad medical conditions. If the pain cannot be relieved after one or two minutes, massage can be continued for 10 minutes.

6. LASER THERAPY

Points: Xiaguan (ST7), Jiache (ST6), Hegu (LI4), Neiting (ST44), Zusanli (ST36), Taixi (KI3) and Kunlun (BL60).

Technique: Apply 3-25 mW He-Ne laser on each point for five minutes, two to four points each time.

[REMARKS]

1. Acupuncture treatment for toothache is very effective. It can relieve pain quickly and the effect will last a long time. It also has the function of strengthening the effect of painkillers.

2. For the pain due to the infection of dental caries, necrotic pulpitis, and difficulties with growing wisdom teeth, the root cause of the disease should be also treated. For pain due to dental caries, the ancient method is to apply moxibustion on Jianyu (LI15) or Yangxi (LI5). If the patient is afraid of needling, Hegu (LI4) or Sanjian (LI3) can be pressed strongly with the thumb for several minutes, and the pain should be relieved.

3. In folklore, people used to drop heated alcohol into the ear to stop the toothache. Nowadays, people use a cotton ball with 70% alcohol and apply on the external ear tract, which does have a certain effect.

CHAPTER SIX
DERMATOLOGY

ACNE

[INTRODUCTION]

Acne is normally seen among young people, and normally disappears naturally with maturity. This disease is caused by the wind and heat in the lung meridian smoking and steaming the skin; or it is caused by overeating greasy or spicy food, when there is an accumulation of heat and damp in the stomach and spleen, which emerges to attack the skin; or disorder of the Governor Vessel and Conception Vessel, which leads to the dysfunction of dispersal and eventual execration of the skin. Modern medicine believes that this disease is due to hypersteatosis with secondary bacterial infection. The treatment principle is to dispel the wind from the lung, resolve the dampness and heat, soothe the liver *qi* and remove stagnation, and regulate the Governor Vessel and Conception Vessel. The points are mainly taken from Hand Taiyin, Hand Yangming, Governor Vessel and Conception Vessel, such as Feishu (BL13), Lieque (LU7), Quchi (LI11), Hegu (LI4), Zusanli (ST36), and Zhongwan (CV12). Reducing needling technique is applied here.

[CLINICAL EXPERIENCE]

1. CONVENTIONAL ACUPUNCTURE

(1) Regulating the Heart and the Lung
Points: Xinshu (BL15), Feishu (BL13), Shaofu (H8), Yuji (LU10), Quchi (LI11) and Xuehai (SP10).

Technique: Apply quick needling technique on Xinshu (BL15) and Feishu (BL13), withdrawing the needle right after the arrival of *qi*. Apply even needling technique on the rest of the points. The needles are retained for 20-30 minutes, and 10 treatments form one course.

(2) Combination of Local Point and Distal Point

Points: Local-Xiaguan (ST7), Jiache (ST6), Zanzhu (BL2), Distal-Zusanli (ST36), Hegu (LI4), Fenglong (ST40), Sanyinjiao (SP6), Guanxia (Ex, 0.5 *cun* below CV4) and Lingong (Ex, 2.5 *cun* lateral to Guanxia)

Technique: Apply mild stimulation with the twisting method on local points, and strong stimulation with twisting needling technique on distal points. The needles are retained for 20-30 minutes. Select only one side of Zusanli (ST36) and Fenglong (ST40) at the beginning. The treatment is given everyday, 10 treatments forming one course. If the symptoms are improved, the treatment can be given once every other day, with a three to five-day break between courses.

(3) Puncturing a Pair of Points

Points: Quchi (LI11) and Hegu (LI4).

Technique: Insert the needle with the rotating method for both points; even stimulation should be applied. The needles are retained for 20-30 minutes after *qi* arrives. The needles are manipulated three to four times intermittently with the technique of lifting, thrusting, rotating and twisting. The treatment is given once a day, 10 treatments in one course.

2. MOXIBUSTION

Points: Quanjian (the top point of the small head of the third metacarpal bone)

Technique: Apply hanging moxibustion technique with moxa stick for five to seven minutes, once or twice a day, and 10 times in one course.

3. AURICULAR THERAPY

(1) Needle-embedding in the Auricular Points

Point: ① Diaphragm and Lung. ② Endocrine

Technique: Embed the thumbtack needle in the auricular points after sterilization, selecting one pair of the points every time, and fixing it with a plaster. The patient should press the points several times everyday, changing the points every two days. Five sessions form one course.

(2) Bleeding Method

Points: ① Heat Blood, and groove for lowering blood pressure. ② Endocrine and Sub-cortex.

Technique: Bleed the points with a three-edged needle after sterilizing the points. Select one pair of points each time, taking the two ears alternately. The treatment is given once every other day, 10 treatments in one course.

4.   PRICKING METHOD

Point: Reflective point of the back

Technique: Use the palm to rub the area, 0.5-3 *cun* literal to the 1st to 12th thoracic vertebra, several times; then look for the reflective points (similar to a papular eruption, a little bit higher than the skin; the color is white or brown, or dark red, or slightly red, and it does not fade by pressing). After sterilization of the reflective point, use a three-edged needle to prick the tissues under the points, squeezing out a small amount of blood, and then covering the injured area and fixing with plaster. Prick one or two points each time. The treatment is given once every five to seven days.

5.   COMBINED TREATMENT

(1) Pricking and Cupping Method

Points: The mid line (GV meridian) and Huatuojiaji Points (Ex-B2) from the level of T1-T7

Technique: Select three points to prick the area from the level of T1, T3, T5, using a three-edged needle to prick the subcutaneous tissues, then apply cupping for 10 minutes to cause more bleeding. At the end, wipe the pricked points with garlic and cover them with gauze. The second time, select two to four Jiaji points (Ex-B2). The points mentioned above must be used alternately. For severe case of acne, the treatment should be given twice a week, but once a week for mild cases. Ten treatments form one course.

(2) Combination of Acupuncture and Herbs

Points: Hegu (LI4) and Houxi (SI3) penetrating to Laogong (PC8)

Technique: Reducing needling technique is applied for every point; a few drops of blood should be squeezed out after removing the needles. The needles should be retained for 15 minutes. The treatment should be given once a week, and one package of Chinese herbs can be combined once every other day. Ingredients: Mahuang (ephedra) 15 g, apricot kernel 15 g, Fangfeng (saposhnikoria root) 15 g, plaster stone 50 g, Cangzhu (atractylodes rhizome) 50 g, Job's tears 50 g, Danggui (Chinese angelica root) 20 g, Chuanxiong 20 g, Shengdi (rehmannia root) 20 g, Chishao (red poeny root) 20 g, Gancao (licoric root) 10 g. Modification should be made according to the symptoms. Twenty treatments form one course.

[REMARKS]

1. Acupuncture is very effective to treat this disease, and the pricking and cupping method has immediate effect.

2. The fat, sugar and irritants food such as cigarettes, alcohol, beef, mutton and shrimp should be avoided.

ALOPECIA AREATA

[INTRODUCTION]

Alopecia areata refers to the sudden loss of hair in a certain area of the scalp, where the patient is unaware of any symptoms. At the beginning, there is only loss of hair in a localized, isolated part of the scalp in a round or elliptical shape. The scalp is bright and with a very clear border. But with the development of the disease, more hair, larger and more widespread areas will be affected. In severe cases, the whole head will be involved, and that means most, or all, of the hair will fall off. This is known as a "bald head." Sometimes, even all the hairs of the body will be affected, such as, eyebrow, mustache and beard, axillary hair and pubic hair. This is called "general loss of hair." The disease is caused by liver and kidney deficiency, insufficient blood nourishing the head, so that the pathogenic wind can attack the body by taking advantage of the opened pores; or it is caused by the improper food intake, and accumulation of heat in the spleen and stomach, which lead to dryness of the blood due to excessive wind; or abnormal emotional changes leads to liver *qi* stagnation, so that the hair cannot be well nourished due to both *qi* and blood stagnation. The treatment principle should be to nourish the blood and dispel the wind; regulate the spleen and the stomach; activate the blood circulation and remove blood stasis and sooth liver *qi*. The following points are selected, such as Xuehai (SP10), Quchi (LI11), Hegu (LI4), Shousanli (LI10), Zusanli (ST36), Taichong (LR3), Taixi (KI3), and Ah-shi points.

[CLINICAL EXPERIENCE]

1.   CONVENTIONAL ACUPUNCTURE

(1) Superficial Acupuncture

Points: Ah-shi point, Baihui (GV20), Fengchi (GB20), Quchi (LI11), Hegu (LI4) and Taichong (LR3).

Technique: Use a one-*cun* needle (Size: No.28) to puncture Ah-shi points shallowly until bleeding, which is known as "superficial acupuncture" in the *Internal Classics*; the rest of points are punctured with even needling technique, and the needles are retained for 20 minutes. The treatment is given once a day and there are 20 sessions in one course.

(2) Selecting the Points According to the Differentiation of the Syndromes

Points: Ah-shi point, Feishu (BL13), Geshu (BL17) and Shenshu (BL23).

Technique: Use the surrounding method to puncture the Ah-shi point obliquely with the tip of the needles toward the center. The rest of the points should be punctured with filiform needles with even needing technique. These four points form the basic prescription. The lung dominates the hair and skin; Geshu (BL17) is the confluence of the blood; the kidney is the congenital foundation in storing the essence and producing the blood; and the hair is called the terminal part of the blood. According to the affected area, more points can be added: On the forehead, Hegu (LI4) and Neiting (ST44) should be added; on the side of the head, Waiguan (TE5) and Zulinqi (GB41) should be added; on the occiput region, Houxi (SI3) and Shenmai (BL62) should be added; on the top of the head, Taichong (LR3) or Xingjian (LR2) and Zhongfeng (LR4) should be added. If the disease is caused by wind, Fengchi (GB20) and Fengmen (BL12) should be added; if it is caused by the accumulation of heat in the stomach and the spleen, Pishu (BL20), Weishu (BL21) and Quchi (LI11) should be added; if the disease is caused by liver *qi* stagnation, Ganshu (BL18) and Taichong (LR3) should be added; and if it is caused by deficiency of the liver and the kidney, Taixi (KI3) and Ququan (LR8) should be added. All the combined points should be punctured with even needling technique. The needles are retained for 20-30 minutes. The treatment is given once a day. Select five to seven points each time, taking 30 treatments as one course.

(3) Three Needles on the Head

Points: Main points: Fanglao [Ex, one *cun* behind Baihui (GV20)], Jiannao [Ex-bilaterally, 0.5 *cun* below Fengchi-(GB20)]. Supplementary points: Touwei (ST8) should be added for loss of hair on the temple region; Dazhui (GV14) is added for itching; Shangxing (GV23) is added for oily skin.

Technique: Puncture the main points with reinforcing needling technique and combine the points with reducing needling technique. The needles are retained for 15-30 minutes. Apply sparrow-pecking needling technique during the removal of the needles. The treatment is given once a day, 10 treatments in a course. It will take several months for the whole treatment to be completed.

(4) Puncturing Shengfa Point (Ex)

Points: Shengfa point [Ex, the mid point of Fengchi (GB20) and

Fengfu (GV16)], Baihui (GV20) and Touwei (ST8). Supplementary points: Shangxing (GV23), Taiyang (Ex-HN5), Fengchi (GB20), Yuyao (Ex-HN4) penetrating to Sizhukong (TE23), Anmian point [Ex, the mid point of Hegu-(LI4) and Sanjian-(LI3)].

Technique: Take the main points every time and select two or three supplementary points each time, puncture the main points with reinforcing needling technique and the combined points with reducing needling technique. The needles are retained for 30 minutes, with manipulation two or three times during retention. The treatment is given once a day, and 10 treatments form one course. This therapy is used to treat the total and general baldness.

2. AURICULAR THERAPY

Points: Lung, Kidney, Liver, Forehead, Ear-Shenmen, Occiput, Endocrine, Sub-cortex and Sympathetic Nerve.

Technique: Select three to five points each time, puncture them perpendicularly with the filiform needles. The needles should be retained for 30 minutes, and manipulated three to five times. The treatment is given once a day, taking the above-mentioned points alternately; or the seed-pressing method can be applied. Ten treatments form one course.

3. PLUM BLOSSOM NEEDLE THERAPY

Points: The reflective points (or reflective thing) on the back, of the neck, lumbar sacrum area, Taiyuan (LU9), Neiguan (PC6) and the area of hair loss.

Technique: First of all, check the back with the hand on both sides of the spinal column to see if there are positive and reflective things in the cord, nodule, or soft vesicular form; or if there are positive and reflective areas of soreness, pain or numbness. Then apply a plum blossom needle to tap these regions equally and densely from the border to the center. Each area should be tapped for about five minutes. Select the reflective area on the back and the hair loss area every time, as well as one of two other areas or points. The treatment is given once a day, 10 treatments in a course.

4. BLEEDING THERAPY

Points: Taiyang (Ex-HN5) and Quze (LU5)

Technique: Use a three-edged needle to prick each point to obtain three to five drops of blood. This therapy is given twice a week. Extract only one to three drops of blood for the aged and a weak patient. Ten sessions form one course.

5. COMBINED THERAPY

(1) Plum Blossom Needle and Hanliancao Tincture

Point: Hair loss area

Technique: Use a plum blossom needle to tap the hair loss area until the skin turns red. This treatment is given twice a day. Apply "Hanlian tincture" on the affected area three times a day (morning, noon, and evening). If the new-growing hair is increasing obviously, the tincture needs only to be applied twice a day, along with tapping with the plum blossom needle once a day until patient recovers. The preparation of Hanlian tincture: Hanliancao (dry whole grass) 20 g, (fresh grass, with double the amount). Wash the grass carefully with water and steam for 20 minutes; once it gets cold, soak it in 22 grams of 75% alcohol for three days in winter and two days in spring, summer and autumn. Use a piece of cloth as a filter to get the liquid; the tincture, which looks like coffee, is then achieved. The liquid should be stored in a bottle. Apply Hanlian tincture on the affected area with a cotton stick. In 11 treated cases of alopecia areata, 10 patients were cured and one case was effective. The new hair started to grow after four to seven days of treatment.

(2) Plum Blossom Needle Combined with Moxibustion with Moxa Stick and Fresh Ginger

Point: The hair loss area

Technique: Shave the hair around the hair loss area. After sterilization, tap the affected area with a plum blossom needle until a little blood is drawn. Then, rub fresh ginger or dried ginger until patient has a burning sensation in the localized area. Finally, moxibustion with moxa stick is applied for three to five minutes. The treatment is given once a day, and should be continuous. Six cases of this disease were treated, and all of the patients were cured.

[REMARKS]

1. Acupuncture is very effective for treating alopecia areata, but the treatment should be persisted in for a long time.

2. During the treatment, the patient should keep a good mood. Vexation, pessimism sadness, and anger are forbidden.

3. A light diet should be taken. No spicy and aromatic and greasy foods are allowed.

CUTANEOUS PRURITUS

[INTRODUCTION]

Cutaneous pruritus refers to the severe itching of the skin without any primary skin injury. The itching occurs from time to time and is especially getting severe during the night. There are scrape marks, blood scabs and pigmentation due to the patient scratching the skin. There are general and local, two types of cutaneous pruritus. It often occurs on aged people and the young who have chronic disease. The disease occurs because: If there is blood deficiency, wind and dryness, then the skin cannot be well nourished; or there is internal retention of dampness and heat leading to the disharmony of the *ying qi* and the defensive *qi* of the skin; or constitutional blood heat produces wind, then the excessive wind causes the itching; or the body is attacked by exterior pathogenic wind leading to lack of nourishment to the skin. The treatment principle is: To dispel the wind, nourish the blood, moisten the dryness, clear away the heat, and remove the dampness. Select the points from Hand and Foot Yangming meridians, Foot-Taiyin meridian, such as: Hegu (LI4), Quchi (LI11), Waiguan (TE5), Xuehai (SP10), Sanyinjiao (SP6), Zusanli (ST36) and Ah-shi points.

[CLINICAL EXPERIENCE]

1. CONVENTIONAL ACUPUNCTURE

(1) Penetrating Acupuncture

Points: Quchi (LI11) and Sanyijiao (SP6).

Technique: Puncture Quchi (LI11) penetrating to Shaohai (SI8), and Sanyijiao (SP6) penetrating to Xuanzhong (GB39); apply rotating and even needling technique for all the points, the needles being manipulated quickly for a short time. The needles are retained for 20-30 minutes, 10 sessions in one course. This method is very effective for treating general cutaneous pruritus.

(2) Puncturing Obliquely

Points: Xuehai (SP10) and Chengshan (BL57)

Technique: Puncture Xuehai (SP10) obliquely at a 45° angle upward, 0.5-0.8 *cun* deep; puncture Chengshan (BL57) obliquely at a 30° angle upward, 0.5-1 *cun* deep; and apply the rotating method for both points. The needles should be retained for 15-30 minutes and manipulated once every five to 10 minutes. During retention, the patient should use a moxa stick on the itching area for 15 to 30 minutes by himself. This method is good to treat local cutaneous pruritus on the areas, such as, scrotum, perineum or the anus. The treatment is given once a day, 10 times in one course.

(3) Treatment on the Basis of Differentiation of the Syndromes

Points: Main points: Xuehai (SP10), Sanyinjiao (SP6) and Quchi (LI11). Add Xuanzhong (GB39), Yinlingquan (SP9) and Fengchi (GB20) if the disease is caused by wind deficiency and wind dryness. Add Fengchi (GB20), Fengfu (GV16) and Zusanli (ST36) if the disease is caused by blood heat, wind and dryness. Add Ligou (LR5), Fenglong (ST40) and Xingjian (LR2) if the disease is caused by damp heat.

Technique: Apply even needling technique on the main points, selecting the combined points according to the symptoms. The treatment principle is to tonify the deficiency and reduce the excess. The needles are retained for 30 minutes, and the treatment is given once a day, 10 sessions making up one course.

2. BLEEDING THERAPY

Point: Sifeng (Ex-UE10), bilateral.

Technique: Prick Sifeng (Ex-UE10) with a three-edged needle to cause a little yellow and white sticky liquid to emerge. This therapy is given once a day, and three times in one course.

3. MOXIBUSTION WITH MOXA STICK

Point: Affected area

Technique: Apply the burning moxa stick hanging on the affected area for 10-15 minutes, until the skin turns deep red. This therapy is given twice a day, over two or three days. This method is good to treat local cutaneous pruritus.

4. AURICULAR THERAPY

(1) Acupuncture with Filiform Needle

Points: Lung, Ear-Shenmen, Allergic Point, Endocrine and related sensitive area.

Technique: Puncture the points with a 0.5-*cun* filiform needle quickly, stimulating the point strongly and retaining the needle for 20 minutes. Apply mild stimulation for the patient who has a weak constitution, embedding the needle for three to four hours. This therapy is given once a day, 10 times in one course.

(2) Bleeding Method on the Back of the Ear

Point: Vein in the back of the ear

Technique: Use a sterilized three-edged needle to prick the vein on the back of the ear after sterilization of the local area, causing a little bleeding and waiting for it to stop naturally. Bleed one to three parts on the ear each time, taking two ears alternately. The treatment is given once every other day, six treatments in one course.

5. HYDRO-ACUPUNCTURE

Point: Changqiang (GV1)

Technique: Inject with the mixture of 0.2 ml 2.5% procaine and 1 ml vitamin B_{12} while the patient is lying on the stomach. Use a No.16 syringe needle to inject 15-20 ml injection into the upper part of the depression between the coccyx and the anus. The patient should have a needling sensation. The treatment is given once every three days, 10 sessions making up one course. This method can stop itching.

6. LASER THERAPY

Points: Quchi (LI11), Hegu (LI4), Xuehai (SP10), Sanyinjiao (SP6) and Yinlingquan (SP9).

Technique: Apply the laser on each point for five minutes. The treatment is given once everyday. It is good for treating general cutaneous pruritus.

[REMARKS]

1. Acupuncture has certain effect for treating this disease, and is especially effective to stop itching.

2. Pay attention to and prevent the causative factors. If the disease is caused by food, then greasy food, seafood and alcohol should be avoided.

3. Do not scratch the itching area; do not rub and wash it with hot water; and do not use soap with strong alkali content.

URTICARIA

[INTRODUCTION]

Urticaria refers to the skin disease in which a fresh red or pale rash appears on the skin combined with itching. It is also called "wind rash," or "hidden rash," because it appears from time to time. Most patients can be cured after an acute occurrence, but a few patients will see a recurrence of the disease after several months or many years without being cured completely. If the striae of the skin is loose, defensive *qi* is not consolidated; then pathogenic wind cold and wind heat will accumulate and attack the skin; or if the patient who has a congenital condition that does not tolerate rich food or seafood, or there are parasites in the intestine, then the intestine and the stomach will not be in a harmony, so that there will be retention of dampness and heat eventually reaching the skin; or if the patient has congenital weak constitution, so that the prolonged illness causes blood deficiency and dryness, this will result in lack of nourishment to the skin; or if there are abnormal changes in the seven emotions, the irregular movement of the Governor Vessel and Conception Vessel, and deficiency of the blood, then the liver and kidney will not be well nourished, so wind and dryness are produced and accumulate in the skin. The treatment principle is to dispel the wind, reduce the heat and regulate *qi* and the blood. The points are mainly chosen from the Hand and Food Yangming meridians, Food Taiyin meridian, such as, Quchi (LI11), Hegu (LI4), Xuehai (SP10), Geshu (BL17), Fengshi (GB31), Fengchi (GB20) Zusanli (ST36), Sanyinjiao (SP6). Apply even or reducing needling technique.

[CLINICAL EXPERIENCE]

1. CONVENTIONAL ACUPUNCTURE

(1) Puncturing Single Point: Dazhui(GV14)

Technique: Puncture Dazhui (GV14) 1.0-1.2 *cun* deep, apply strong stimulating technique; retain the needle for 15 minutes, and manipulate once every five minutes. Three treatments form one course. The treatment is given once or twice a day, and normally the itching feeling will be reduced or stopped. The rash will get smaller and the color will become lighter after acupuncture treatment.

(2) Penetrating Acupuncture

Points: ① Shendao (GV11) penetrating to Zhiyang (GV9), Xuehai (SP10) and Sanyinjiao (SP6). ② Dazhui (GV14) penetrating to GV 12, and Quchi (LI11).

Technique: Take two groups of points alternately, using a 125 mm-long needle of 0.9 mm diameter to puncture the point. After the arrival of *qi,* retain the needles for two hours, stimulating the rest of the points strongly without retention. The treatment is given once every day over seven days. There should be a break of three days before the next course.

(3) Selecting the **Point** *According to the Location of the Disease*

Points: Fengchi (GB20), Quchi (LI11), Xuehai (SP10) and Sanyinjiao (SP6)

Technique: If the rash appears above the waist, puncture Quchi (LI11) and Fengchi (GB20); if the rash appears below the waist, puncture Xuehai (SP10) and Sanyinjiao (SP6); if the rash appears on the whole body, puncture all four points. After the arrival of *qi,* the points should be stimulated moderately or strongly for one to two minutes, and retained for one minute. The needles can be removed after three repeats of this method. The treatment is given once a day.

(4) Puncturing Back-shu Point

Point: Dachangshu (BL25)

Technique: For acute type, the treatment is given once a day; for chronic type, once every other day. More reducing and less reinforcing needling technique should be applied for the acute type and more reinforcing and less reducing technique should be applied for the chronic type. The needles are retained for 20-30 minutes. The effective rate is 96.51% for the acute type and 75.92% for the chronic type.

2. MOXIBUSTION

(1) Moxibustion with Moxa Cone and Ginger

Points: Hegu (LI4), Yangchi (LI5), Xingjian (LR2) and Jiexi (ST41).

Technique: Apply moxibustion with moxa cone and ginger, taking five moxa cones for each point every time; the size of the moxa cone should be as big as a wheat grain. The treatment is given once or twice a day until the symptoms are relieved.

(2) Warming Moxibustion with Moxa Stick

Points: Hegu (LI4), Quchi (LI11), Xuehai (SP10) and Zusanli (ST36)

Technique: Apply moxibustion for five to 15 minutes on each point every time. The treatment is given once or twice a day, six treatments forming a course.

3. AURICULAR THERAPY

(1) Embedding Needle Method

Points: Urticaria area, Lung, Heart, Adrenal, Occiput, Ear-shenmen.

Technique: Using a 0.3-*cun* needle to puncture the point after sterilization. When there is a sensation, apply the reducing thrusting needling technique to embed the needle in one side of the ear, fixing with a plaster to keep it in place for 72 hours. Change to the other ear on the third day.

(2) Medicine Injection

Points: Endocrine and urticaria area.

Technique: Take 1 ml chlor-trimeton injection (contains 10 mg), which is diluted with 2 ml of injected water, and inject 0.1 ml of it into each of the above-mentioned points once a day.

(3) Cutting Bleeding Method

Points: The vein on the back of the ear and the sensitive point on the ear

Technique: Use a sterilized three-edged needle to prick the vein on the ear to cause bleeding. Take a small knife to cut the reflective auricular area or the sensitive point. The point should be cut once every three days; and the effect should appear after several treatments.

4. BLEEDING THERAPY

Point: Houxi (SI3)

Technique: Use a three-edged needle to prick Houxi (SI3) to cause slight bleeding. Zusanli (ST36) and Quchi (LI11) should be punctured at the same time with strong and quick stimulation. The needles are not necessarily retained. The treatment is given once every other day, five sessions in one course.

5. CUPPING THERAPY

Point: Shenque (CV8)

Technique: Use the holding fire cupping method. Apply one plastic lid that is a little bit bigger than the umbilicus on that place (Shenque-CV8); place a cotton ball with alcohol on the lid, and burn the cotton, using the cup to cover it rapidly. Remove the cup when it is no longer tight. Repeat this cupping therapy three times. The treatment is given daily for three days. One or two treatments will be enough for mild cases, but four courses may be needed for a severe case.

6. LASER THERAPY

Points: If there is disharmony of the Governor Vessel and the Conception Vessel, select Sanyinjiao (SP6) and Xuehai (SP10); if there is deficiency of *yin* and blood, select Sanyinjiao (SP6) and Zusanli (ST36); and if there is coldness, select Zusanli (ST36) and Quchi (LI11).

Technique: Apply the laser with 1 mW power and 2 mm diameter; the distance between the points should be 10 cm. Select the above-mentioned points according to the differentiation of the symptoms. The treatment is given once a day, taking the points of left and right side alternately over 10 sessions.

[REMARKS]

1. Acupuncture treatment for urticaria is very effective. The cupping method has the immediate effect.

2. This disease is usually related to an allergy. Hence if possible, the sensitizing agent should be identified and avoided.

3. Fish, shrimp, crab, spicy food, onion, garlic and alcohol are forbidden.

ECZEMA

[INTRODUCTION]

Eczema is a common skin disease, which has erosion and itching as the main symptoms. It injures the skin uniformly and is distributed symmetrically. It occurs repeatedly and it is easy to change into the chronic type. It can happen at any age, to either sex and on any part of the body. Modern medical science considers the disease is related to allergy. According to the traditional Chinese medicine, the acute type is due to pathogenic wind, damp and heat attacking the skin; the chronic type is mainly due to spleen deficiency failing to fulfill the function of transportation and the prolonged retention of dampness producing heat; the prolonged chronic type is mainly due to long-term illness injuring *yin* and blood, the blood deficiency producing wind and dryness that leaves the skin with a lack of nourishment. The treatment principle is to dispel the wind, reduce the heat, strengthen the spleen, and moisten the dryness. Select the main points from the Governor vessel, Hand and Foot Yangming meridians and Foot Taiyin meridian. Points: Dazhui (GV14), Quchi (LI11), Hegu (LI4), Xuehai (SP10), Zusanli (ST36), Sanyijiao (SP6) and Neiguan (PC6). Apply the reducing needling technique on acute stage outbreaks, even needling technique on the delayed stage, and reinforcing needling technique in the chronic stage.

[CLINICAL EXPERIENCE]

1.   CONVENTIONAL ACUPUNCTURE

(1) Puncturing Yuan-primary Point and Xi-cleft Point

Points: The Yuan-primary point and Xi-cleft point of the meridians that belong to the affected area; combined with Xuehai (SP10), Pishu (BL20), Xinshu (BL15), Quchi (LI11), Weizhong (BL40), Geshu (BL40) and Sanyijiao (SP6).

Technique: Puncture the Yuan-primary point and Xi-cleft point with reducing needling technique; the needles are retained for 30 minutes. Select two to three pairs of the combined points each time. The treatment is given once a day, seven sessions in one course.

(2) Puncturing Jing-well Point

Points: Main points: Quchi (LI11), Huantiao (GB30), Yanglingquan (GB30), adding Hegu (LI4) for the face; Waiguan (SJ5) for the head; Weizhong (BL40) for the lumbar and back region; Zusanli (ST36) and Xuehai (SP10) for the chest and abdomen.

Technique: Puncture Huantiao (GB30) 1.5-3 *cun* deep perpendicularly, apply thrusting and lifting needling technique. Puncture

Weizhong (BL40) 0.5-0.8 *cun* deep perpendicularly with rotating needling technique, stimulating both points shortly and rapidly. Puncture Quchi (LI11) penetrating to Shousanli (LI10) subcutaneously; puncture Yanglingquan (GB34) subcutaneously downward about 1.5-2 *cun* deep; puncture Zusanli (ST36), penetrating in the direction of Shangjuxu (ST37) subcutaneously; puncture Xuehai (SP10) subcutaneously upward about 1-1.5 *cun*. The needles should be retained for one or two hours for all four points. No other needling technique should be applied during the insertion and retaining of the needles. The treatment is given once a day, 10 times in one course. In order to improve the effect of the treatment, moxibustion with moxa stick can be combined on Quchi (LI11), Xuehai (SP10), and Yanglingquan (GB34) for 10-20 minutes.

(3) Puncturing the Meeting Point of Yang

Points: Dazhui (GV14, the meeting point of Yang), Feishu (BL13), combined with the points according to the differentiation of the symptoms.

Technique: The lung dominates the skin and hair, therefore Feishu (BL13) can reduce the heat from the lung; Dazhui (GV14) is the meeting point of *yang*, and *yang* dominates the exterior part of the body, so Dazhui (GV14) can dispel the pathogenic factor from the exterior of the body. That is the reason why these two points are taken as the main points. Select Hegu (LI4), Yinlingquan (SP9) and Sanyijiao (SP6) for the damp heat type; Yinlingquan (SP9), Zusanli (ST36) and Sanyijiao (SP6) for the type of spleen deficiency combined with dampness; Xinshu (BL15), Geshu (BL17), Ganshu (BL18), Xuehai (SP10) and Hegu (LI4) for the type of blood deficiency that is combined with wind and dryness. Select two main points and two or three supplementary points every time. Puncture with a filiform needle with reducing needling technique, and retain it for 15-20 minutes. The above-mentioned points can also be chosen for infantile eczema, but puncturing shallowly without retaining of the needles. The treatment is given once a day, 10 times in one course.

(4) Puncturing Extraordinary Points

Point: One *cun* above Chengshan (BL57)

Technique: The patient should stand straight and lift the arms straight upward, stepping with the tip of the feet and lifting the heel, so that the gastrocnemius is contracted, Chengshan (BL57) is located on the top of the lambdoid, and this point is located one *cun* above Chengshan (BL57). Puncture this point with the tip of the needle pointing upward, normally about 1.5-2 *cun* deep, and rotate the needle about 180° after the arrival of *qi* until the sensation reaches the scrotum. The needles are retained for 30 minutes, with the points stimulated every five minutes. Hegu (LI4) and Baichongwo (Ex) can be added to improve the effect. This method is good for treating scrotum eczema.

2. MOXIBUSTION

(1) Warming Moxibustion with Moxa Stick

Points: Main points: Quchi (LI11) and Xuehai (SP10). Supplementary points: Jianyu (LI15), Huantiao (GB30), Hegu (LI4), Baihui (GV20), Dazhui (GV14), Ah-shi point, and the extreme itching point.

Technique: Apply hanging moxibustion with moxa stick. The patient should not feel any pain, but only a warm sensation. It is better to have a small blister appear after moxibustion. Less moxibustion applied on the head and face in order to avoid blistering and pus. The treatment is given once or twice a day. Alternatively, apply moxibustion when the itching begins for 10 minutes on each point every time, selecting two to five points. Extremely severe itching and other symptoms can be relieved or stopped right away after the moxibustion treatment.

(2) Steaming Moxibustion

Point: Affected area

Technique: Difuzi (broom cypress fruit) 30 g, Shechuangzi 30 g, Kushen (flarescent sophora root) 15 g, Baixianpi (dittany bark) 15 g, Huajiao (Chinese prickly ash) 9 g and alum 3 g, are boiled in water for 30 minutes. Place the decoction in a basin and steam the affected area, followed by washing when the decoction is no longer hot. The treatment is given once a day. It is a good way to treat prolonged chronic eczema that is difficult to cure.

3. BLEEDING CUPPING THERAPY

Point: Affected area

Technique: Use a plum-blossom needle to prick the affected area and cause slight bleeding; or use a three-edged needle to prick the affected area divergently until bleeding, and then apply cupping for 10 minutes. The treatment is given once a day, selecting two or three affected areas each time. Ten sessions form one course.

4. AURICULAR THERAPY

Points: ① Lung, Ear-shenmen, Adrenal, allergic area, and reflective point of the affected area. ② Liver, Spleen and Sub-cortex.

Technique: Select points of the first group for acute eczema, and points from the second group for chronic type, using a filiform needle to puncture the point with even needling technique. The needles are retained for one or two hours. Treat the two ears alternately. The seed-embedding method can be also applied, once a day, 10 times in one course.

5. ELECTRIC ACUPUNCTURE

Point: The area around injured skin

Technique: After sterilizing with alcohol, puncture the affected area along the border horizontally to the depth of the tissues layer. According to the size of the affected skin, two to six needles can be used. Connect the electricity to the filiform needles, making sure the intensity and frequency are within the tolerance range of the patient. The treatment is given for 20 minutes for each time, one treatment a day or every other day.

6. HYDRO-ACUPUNCTURE

(1) Phenergan Therapy

Point: Changqiang (GV1)

Technique: Take 12.5 mg phenergan with 1 mg vitamin B_1 to inject into Changqiang (GV1). This injection is given once every three days, and two treatments comprise one course.

(2) *Vitamin Method*

Points: Zusanli (ST36) and Quchi (LI11).

Technique: Select the points bilaterally, injecting 0.1 mg vitamin B_{12} into each point. This injection is given once a day, 10 times in one course, with a break of five to seven days between courses. Fifty cases of intractable eczema were treated, and the general effective rate was 96%. The immune function was tested in 17 cases before and after treatment, the functions of most of the immune cells had improved.

[REMARKS]

· 1.   It is better to use combined treatment for treating this disease. Normally, herbal medicine are combined, such as phellodendron bark, burnet root, green Chinese olive, tea, Chinese gall and Jiuliming. Cook the herbs with water, wash or apply it on the affected area externally. Liuyi powder, Ermiao Powder can be used as well.

2.   If the patient has general itching of the whole body, puncture the Zhiyang point for stopping the itching [one *cun* above Zhouliao (LI12)], bleeding the back of the ear.

3.   For acute type, wash with hot water, and irritating soap are forbidden. No matter whether it is the acute or the chronic type, scratching should be avoided. Food, such as spicy products, seafood, beef, and mutton, are forbidden, and light food should be taken instead.

HERPES ZOSTER

[INTRODUCTION]

Herpes zoster refers to a bunch of small herpes distributed along one side of the peri-nerves. The main symptoms: Purulent liquid fills the herpes; there is redness around the affected area; pain, with or without burning sensation. The disease occurs mostly around the waist region, and the herpes always appears in a group and in the shape of a belt. The disease is mainly caused by excessive fire of the gall bladder and liver due to abnormal emotional changes, or heat due to prolonged spleen deficiency and accumulation of dampness; or herpes caused by the blockage of the Ying and defensive *qi* of the skin due to exogenous pathogenic wind and heat. The treatment principle is to dispel the wind, reduce the heat, and remove the dampness. Select the points mainly from Foot Shaoyang, Hand Yangming, Foot Jueyin, and Food Taiyin meridians. The main points are Waiguan (TE5), Quchi (LI11), Sanyinjiao (SP6), and Yanglingquan (GB34) and Taichong (LR3). Apply reducing needling technique, the needles retained for 30 minutes, and the treatment given twice a day.

[CLINICAL EXPERIENCE]

1. CONVENTIONAL ACUPUNCTURE

(1) Puncturing "Sheyan Point"(Ex, the eyes of the snake)

Point: Sheyan point (Ex, located besides the Dagukong point, refers to the two joints of the thumb on the dorsal aspect, two points on one thumb)

Technique: After the usual sterilization, take a No.26, one-*cun* needle to puncture the points 0.3 *cun* deep, inserting the needle into the joint cavity along the space of the bones, and removing it after small rotation. Squeeze the point until the sticky yellow liquid emerges, one or two drops for each point. Puncture the affected side point on the finger the first time, and the other side the second time. The treatment is given once a day, and it should be repeated on the third and fourth days. Normally, the pain can be relieved after half-an-hour of treatment; the development of the affected area will be stopped after 24 hours, and become dry after 48 hours.

(2) Surrounding Acupuncture

Point: Main points: Surrounding points (4-8 points 0.5-1 *cun* from the herpes on the affected area). Supplementary points: Add Zhigou (TE6), Waiguan (TE5), Hegu (LI4) and Quchi (LI11) if the herpes appears above the waist (including the head and face); and add Taichong (LR3) and Sanyijiao (SP6) if the herpes appears below the waist.

Technique: Apply thrusting, lifting and rotating needling technique for every point. The tip of the needle should be toward the center of the herpes, puncturing the surrounding points at an angle of 25°. A gentle sensation of soreness, numbness, distention and heaviness should be achieved. There should be strong stimulation for the points on the four extremities, and soreness, numbness, distention and heaviness must radiate to the distal area. The needles are retained for 30-40 minutes. For severe pain, or while the disease is still developing, the treatment must be given twice a day. If the pain is relieved and the herpes is getting better, the treatment is given only once a day. If the pain disappears, and the crust is formed and is falling off, the treatment can be stopped.

(3) Puncturing Jiaji (Ex-B2) Points

Points: The related Jiaji points (Ex-B2). If the herpes appears above the waist, Hegu (LI4), Quchi (LI11) and Waiguan (TE5) of the same side should be added; if the herpes appears below the waist Zusanli (ST36), Xiaxi (GB43), and Taichong (LR3) of the same side should be added.

Technique: Apply reducing needling technique for each point. The treatment is given once a day. A total of 25 cases were treated, of which 24 were cured. From the observation of the clinical test statistics, acupuncture does have the function of strengthening the immunity of the non-special cells of the human body.

2.   MOXIBUSTION

(1) Brightening Moxibustion

Point: Ah-shi point

Technique: Apply two moxa cones as big as wheat grain on the first herpes and the region where it is most prevalent. Burn the moxa and remove it when the patient feels pain, blowing away the unburned part of the moxa cone. Apply one moxa cone on one or two distal area respectively. The treatment is given once a day, and a cure is usually achieved after three to five days.

(2) *Moxibustion on the Zhizhu Point (Ex, Spider Point)*

Point: Zhizhu point (Ex-spider point). The patient should sit up straight and the doctor stands behind. The doctor uses a thin thread to measure the size of the patient's head, and then uses a cut piece of this exact size on the neck from front to behind. The doctor pulls the thread backward along the mid line of the thoracic vertebra, the point at which the meeting ends of the thread arrive is the spider point).

Technique: After finding the point, apply one moxa cone as big as a date kernel. The pain will be greatly relieved after moxibustion. The redness, swelling and puncturing pain will disappear after three days, the crust will fall off and the patient will be cured.

(3) *Surrounding Moxibustion*

Technique: Hold the burning moxa stick near the affected area, apply it until the skin around the herpes turns red. Then, apply it on Xinshu (BL15) and Feishu (BL13) until the skins turn red as well. Normally, the moxibustion should be applied for 30-40 minutes and once a day. The herpes will be absorbed or disappear gradually after the surrounding moxibustion treatment. There is no sequelae pain.

(4) *Cotton Moxibustion*

Point: Affected area

Technique: Ask the patient to expose the back. Take one piece of thin purified cotton, as thin as possible (a thick piece cannot be compressed to make it thin). There must be no hole or space in the cotton, otherwise the result of the treatment will be affected. Apply the cotton in the same size of the affected area on the herpes. The doctor then takes a match to burn one side of the cotton, which will be burned off right away. The patient will feel a little pain, but this should be ignored. For most patients, the color of the herpes will get darker and will get smaller or disappear. The pain will be relieved on the second day of treatment. There is no necessity to repeat the treatment, although in some cases, up to four treatments may prove necessary for a full cure.

3. THICK NEEDLE THERAPY

Point: Shendao (GV11) penetrating to Zhiyang (GV9)

Technique: Use a needle of 1.0 mm diameter and 3 *cun* thick to puncture Shendao (GV11) penetrating to Zhiyang (GV9). The needles should not be manipulated, but they are retained for four hours. The treatment is given once every other day. This method has the function of promoting the channels and meridians, reducing inflammation and stopping pain. Normally, the pain will be greatly relieved after the needling.

4. BLEEDING CUPPING METHOD

(1) Cupping in a Row
Point: Ah-shi point
Technique: Prick the skin where the herpes have accumulated until slight bleeding occurs. Apply flashing cupping technique on each side of the affected area, and then cup on the herpes area in a row, keeping it there for 10 minutes.

(2) Combined Points Therapy
Points: ① Dazhui (GV14), Ganshu (BL18) and Ah-shi point. ② Shenzhu (GV12), Pishu (BL20) and Ah-shi point.
Technique: Select one group of the above points each time. The treatment is given once every day or every other day. Pricking the points first causes slight bleeding, after which the cupping method is applied for 10 minutes.

5. PLUM-BLOSSOM NEEDLE THERAPY

Technique: Stimulate different part of the body according to the different affected area, including general stimulation (stimulating the parallel line 2 cm wide from the spine) and local stimulation (tapping the circle which is about 1 cm to the border of the herpes). The affected area must not be tapped. Strong stimulation is applied for a normal case and even stimulation for a special case. Each area should be tapped three to five times. The treatment is given twice a day.

6. AURICULAR THERAPY

(1) Acupuncture therapy
Points: Ear-shenmen, Lung, Sub-cortex, Endocrine, and related

point.

Technique: Apply strong stimulation technique. The needles are retained for two hours, and the treatment is given once or twice a day, or once every other day for mild cases, 10 treatments in one course. A total of 112 cases of herpes zoster were treated by this method, and all were cured after three treatments.

(2) Moxibustion

Point: Liver, Kidney, Ear-shenmen and related area.

Technique: Apply moxibustion with moxa stick on the above-mentioned points, five minutes for each point. The treatment is given twice a day. The pain can be relieved or stopped after one moxibustion treatment normally.

7. LASER THERAPY

Point: Affected area

Technique: Apply 7-25 mw He-Ne laser therapeutic apparatus with divergent focus on the local area. The result is also good.

[REMARKS]

1. Acupuncture therapy is very effective for treating this disease.

2. If the herpes is broken, gentian violet should be applied to avoid the infection. If there is too much secretion from the herpes, the local skin should be cleaned according to surgical procedure once a day, and the area should be covered by sterilized gauze after cleaning.

3. No spicy food, seafood, such as fish, shrimp or crab, and other foods likely to irritate are allowed.

4. There are many different therapies that can be applied for the disease, the rule of selecting the points are: ① Local point (Ah-shi point) or nearby point. ② Distal points: Shenzhu (GV12), Feishu (BL13), Quchi (LI11), Hegu (LI4), Xuehai (SP10), Sanyinjiao (SP6), Zusanli (ST36) and so on. ③ The root of the nerve which controls the affected skin—Jiaji point (Ex-B2). ④ More points can be added according to the symptoms. Normally, the reducing needling technique should be applied.

NEUROLOGICAL DERMATITIS

[INTRODUCTION]

Neurological dermatitis often occurs on the neck, nape, elbow, popliteal and sacrum, and is distributed symmetrically. Because it looks like the skin of the ox neck, thick and hard, it is called "ox skin ringworm" in traditional Chinese medicine. The main symptoms are: flat papular connecting to one big area; the skin becoming thicker and desquamated; extreme severe itching of the local area, especially at night; and no pain from scratching. The disease is due to the wind, heat and damp accumulated in the channels and meridians of the skin, leading to lack of nourishment; or to prolonged blood deficiency producing dryness. The disease can become severe if there is abnormal emotional stress, causing disharmony of *qi* and blood. The discomfort of clothing, especially collars, or scratching can all induce the problem or make the disease more severe. The treatment principle is to dispel the wind, remove the dampness, reduce the heat, nourish the blood and moisten the dryness and stop the itching. Select the points mainly from Hand Yangming and Foot Taiyin meridians, such as Quchi (LI11), Xuehai (SP10), and Zusanli (ST36) and Ah-shi point. Apply even needling technique. The needles are retained for 20-30 minutes; the treatment is given once a day, 10 times in one course.

[CLINICAL EXPERIENCE]

1. CONVENTIONAL ACUPUNCTURE

Point: Affected skin broken area

Technique: Insert a 1.5-*cun* needle (Size: No.28) from the border of the skin broken area to the center subcutaneously, about 0.5-1 *cun* deep. Between 10 and 30 needles should be used each time. At the end, puncture one to three needles perpendicularly in the center of the broken skin area about 0.3-0.5 *cun* deep. No retention is required. The treatment is given twice a week, 10 times in one course.

The method is good to treat local, limited ox skin ringworm.

2. MOXIBUSTION THERAPY

(1) Moxibustion with Moxa Cone on the Skin

Point: Ah-shi point of the affected area

Technique: Apply garlic juice (or oil) on the affected skin, and place a burning moxa cone on it. The size of the cone should be as big as a wheat grain or the head of a match. The distance between each moxa point should be 1.5 cm. The number of many points that should be selected depends on the size of the affected skin. Apply one to three cones on each point every time. When the moxa cone is burned off, remove the ash and cover the point with sterilized gauze. In order to relieve the burning pain, the moxa area can be lightly patted, or the affected skin can be punctured with two-*cun* filiform needles subcutaneously (one needle in an upward direction and one needle down), and connected with the anesthetic apparatus. The moxibustion treatment is given once every 10 days until the skin turns normal. Normally, after moxibustion, the skin that has been subjected to moxibustion becomes dry and turns burning yellow; a crust will form and fall off after two or three days. A few of the Moxa points will have small blisters after moxibustion, and this will form a dry crust and fall off in two or three days; no scar will be left in either case. This method is good at treating local neurological dermatitis, but not the general type. A total of 120 cases were treated, 89% of which were effective. The effect can be seen after one to three treatments.

(2) Warming Moxibustion with Herbal Moxa Stick

Point: Ah-shi point

Technique: Prepare the herbal moxa stick with old moxa wool, and a thin powder made from Baizhi (dahurian angelicaroot) and Cangzhu (the rhizome of Chinese atractylodes) 150 g for each, Sulphur 60 g. This should be applied with the warming moxibustion technique on Ah-shi points. The moxibustion is applied for 15-30 minutes every time and once or twice a day. One treatment course lasts seven to 10 days. For a large affected area, a moxa box can be applied.

3. BLEEDING METHOD

Points: Quze (PC3) and Weizhong (BL40).

Technique: Prick the two points with a three-edged needle until a few drops of blood appear. The treatment is given once a day, three times in one course.

4. ELECTRIC ACUPUNCTURE THERAPY

Points: Affected area, Hegu (LI4), Quchi (LI11), Zusanli (ST36), Xuehai (SP10) and Sanyinjiao (SP6)

Technique: Puncture one needle on four sides of the affected area respectively. The direction should be toward the center, and the tips of the needles should meet in the center of the affected area. Connect the electricity to the handles of the needles, using a frequency of 500-600 times/min. The needles are retained for 15-20 minutes. Apply normal even needling technique for the rest of the points. The treatment is given once daily or once every other day, 10 times in one course, with a three-day interval between each course.

5. CUTANEOUS NEEDLE

Points: ① General stimulation: The location is on both sides of the spine (BL meridian area). ② Special stimulation: The area of positive things is beside the spine. ③ Local stimulation: the local affected area and the nearby area.

Technique: Tap the above-mentioned area with a plum blossom needle with even strength for about 10-20 minutes until there is slight bleeding. The treatment is given once daily, 10 times in one course. The method is good for treating diffuse neurological dermatitis.

6. EMBEDDING THREAD METHOD

Points: Apply mainly to the affected area, such as Weizhong (BL40) on popliteal area, Quchi (LI11) on the elbow, Dazhui (GV14) on the nape, Tianding (LI17) and Futu (LI18).

Technique: Embed the surgical catgut crosswise on the point (be careful not to injure the big blood vessels). Symptoms, such as shivering or fever, can be seen in two or three days after the surgery, and this should be treated properly according to the symptoms. More than 10 days after the surgery, the itching will gradually stop, and the affected skin will be desquamated; and the color will change from red to dark purple, and slowly turn to normal skin color.

7. POINT APPLICATION

Point: Ah-shi point (affected area)

Technique: Take a proper amount of garlic and make into a paste, apply it on the affected area, and cover it with gauze fixed with plaster. The application should be kept on for a day every time, and the treatment is given once every seven to 10 days, three times in one course.

8. AURICULAR THERAPY

Points: Lung, Ear-shenmen, Adrenal, Subcortex, Liver, and the related affected area.

Technique: Puncture with even stimulation. The needles are retained for one hour, embedding Wangbuliuxing seed after their removal.

9. COMBINED THERAPY

(1) Bleeding Cupping Method

Point: Ah-shi point

Technique: Tap Ah-shi points on the affected area with a cutaneous needle until there is slight bleeding; then apply cupping for 10 minutes. The treatment is given once a day, 10 times in one course.

(2) Plum Blossom Needle and Moxibustion

Point: Ah-shi point

Technique: After sterilization of the local area, tap the affected area in a circular manner from its border to the center with a plum blossom needle. The method is repeated two or three times every time until the skin bleeds slightly. Then, apply moxibustion with a moxa stick on the tapped area. Normally, the patient has no itching sensation at the beginning of the moxibustion treatment, but after five to 15 minutes this will appear in varying levels of intensity. The treatment should continue until the itching disappears. If the patient feels itchy from the very beginning of the moxibustion treatment, it should also continue until the itching disappears. The treatment is given once a day, seven treatments in one course, and an interval of two days between courses. Use this method once every other day if the symptoms are relieved until the patient is cured.

[REMARKS]

1. Acupuncture is pretty effective to treat this disease.
2. The affected skin should not be scratched and washed with hot water, and irritating medicine should not be taken.
3. No spicy food or seafood is allowed; more light food and vegetables should be taken.

VITILIGO

[INTRODUCTION]

Traditional Chinese medicine believes that this disease is mainly caused by the blockage of the meridian due to an attack of exterior pathogenic wind, or chemical pollution, or traumatic injury. The disease can be also caused by abnormal emotional changes, the disharmony of *qi* and blood injuring the liver, kidney, and dysfunction of the spleen for transportation; blood deficiency will cause disharmony of Ying and defensive *qi,* so the skin is not well nourished. The treatment principle is to dispel the wind, moisten the dryness, strengthen the spleen, regulate and activate blood circulation. Select the points mainly from the Hand and Foot Yangming meridian, Foot Jueyin meridian, Foot Shaoyin meridian, such as, Quchi (LI11), Hegu (LI4), Xuehai (SP10), Zusanli (ST36), Sanyijiao (SP6), Taichong (LR3) and Taixi (KI3). Even needling technique should be applied, and the needles are retained for 30 minutes. The treatment is given once a day, 10 times in one course.

[CLINICAL EXPERIENCE]

1. CONVENTIONAL ACUPUNCTURE

(1) Surrounding Method
Point: Affected area

Technique: Puncture the affected area from the border to the center horizontally, apply even needling technique. The number of needles depends on the size of the affected area. Use two to six needles each time, and retain them for 30 minutes. The treatment is given once a day, 10 times in one course.

(2) Selecting Points According to the Differentiation of Syndromes
Points: Quchi (LI11), Hegu (LI4), Xuehai (SP10), Sanyijiao (SP6) and Ah-shi point. Supplementary points: Add Fengchi (GB20) and Fengmen (BL12) for pathogenic wind attacking the exterior part of the body; add Tianshu (ST25) and Fenglong (ST40) for accumulation of damp heat; add Taichong (LR3) and Shanzhong (CV17) for liver *qi* stagnation; add Ganshu (BL18), Shenshu (BL23) and Taixi (KI3) for liver and kidney deficiency; and add Geshu (BL17) and Shanzhong (BL17) for blood stagnation blocking the meridians.

Technique: Apply even needling technique for the main points and the surrounding method for Ah-shi point; take the combined points according to the differentiation of the syndromes, tonifying the deficiency and reducing the excess. All the needles are retained for 20-30 minutes. The treatment is given once a day, 10 times in one course.

2. MOXIBUSTION

(1) Moxibustion with Moxa Cone and Garlic
Point: Affected area.

Technique: Take a proper amount of garlic, smash it and apply 0.2-0.3 cm thick on the affected area. Place a moxa cone in the size of a broad bean on it. Three to five moxa cones should be applied. The treatment is given once a day, 10 times in one course.

(2) Hanging Moxibustion with Moxa Stick
Point: Affected area

Technique: Focus the burning moxa stick on the white patch, the distance between the moxa stick and the skin depends on the tolerance of the patient. If the white patch is small on the head and the face, a piece of paper with a hole in the size of the white patch should be placed on top of it. This method can prevent the local skin from turning dark. If the white patch is very big, then moxibustion can be applied, circle-by-circle, from outside to inside. If there are many white patches distributed divergently, then moxibustion should be applied group by group. The white patch should have strong blood congestion (pink color) after the treatment. This treatment is given once a day, 10 times in one course.

3.   BLEEDING METHOD

Points: Quchi (LI11), Quze (PC3) and Weizhong (BL40)

Technique: Prick the points with a three-edged needle to draw one to three drops of blood. The treatment is given once a day, five times in one course. The method is good at treating prolonged vitiligo or that due to blood stagnation.

4.   PLUM BLOSSOM NEEDLE

Point: White patch area

Technique: Tapping the affected area with the plum blossom needle from outside to inside until the blood spot coming out, tapping about 10 minutes. If there are many white patches and spread divergently, it should be tapped group by group. The treatment is given once a day, 10 times making up one course.

5.   FIRE NEEDLE THERAPY

Point: Affected area

Technique: Burn the tip of the fire needle on the alcohol lamp until it gets red, and then prick the affected area rapidly, 0.1 cm deep; repeat this several times, normally selecting six to eight points on the white patch one cm in size. The treatment is given once a week. Sterilization should follow the therapy to prevent infection.

[REMARKS]

1.   This disease is very difficult to treat.

2. External application should be under the guidance of the doctor, otherwise the disease will get severe.

3. No fish or irritating foods are allowed.

ERYSIPELAS

[INTRODUCTION]

Erysipelas is a kind of acute infective skin disease, because the skin will turn red suddenly; the color is bright red, so it is also called "cinnabar toxin." The disease is caused by the accumulation of damp heat in the stomach and spleen flowing downward to the lower leg; or the accumulation of heat in the blood due to the exogenous pathogenic wind and heat; or the pathogenic factor invading the skin through injury to the derma mucosa. If it occurs on the head and face it is mainly due to the wind heat; on the waist and hip region, mainly due to the liver fire; on the lower extremity, mainly due to the damp heat. Treating principle is: dispelling the wind and the heat, removing the damp and the heat, cooling the heat in the blood, and relieving the pathogenic heat. Selecting the points mainly from Hand and Foot Yangming, Foot Taiyin meridians, such as, Hegu (LI4), Quchi (LI11), Zusanli (ST36), Xuehai (SP10), Weizhong (BL40), Ah-sh point, reducing needling technique should be applied.

[CLINICAL EXPERIENCE]

1. CONVENTIONAL ACUPUNCTURE

Points: Main points: Diji (SP8), Xuehai (SP10), Sanyinjiao (SP10) and Taichong (LR3). Supplementary points: add Touwei (ST8), Hegu (LI4) and Yifeng (TE17) if the disease is on the head and face; add Zhigou (TE6), Qimen (LR14) and Yanglingquan (GB34) if the disease is under the hypochondriac region or on the waist and hip; add Fenglong (ST40) and Neiting (ST44) if the disease is located on the lower extremities; and add Shenzhu (GV12) for infants.

Technique: Select three to five points on the affected side each time, apply the thrusting, lifting, and rotating needling technique combined with slow and rapid reducing technique. Retain the needle for 20-30 minutes, manipulating every 10 minutes. If there is redness, pain and swelling of the local area, prick with a three-edged needle until blood comes out. The treatment is given once a day, three times in succession.

2. BLEEDING METHOD

(1) Puncturing Sifeng Points (Ex-UE10)

Point: Sifeng points (Ex-UE10)

Technique: After regular sterilization, prick the Sifeng points (Ex-UE10) quickly with a three-edged needle, squeezing out the sticky liquid. Select the points of the affected side. If the disease is located in the middle, puncture the points on both side of the hands. For a mild case, it is enough to puncture one point on the middle finger only.

(2) Bleeding method

Points: Affected area, Xuehai (SP10) and Yinbai (SP10).

Technique: Find the congested small vessels with dark purple color under the affected skin. After sterilization, insert the round-sharp needle (or No.28, 0.5-*cun* filiform needle) into the blood vessels. Take the needle out slowly, waiting for the dark blood to appear, and prick four or five times in all. If the small vessels are not obviously congested, select the vein that can be seen. Puncture Xuehai (SP10) and Yinbai (SP1) at the same time. Shake to enlarge the needle holes while withdrawing, squeezing out a few drops of the blood. The treatment is given once a day or every other day. Normally the disease can be cured after three to seven days.

(3) Bleeding the Jing-well Point

Points: Lingtai (GV10), Weizhong (BL40) and Ah-shi point.

Technique: Bleed the points with a three-edged needle to draw two to three drops of blood once a day, five times in one course.

(4) Bleeding and Cupping Method

Technique: Bleed the red and swollen area with a three-edged needle or small eyebrow-shaping needle. Let the blood come out, adding cupping when necessary. The treatment is given once or twice a day, five to 10 times forming one course.

3. AURICULAR THERAPY

Points: Ear-shenmen, Adrenal, Sub-cortex and Occiput.

Technique: Select two or three points every time, apply moderate or strong stimulation; and retain the needle for 30-60 minutes. The treatment is given once a day, five times in one course. It is very effective to stop pain and reduce inflammation.

[REMARKS]

1. Through clinical observation, acupuncture can control the development of the inflammation and relieve the symptoms of erysipelas in the acute stage, the hemogram returning to normal after two to three days.

2. If the complicated infection forms ulceration, or develops into septicemia or pyemia, a combination of Chinese and Western therapy must be considered.

PSORIASIS

[INTRODUCTION]

Psoriasis is normally seen in chronic skin disease. The characteristics of the disease are red marks with a clear border in different sizes, covered by white scales. If the scales are removed, the bleeding spot can be seen, so Chinese medicine calls it "white rust." It occurs often in winter and spring, and the disease is recurrent and very difficult to cure. It usually appears on the scalp, four extremities and the entire body. Psoriasis is mainly caused by blood heat, dryness and stagnation, which are due to the struggling of the exterior pathogenic wind and the anti-pathogenic *qi* in the skin; or it is caused by spleen and the kidney deficiency, disharmony of the blood and the imbalance between *yin* and *yang*. It is also related to improper food intake, over-eating rich flavored food, and abnormal emotional changes. The treatment principle is to clear away the heat, cool and nourish the blood, moisten the dryness, activate the blood circulation and regulate the Governor and Conception Vessels. Select the points mainly from Hand and Foot Yangming meridians, Foot Taiyin meridian and conception vessel, such as, Dazhui (GV14), Quchi (LI11), Hegu (LI4), Xuehai (SP10), Yinlingquan (SP9), Sanyinjiao (SP6) and Zhongji (CV3), apply the reducing needling technique and retain the needle for 30 minutes. The treatment is given once a day and 10 treatments make up one course.

[CLINICAL EXPERIENCE]

1. CONVENTIONAL ACUPUNCTURE

(1) *Spiral Dragon Acupuncture*
Point: Huatuojiaji (Ex-B2, T1-L5)

Technique: After sterilization, puncture the Jiaji (Ex-B2) points perpendicularly and bilaterally about 1-1.5 *cun* deep according to the spiral dragon needling technique. Apply the even method with rotating technique, retaining the needle for 30 minutes. The treatment is given once a day, 10 times in one course. Huatuojiaji points (Ex-B2) are connected to the Governor Vessel and share the same source with the thoroughfare meridian and Conception Vessel; it is also related to the urinary bladder meridian and internally connected with the kidney meridian. Therefore, by puncturing these points, *yin* and *yang* can be adjusted, *qi* and blood can be harmonized, skin and muscles can be moistened, and the Zang and Fu organs can be regulated.

(2) *Selecting the Points Partly*
Points: Main points: Quchi (LI11), Xuehai (SP10) and Sanyinjiao (SP6). Supplementary points: Add Yingxiang (lI20) and Suliao (LI25) if the disease is located on the head and face; add Zhigou (TE6), Fengchi (GB20) and Hegu (LI4) if the disease is located on the upper extremity; add Zusanli (ST36) and Zhigou (TE6) if the disease is located on the lower extremity; add Dazhui (GV14) and Hegu (LI4) if

the disease is located on the whole body.

Technique: Apply reducing needling technique for all the points, retaining the needle for 30 minutes and manipulating several times intermittently. The treatment is given once a day, 10 times in one course. A total of 41 cases of psoriasis were treated, of which 26 were cured, 11 were obviously effective, and five were effective.

2. MOXIBUSTION

Point: Affected area

Technique: Take a proper amount of garlic, removing the skin and smashing it into the paste about 0.3 cm thick. Apply and place a moxa cone in the size of a broad bean or date kernel on it. If the affected area is very big, more moxa cones can be applied every 1.5 cm in between. Apply moxibustion on the point until the patient feels itching and pain that cannot be borne anymore. Sometimes, there will be blister on the local area after the moxibustion treatment. This can be covered with sterilized gauze and fixed with plaster in order to avoid infection. The treatment is given once every other day or two times a week, seven to 10 treatments in one course.

3. AURICULAR THERAPY

(1) Cutting Therapy on the Ear Point

Point: Auricular concha and the inferior antihelix crus, or the mid point of the back of the ear.

Technique: After regular sterilization of the local area, use a surgical knife to cut one of the above-mentioned points about 3-5 mm long and 0.1 cm deep, causing four to five drops of blood (for a severe case, more blood can be let out). Then, cover the cut with non-bacterial dry cotton. The treatment is given once every four to seven days, cutting both ears every time. During the period of treatment, no beef, mutton, egg, sea fish, and spicy food are allowed.

(2) Auricular Hydro-acupuncture

Points: Lung, Adrenal, Endocrine, Liver, Spleen and Occiput.

Technique: Select two to three points. Vitamin B_1, Angelica injection or 0.5-1% of Novocain should be injected, 0.1-0.5 ml for each point. Treat the ears alternately once a day.

(3) Auricular Point Bleeding Therapy

Points: The upper, middle and lower veins on the back of the ear, urticaria point.

Technique: Select two or three points and use a thick filiform needle or three-edged needle to prick and draw about three drops of blood. This method is very effective to stop the extreme itching of "white crust." The treatment is given once daily.

(4) Acupuncture with Filiform Needle

Points: Lung, Endocrine, Ear-shenmen, Occiput, Adrenal, Liver, Spleen, Brain and Heart.

Technique: Select three to five points, and use a filiform needle to puncture perpendicularly, applying reducing needling technique with strong stimulation. Retain the needle for 30-60 minutes. The treatment is given once a day, 10 times in one course. Puncture the ears alternately. Seed application on the point can also be applied.

4.   THREE-EDGED NEEDLE THERAPY

Points: Zhongkui (Ex), three points of sulcus auriculae posterior (the middle point located on the sulcus auriculae posterior between the back of the auricle and the mastoid process, on the same level with helix cauda; the upper and lower point is 2.5 *cun* to the middle point)

Technique: Prick the sterilized point with a three-edged needle to cause several drops of blood. The treatment is given once a day, seven times in one course.

5.   CUTANEOUS PUNCTURE

Points: Back-shu point on the back, Baliao point (BL32-BL34), Huatuojiaji point (Ex-B2) and Ah-shi point.

Technique: Tap the points strongly for a severe case, with moderate tapping for a mild one, and light tapping on the border of the affected area. There should be slight bleeding for all the types. Tap three to five minutes every time. The points must be cleaned by sterilized dry cotton after the treatment and covered with plaster. The treatment is given once every three to five days and covers five sessions.

6. POINT CATGUT-EMBEDDING THERAPY

Points: ① Geshu (BL17) and Danshu (BL19). ② Geshu (BL17), Danshu (BL19) and Fengmen (BL12) ③ Geshu (BL17), Danshu (BL19), Piwai (EX, 0.5 *cun* literal to Pishu-BL20).

Technique: Using every group of points alternatively, embedding the needle once every two weeks. After local sterilization and local anesthesia, take a No.12 blood transfusion needle and embed No.2 medical surgical catgut (1-1.5 cm), inside the point. Cover it with sterilized material. The method is good to treat psoriasis due to blood heat, wind and dryness.

7. COMBINED THERAPY

(1) Acupuncture, Cupping and Electric Therapy

Points: Dazhui (GV14), Taodao (GV13), Ganshu (LI18), Pishu (BL20) and Jiaji points (Ex-B2) from T5-T6 and L1-L2.

Technique: Take a three-edged needle to prick the first four points (altogether six parts), and then apply cupping for five to 10 minutes; bleed the points of about 0.3-0.5 ml of blood after removing the cups. At the end, puncture Jiaji points (Ex-B2); after the arrival of *qi*, connect the needles with the electricity for 20 minutes. The treatment is given once a day, 10 times in one course.

(2) Laser and External Medicine

Point: Affected area

Technique: Apply the laser therapeutic apparatus on the affected area for 10-15 minutes. Apply tincture of Fufangtujinpi after treatment. The treatment is given once a day, 10 times in one course.

[REMARKS]

1. Acupuncture therapy is very effective for the disease, and the combined therapy will be best.

2. The spicy and aromatic food, such as mutton, beef, fish and shrimp, are forbidden; light vegetables and fruit should be taken instead.

FUNGUS DERMATOLOGICAL DISEASE

[INTRODUCTION]

Fungus dermatological disease has different names according to the location of the disease. If it occurs on the head, it is called "tineatonsure" or "tinea capitis"; on the hand, "tinea unguium"; on the foot, "tinea pedis" or "tinea pedes"; on the finger, "tinea unguium." The main symptoms are: blisters on the affected area connected together; erosion of the skin; extreme itchiness and desquamation after the skin becomes dry. If the disease is located on the nails, they lose their luster and thicken. Traditional Chinese medicine believes that the disease are caused by long time living in a damp place or improper food intake that will affect the spleen and stomach; then the accumulation of heat will attack the skin and cause the disease; or the patient is attacked by the pathogenic wind and dampness, and the damp heat goes down to the lower Jiao and causes the disease. The treatment principle is to strengthen the spleen, remove the dampness, clear away the heat, dispel the wind, detoxify and stop the itching. Select the points mainly from the Hand Taiyin meridian, Hand Yangming meridian and Foot Taiyin meridian, such as Hegu (LI4), Quchi (LI11), Yinlingquan (SP9), Chize (LU5) and Sanyijiao (SP6). Apply the reducing needling technique. and retain the needle for 30 minutes. The treatment is given once a day, 10 times in one course.

[CLINICAL EXPERIENCE]

1. CONVENTIONAL ACUPUNCTURE

(1) Puncturing Hegu (LI4) Point, Ying-Spring Point

Points: Hegu (LI4) and Rangu (KD2).

Technique: Select the points bilaterally. The acupuncture is given once a day, seven times in one course, with three days between two courses. The method is good at treating tinea capitis. More points can be punctured such as Ganshu (LR18), Shenshu (BL23) and Zusanli

(ST36) in order to strengthen the result. The method is effective to treat tinea capitis.

(2) Puncturing the Single Point

Point: Chengshan (BL57) or 0.5 *cun* below it.

Technique: Use a 3-4 *cun* needle to puncture the point two to three *cun* deep. Apply strong reducing stimulation, removing the needle right away after the sensation of the needling goes down to the toes. The treatment is given once a day, four to five times in one course. It is very effective to treat tinea pedes of due to damp heat.

(3) Surrounding Method

Point: Affected area

Technique: Puncture around the affected area, insert the needle 0.3-0.5 *cun* deep. Apply even needling technique, retaining the needle for 30 minutes, manipulating it three times intermittently. If the disease is distributed divergently, select two or three places to treat. The treatment is given once a day, treating the diseased area alternately. Ten sessions form one course.

2. MOXIBUSTION

Points: Affected area, Hegu (LI4) and Quchi (LI11).

Technique: Apply the match moxibustion technique, select the moxa point, burn the match (not letting the wooden stick burn) and extinguish the flame as soon as the match head is consumed. Press it onto the moxibustion point, removing it when it is cold. The point is taken from outside to inside. Moxibustion is given once on every point (5 mm at most between two points). Taking Hegu (LI4) and Quchi (LI11) alternately. The treatment is given once a day for the first two sessions and then after that, every other day. Normally the disease can be cured after 10 treatments. The method is good to treat tinea unguium.

3. ELECTRICAL THERAPY

Point: Yuzhen (BL9)

Technique: Select Yuzhen (BL9) bilaterally, and puncture 4 cm deep perpendicularly until the galea aponeurotica is reached. Apply the electricity with continues wave, frequency of 200 times/min, and retain the needle for 30-40 minutes. The treatment is given once a day, 10 times in one course. A total of 100 cases of tinea pedis were treated by this method, and 46 cases were cured, 29 were obviously effective, 13 got better, and 12 saw no effect. Normally, after one or two acupuncture treatments, the itching can be relieved, the infusion is reduced, and the blister will dry.

4. PLUM-BLOSSOM NEEDLE

Point: Affected area

Technique: Sterilize the affected area with an alcohol-drenched cotton ball. Then tap it with a plum-blossom needle until the skin turns red, and the patient experiences a burning, hot feeling. The tapping can be stopped if divergent bleeding spots appear. Tap heavily if the itching is severe. The treatment is given once a day, but it can be carried out once every other day for mild itching. Five treatments form one course, with a two to three-day break before the next one. Puncture three to five times again if the itching disappears.

5. COMBINED THERAPY

(1) Acupuncture and Moxibustion

Points: Hand: Hegu (LI4) penetrating to Laogong (PC8) and Neiguan (PC6) penetrating to Waiguan (TE5). Foot: Bafeng (Ex-LE10), Yongquan (KI1) and Kunlun (BL60) penetrating to Taixi (KI3)

Technique: Apply twisting and scraping needling technique for all the points. Retain the needle for 15-30 minutes, manipulating every five to 10 minutes. Apply moxibustion with moxa stick on the affected area for 30-60 minutes after removing the needles. Normally, the patient has no itching feeling at the beginning, but this will appear in varying degrees after five to 15 minutes. This will disappear if the moxibustion is continued. The treatment should also be continued if itching is present at the very start until itching disappears. The treatment is given once a day, seven times in one course with an interval of two days before the next one. The treatment can be given once every other day if the symptoms are reduced. The treatment is given until the disease is cured.

(2) The Needling Technique of Setting Fire on the Top of the Mountain Combined with Heat Application

Points: Hegu (LI4) penetrating to Laogong (PC8). Supplementary points: Zhongzhu (TE3), Houxi (SI3) and Baxie (Ex-UE9).

Technique: Puncture Hegu (LI4) penetrating to Laogong (PC8) and apply the needling technique of setting the fire on the top of the mountain, soaking two towels in hot water in order to use alternately and wrapping the patient's hand for 20-30 minutes to cause sweating. This will get rid of the pathogenic wind. If there is pain in the palm, Zhongzhu (TE3) and Houxi (SI3) can be combined with the needling technique, retaining the needle for 20-30 minutes, and making the hand sweat to dispel wind and stop the itching. If the hand is dry and bleeding, or there is infusion coming out of the blister, then Baxie (Ex-UE9) should be added with the needling technique. Apply the ironing warming moxibustion for 20-30 minutes to dispel the wind and activate the blood circulation, remove the dampness and stop the itching. If the skin on the hand has become dry and hard, apply fresh garlic juice and moxibustion for 20-30 minutes in order to activate blood circulation, moisten the dryness, dispel the wind and stop the itching. The method is good to treat tinea unguium.

6. BLEEDING METHOD

Point: The tip of the external malleolus

Technique: After local sterilization, use a three-edged needle to prick the tip of the external malleolus three to five times, until there is slight bleeding. The treatment is given once a day, seven times in one course. The method can treat tinea pedis.

[REMARKS]

1. Acupuncture treatment is good to stop the extreme itching.

2. Comparing acupuncture with external medicine for treating the tinea, the effective rate of the acupuncture group is 80%, while that for external medicine is 33.3%. Therefore, acupuncture treatment does have good effect.

INDEX OF EXTRA ACUPOINTS IN THIS BOOK

Name of point	Location	Acupuncture-moxibustion technique	Indications
Weilexue (Point for stomach comfort)	0.2 *cun* above Shuifen (CV9) and 4 *cun* lateral	Punctured perpendicular for 0.7 to 1 *cun* with intense stimulation	Epigastric pain
Fuxietexiaoxue (Special point for diarrhea)	At the junction between the white and red skin directly below the highest point of the external maniolus	Mild moxibustion with moxa stick	Diarrhea
Jianweixue (Point for the cure of stomach)	Approximately 2 *cun* below Zusanli (ST 36)	Punctured perpendicularly for 1 *cun*	Constipation
Anmian (Soporific)	Between Fengchi (GB20) and Yifeng (TE17)	Punctured perpendicularly for 0.5 *cun*	Insomnia
Jiuzhengxue (Point for curing deviation of mouth and eyes)	At the junction between the white and red skin at the ulnar end of the crease of the metacarpophalangeal joint of the 5th finger	Punctured 1 to 1.5 *cun* toward Hegu (LI 4)	Facial paralysis

Shangshandianxue (Upper thunder lightning point)	3 *cun* lateral to the center of the Adam's Apple and 1 *cun* below, i.e., the posterior border of the sternocleidomastoid muscle	Punctured superficially for 0.2-0.3 *cun*	Scapulohumeral periarthritis
Weiguanxiashu	1.5 *cun* lateral to the lower border of the 8th thoracic spinous process	Punctured superficially 0.5-0.8 *cun*	Diabetes mellitus
Peigen (The root of the indigestion)	3.5 *cun* lateral to the 1st lumbar vertebra	Moxibustion with moxa stick	Jaundice and malnutrition due to indigestion
Naoqing (Clearance of brain)	2 *cun* above Jiexi (ST41)	Punctured superficially 0.2-0.3 *cun*	Underdevelopment of intelligence in young children
Yinfu (mons pubis)	(1 *cun* above the clitoris and 1.5 *cun* lateral)	Punctured obliquely downward for 1-2 *cun*	Pruritus vulvae
Ruquanxue (milk spring point)	Half *cun* anterior to the Jiquan (HT1) and on the anterior end of the axillary fold	Punctured perpendicularly 0.5-0.8 *cun*	Lactation deficiency
Huiguang (brightness of vision)	At the crossing point of the horizontal line along the cricoid cartilage and the longitudinal line from the mastoid process	Punctured perpendicularly 0.3 *cun*	Myopia

Mingchaxue (Point of bright vision)	On the anterior border of the fibula and 8 *cun* above the external mallelos	Punctured perpendicularly 1-1.5 *cun*	Myopia
Xiaoyixue (Point of eliminating the cloudiness)	0.2 *cun* below the midpoint of the lateral orbital margin	Punctured perpendicularly 0.8-1 *cun* between the orbital ridge and the eyeball with the needle tip moving backward, medially and slightly upward	Myopia
Qiuhou (Behind the eyeball)	At the junction between the lateral 1/4 and medial 3/4 of the infraorbitale margin	Punctured perpendicularly 0.5-1 *cun*, large amplitude of manipulation of the needle is inapplicable	Disorders of eyes
Tianting (Natural hearing)	0.5 *cun* below Anmianxue	Punctured perpendicularly 0.5-0.8 *cun*	Deafness and tinnitus
Lingxia (Below Yanglingquan)	2 *cun* below Yanglingquan (GB34)	Punctured perpendicularly 0.8-1 *cun*	Deafness and tinnitus
Lingong (Neighboring the palace)	0.5 *cun* below Guanyuan (CV4) and 2.5 *cun* lateral	Punctured perpendicularly 1-1.2 *cun*	Acne
Fashengxue (Hair-growing point)	The midpoint between Fengchi (GB20) and Fengfu (GV16)	Punctured perpendicularly 0.8-1 *cun*	Alopecia
Baichongwo (Nest of insects)	1 *cun* above Xuehai (SP10)	Punctured perpendicularly 1-1.2 *cun*	Urticaria, eczema, and parasitosis

INDEX OF CHINESE MATERIA MEDICA

(In the alphabetic order according to the names of Chinese Pinyin Pronunciation)

图书在版编目（CIP）数据

针灸临床妙用／郑其伟，钱淳宜编著；杜巍，洪涛等译．
一北京：外文出版社，2002.1
ISBN 7-119-02982-7

Ⅰ.针… Ⅱ.①郑… ②钱… ③杜… ④洪…
Ⅲ.针灸疗法—临床应用—英文
Ⅳ.R246

中国版本图书馆 CIP 数据核字 (2001) 第 091777 号

外文出版社网址：
http://www.flp.com.cn
外文出版社电子信箱：
info@flp.com.cn
sales@flp.com.cn

责任编辑　余冰清
英文编辑　许　荣
封面设计　席恒青
印刷监制　张国祥

针灸临床妙用

郑其伟　钱淳宜　编著

杜巍　洪涛　胡蓉晖
黄晖　陆小贞　王芳　译
王悦　张咏梅

*

ⓒ外文出版社

外文出版社出版
（中国北京百万庄大街24号）
邮政编码　100037
三河市实验小学印刷厂印刷
中国国际图书贸易总公司发行
（中国北京车公庄西路35号）
北京邮政信箱第399号　邮政编码 100044
2002年（大32开）第 1 版
2002年第 1 版第 1 次印刷
（英）
ISBN 7-119-02982-7/R.185(外)
07000(平)
14-E-3489 P